CHRONIC PAIN

A resource for effective
manual therapy

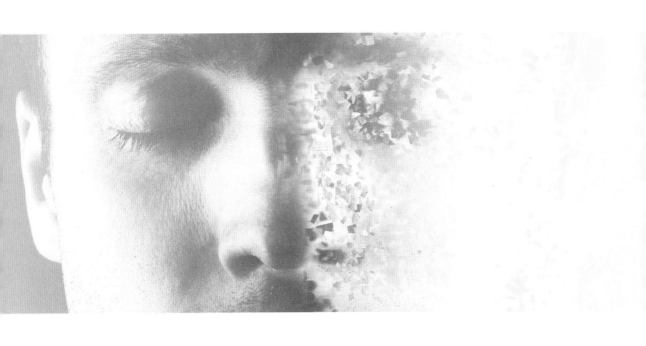

CHRONIC PAIN

A resource for effective manual therapy

Philip AUSTIN BSc (Hons) Ost, MSc, PhD
Researcher and Osteopath,
Honorary Fellow, University of Sydney / University of Edinburgh

Forewords by
Philip Siddall • Michael A Seffinger

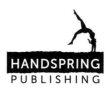

HANDSPRING
PUBLISHING

EDINBURGH

HANDSPRING PUBLISHING LIMITED
The Old Manse, Fountainhall,
Pencaitland, East Lothian
EH34 5EY, Scotland
Tel: +44 1875 341 859
Website: www.handspringpublishing.com

First published 2017 in the United Kingdom by Handspring Publishing

ISBN 978-1-909141-51-3

British Library Cataloguing in Publication Data
A catalogue record for this book is available from the British Library

Library of Congress Cataloguing in Publication Data
A catalog record for this book is available from the Library of Congress

Notice

Neither the Publisher nor the Author assume any responsibility for any loss or injury and/or damage to persons or property arising out of or relating to any use of the material contained in this book. It is the responsibility of the treating practitioner, relying on independent expertise and knowledge of the patient, to determine the best treatment and method of application for the patient.

Commissioning Editor Mary Law
Project Manager Morven Dean
Copy Editor Stephanie Pickering
Cover and Design Direction by Bruce Hogarth, Kinesis Creative
Indexer Aptara, India
Typesetter DSM Soft, India
Printer Melita Press, Malta

The
Publisher's
policy is to use
paper manufactured
from sustainable forests

CONTENTS

FOREWORD by Philip Siddall

Those involved in the treatment of chronic pain need no convincing that pain is not only common, but is also one of the most complex and challenging conditions that we face in clinical practice. It is telling that opioids – drugs that have been used for thousands of years and bring with them both incomplete pain relief and a host of other issues – remain a debated but still large part of the armamentarium for treating pain. Providing the best possible treatment for those living with chronic pain therefore requires a strong foundation in understanding basic pain mechanisms, excellent diagnostic skills, an appreciation of the important role of psychological and environmental factors and an awareness of best-evidence treatment for the many conditions that may be encountered.

Dr. Austin has done a remarkable job in covering so many of these aspects that are central to the effective management of pain. He has also expertly drawn together the various strands that are essential to understanding pain and applying it to clinical practice. This book reflects his many years of work as a clinician combined with a lively enthusiasm for understanding the processes that give rise to our experience of pain. This includes the mechanisms associated with the initial onset in the periphery through to the complex and fascinating changes that we now know occur in the brain. He also brings a breadth of perspective in describing the crucially important role of psychological and environmental factors and what they mean for the assessment and treatment of pain. This is in line with current thinking which recognises that single-modality treatment is enriched and treatment outcomes almost always improved by an approach that focuses not just on the body but also understands and addresses the vital interplay between mind and body in the experience of pain.

Armed with this knowledge, clinical application is paramount. Again, Dr. Austin brings his wide clinical experience to bear in describing the presentation of pain conditions and their treatment. The approach to treatment is both balanced and comprehensive. The evidence for various forms of manual therapy is considered and presented in each of these pain conditions with careful attention to the latest evidence. In addition, other evidence-based options that may be utilised are also helpfully discussed.

For both the person living with pain and the clinician who is aiming to help, chronic pain can be a major challenge. This book will aid enormously those clinicians who are working in the field of chronic pain and particularly those with a focus on manual therapy. The excellent overviews of different conditions, the up-to-date description of underlying pain mechanisms and the presentation of the latest evidence-based treatments provide an invaluable resource for the clinician whose goal it is to improve the lives of people living with pain.

Philip Siddall MBBS MMed (Pain Mgt) PhD FFPMANZCA
Director, Pain Management Service
Greenwich Hospital, Hammond Care, Sydney
Conjoint Professor in Pain Medicine,
University of Sydney, Australia
Sydney, August 2017

FOREWORD by Michael A Seffinger

Patients with chronic pain are seen daily in manual therapy practices across the globe. This condition is one of the most challenging to manage effectively. Recent scientific evidence from biological, social and psychological studies has shed considerable light on the mechanisms underlying this ubiquitous condition. To understand these etiologies enables the clinician to accurately assess and effectively manage each patient. Dr. Austin provides an excellent, cogent and critical review of the scientific literature from the last quarter of a century that serves to inform, enlighten and guide the manual therapist towards the most up to date understanding of how chronic pain manifests and persists, as well as how to break the pain cycle and provide relief. Manual therapy can be a sole treatment approach, or combined with exercise, education, medications and behavioral therapy. This textbook presents clinical outcomes data from a variety of therapeutic approaches to chronic pain management. This vital information will help the manual therapist to select the most proven techniques, and also provide insight into what other health professionals can offer, facilitating networking amongst clinicians and educating patients appropriately.

The addictive and lethal potential of opiate-based analgesic medications that have been used by patients seeking to find relief from chronic pain has long plagued mankind. All too often, patients have met an untimely death due to the overuse of these drugs. Manual therapies provide a relatively safe and effective alternative or adjunctive option to chronic pain management. This text is a timely addition to the literature as it fosters awareness and comprehension of all the factors that are at play in chronic pain conditions, and the variety of approaches necessary to successfully manage these patients. It also provides the necessary scientific basis for a manual therapeutic approach to patients suffering from chronic pain. Dr. Austin aptly identifies where research is lacking, and advises what needs to be done to close the gaps in knowledge so as to better inform clinicians and their patients.

The text itself is written with great clarity, the topic is covered thoroughly, and the information is pragmatic for practicing manual therapists. The illustrations are also clear, very easy to understand and greatly facilitate comprehension. The text boxes highlight essential information to be gleaned from each chapter, and the latest references are well selected and pertinent. The publishers did a masterful job at presenting the information in a reader-friendly manner. The reader will find that this textbook will be used often to engender evidence-based and effective management of this patient population.

Michael A Seffinger DO
Professor, Department of Neuromusculoskeletal Medicine/Osteopathic Manipulative Medicine College of Osteopathic Medicine of the Pacific Pomona, California July 2017

PREFACE

Chronic pain is a debilitating phenomenon that impacts people not only through the suffering caused by any kind of severe bodily pain, but also through its emotional, social, spiritual, vocational, and economic impacts. While it is not possible precisely to determine the extent of the current economic burden of chronic pain on society, its direct and indirect costs in the United States and Europe have been shown to exceed those of many other chronic conditions such as heart disease, cancer, and diabetes. Importantly, it is not only patients who are challenged by chronic pain, but also family, friends, work colleagues, and treating health care professionals. In this regard chronic pain conditions represent a daunting challenge to practitioners who, although they steadfastly attempt to treat these conditions, are, more often than not, left feeling frustrated at their inability to relieve the physical and emotional suffering their clients are experiencing. One major problem lies with the fact that practitioners and patients alike often consider chronic pain as simply a prolonged form of acute pain, and aiming for a cure often delays the implementation of the multidisciplinary approaches more appropriate for chronic pain.

Manual therapy as practiced by physiotherapists, osteopaths, chiropractors, and massage therapists has long been considered important in managing people with chronic pain. Traditionally, manual therapy focuses on biomechanical dysfunction as a source of pain, and treatment is aimed at promoting and relieving pain in musculoskeletal structures. Importantly, recent experimental data show that manual therapy also activates inhibitory peripheral and central nervous system responses in chronic pain conditions. However, these findings have not been replicated in clinical studies. There are two reasons for this:

- the reductions in pain are short-lived because of other endogenous and exogenous confounding factors

- manual therapy-based clinical trials have lacked methodological rigor due to the heterogeneity of sampling and types of treatments employed and the use of multiple types of outcome measure.

Manual therapy is not alone in lacking supportive clinical results. Various psychological and pharmaceutical approaches are recommended for many chronic pain conditions despite a lack of evidence that they have significant therapeutic effect. The mechanism of action of many drugs is not completely understood, yet despite their potential for unwanted side-effects they are widely prescribed for long-term use for people with chronic pain. Manual therapy is generally safer than medication and has fewer adverse effects. Many patients also prefer to have therapy involving human touch rather than having to rely on taking drugs. Thus, the possible inhibitory effects of manual therapy on peripheral and central nociceptive and pain pathways may play a critical role in the personal experience and patient satisfaction. Each chapter in this book describes clinical and research areas showing strong validation for the use of manual therapy. Where there is little proof of effectiveness the chapter suggests what types of research are needed to increase validation.

Chronic Pain – a resource for effective manual therapy has been written to help manual therapists involved in the care of chronic pain patients. It aims to describe effective diagnosis and management in manual therapy settings. The content is based on best available epidemiological, clinical, and experimental evidence. Although the evidence-based practice model has met with resistance in many clinical fields it is important to underline a judicious use of current best evidence when making decisions about the management of individual patients. However, we need to recognize the importance of patient beliefs, values, and personal preferences in the clinical decision-making process.

The text is divided into three sections that cover the basic peripheral, spinal, and brain pain mechanisms; the epidemiology, psychology, and evaluation of chronic pain and the efficacy of manual therapy for chronic pain conditions; and the clinical presentations of chronic pain. It is written so that readers can easily cross-reference between chapters to first, understand associations between factors involved in the onset and maintenance of chronic pain and second, apply this understanding to the effective management of people with chronic pain. I hope the book will provide a reflective, unbiased, easy-to-follow approach to the understanding of this debilitating condition.

Philip Austin
Sydney, Australia
May 2017

GLOSSARY

5-HT	Serotonin

A

ACC	Anterior cingulate cortex
ACT	Acceptance and commitment therapy
ACTH	Adrenocorticotropic hormone
AMPA receptor	S-alpha-amino-3-hydroxy-5-methyl-4-isoxazolepropionic acid receptor
ANS	Autonomic nervous system
ASIC	Acid sensing ion channel
ATP	Adenosine triphosphate

B

BDI	Beck Depression Inventory
BDNF	Brain-derived neurotrophic factor
BK	Bradykinin
BPS	Biopsychosocial

C

Ca^{2+}	Calcium ion
Ca $\alpha_2\delta$	calcium channel alpha-2-delta subunit
CaMK	Calmodulin-dependent protein kinase
CBT	Cognitive behavioural therapy
CeA	Central nucleus (amygdala)
CGRP	Calcitonin gene-related peptide
cAMP	Cyclic adenosine monophosphate
cGMP	Cyclic guanosine monophosphate
CGRP	Calcitonin gene related peptide
CLBP	Chronic low back pain
CNS	Central nervous system
COX	Cyclooxygenase
CP	Chronic pain
CPM	Conditioned pain modulation
CPSP	Central post stroke pain

CREB	cAMP-response-element-binding protein
CRH	Corticotropin releasing hormone
CRPS	Chronic regional pain syndrome
CS	Central sensitisation
CSD	Cortical spreading depression
CT	Computer tomography
CTTH	Chronic tension headaches
CVP	Chronic visceral pain
CWP	Chronic widespread pain

D

DAG	Diacylglyceride
DASS	Depression Anxiety and Stress Scale
DCs	Dorsal columns
DH	Dorsal horn
DN4	Douleur Neuropathique en 4
DNIC	Diffuse noxious inhibitory control
DRG	Dorsal root ganglion

E

EMG	Electromyography
ENS	Enteric nervous system
ERK	Extracellular signal-regulated kinases

F

FABQ	Fear Avoidance Beliefs Questionnaire
FACIT-Sp	Functional Assessment of Chronic Illness-Spiritual Wellbeing
FD	Functional dyspepsia
FGIDs	Functional gastrointestinal disorders
fMRI	Functional magnetic resonance imaging
FPS	Faces Pain Scale

G

GABA	Gamma-Aminobutyric acid
GFAP	Glial fibrillary acidic protein
GI	Gastrointestinal
GMI	Graded motor imagery
GPCR	G protein-coupled receptor

H

Hi	Histamine
HIV	Human immunodeficiency virus
HPA axis	Hypothalamic-pituitary-adrenal axis
HVLA	High-velocity-low amplitude manipulation

I

IASP	International Association for the Study of Pain
IBS	Irritable bowel syndrome
ICHD	International Classification of Headache Disorders
IGLEs	Intraganglionic laminar endings
IL	Interleukin
IMAs	Intramuscular arrays
IP$_3$	Inositol triphosphate

L

LA	Lateral nucleus (amygdala)
LANSS	Leeds Assessment of Neuropathic Symptoms and Signs
LEA	Lower educational attainment
LPA	Lysophosphatidic acid
LTP	Long term potentiation
LVLA	Low-velocity-low amplitude manipulation

M

mGlu receptor	Metabotropic glutamate receptors
Mg^{2+}	Magnesium ion
MBSR	Mindfulness-based stress reduction
MCS	Motor cortex stimulation
MORs	mu-opioid receptors
MPQ	McGill Pain Questionnaire
MSPQ	Modified Somatic Perceptions Questionnaire

N

Na$^+$	Sodium ion
NGF	Nerve growth factor
NK1 receptor	Neurokinin 1
NMDA receptor	N-mythyl-D-aspartate receptor
NO	Nitric oxide
NPS	Neuropathic Pain Scale
NRS	Numerical Rating Scale
NSAIDs	Non-steroidal anti-inflammatory drugs
NTS	Nucleus tractus solitarius

O

OA	Osteoarthritis
ODI	Oswestry Disability Index

P

PAG	Periaqueductal gray
PASS	Pain Anxiety Symptom Scale
PC	Pain catastrophising
PCC	Posterior cingulate cortex
PCS	Pain Catastrophising Scale
PESQ	Pain Self-Efficacy Questionnaire
PFC	Prefrontal cortex
PKA	Protein kinase A

PKC	Protein kinase C		**STAI**	State-Trait Anxiety Questionnaire
PGE2	Prostaglandins E2		**StEP**	Standardised Evaluation of Pain
PQAS	Pain Quality Assessment Scale		**STT**	Spinothalamic tract
PSNS	Parasympathetic nervous system			
PTSD	Post-traumatic stress disorder			
PVAQ	Pain Vigilance and Awareness Questionnaire			

T

PKC Protein kinase C
PGE2 Prostaglandins E2
PQAS Pain Quality Assessment Scale
PSNS Parasympathetic nervous system
PTSD Post-traumatic stress disorder
PVAQ Pain Vigilance and Awareness Questionnaire

Q

QST Quantitative sensory testing

R

rACC Rostral anterior cingulate cortex
RAIC Rostral agranular insular cortex
RCT Randomised controlled trial
RMDQ Roland Morris Disability Questionnaire
RVM Rostroventral medulla

S

S1 Primary somatosensory cortex
S2 Secondary somatosensory cortex
SC Spinal cord
SE Self-efficacy
SES Socioeconomic status
SF-36 Short-form 36
SMT Spinomesencephalic tract
SNRI Serotonin-norepinephrine reuptake inhibitor
SNS Sympathetic nervous system
SRD Subnucleus reticularis dorsalis (caudal medulla)
SRT Spinoreticular tract
SSRI Serotonin reuptake inhibitor

T

TACs Trigeminal autonomic cephalalgias
TCA Tricyclic antidepressant
TENS Transcutaneous electrical stimulation
TMDs Temporomandibular disorders
TMJ Temporomandibular joint
TNF-α Tumour necrosis factor-alpha
TRP Transient receptor potential
TTX Tetrodotoxin

V

VAS Visual analogue scale
VGCC Voltage gated calcium channel
VGSC / Na$_v$ Voltage gated sodium channel
VLO Ventrolateral orbital cortex
VPI Ventral posterior inferior nucleus (thalamus)
VPL Ventral posterolateral nucleus (thalamus)
VPM Ventral posteromedial nucleus (thalamus)
VR Virtual reality
VRS Verbal Rating Scale

W

WDR Wide dynamic range neuron (spinal cord)
WOMAC Western Ontario and McMasters Universities Osteoarthritis Index

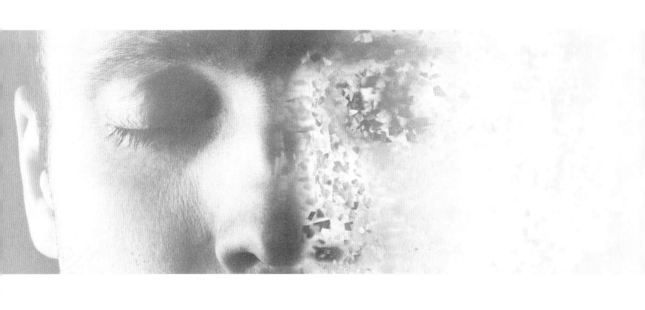

SECTION 1
Basic pain mechanisms

Introduction

Primary afferent nociceptors are the first integral part of the pain pathway. These sensory neurons detect actual or potential tissue damage and are widespread throughout skin, muscle, connective tissue, blood vessels, and viscera.[1] Like all parts of the pain pathway, peripheral pain mechanisms are not hardwired, but are continually modulated by changes in pain processing after inflammation or injury.[2] Injury to tissues, whether caused by disease, inflammation, trauma, or provoked by therapeutic intervention, generates noxious stimuli. These stimuli cause the breakdown of local cells, resulting in the liberation of a flood of chemical mediators which then contribute to and facilitate changes in pain processing. Peripheral pain mechanisms are both specialized and diverse where different classes of nociceptive cells are based on their response properties (e.g., mechanical and heat). Neurons may also express different receptors and chemical mediators and project to different areas of the dorsal horn in the spinal cord.[2]

This chapter first describes the structure and specific function of peripheral afferent nociceptors and the conduction of pain signals to the dorsal horn in normal conditions. Peripheral sensitization is then explained, specifically the role of proinflammatory mediators and their effect on the musculoskeletal system. Lastly, treatment approaches specific to peripherally sensitized tissue are reviewed.

Primary afferent nociceptors

Structure and function

Primary afferent neurons are pseudounipolar, which by definition means that they consist of one axon that has split into two branches: one running to the periphery and the other to the spinal cord.[3] The peripheral processes of these neurons ramify profusely and innervate a wide range of tissues where they lose their perineural sheath, while their central processes project to the spinal cord.[1] As opposed to large-diameter myelinated afferent fibers that have specialized terminal endings (e.g., Ruffini nerve endings), nociceptive afferent fibers have structurally 'free' endings (unspecialized and not capsulated). Peripheral nociceptive afferent neurons have two functions. First, they act as a transducer of mechanical, chemical, and thermal input to the spinal cord, and second, they release neurotransmitters in response to injury (e.g., substance P and calcitonin gene-related peptide (CGRP)), which then contribute to peripheral inflammatory processes.

All primary afferent neurons have a similar shape, but they come in a range of sizes. Generally, primary afferent neurons with large cell bodies and which are heavily myelinated conduct very quick action potentials in response to innocuous mechanical stimulation such as vibration and two-point discrimination. These Aβ fibers are associated with muscle spindle function and can conduct action potentials over 100 ms[-1]. Nociceptors fall into two main classes. The first are lightly myelinated (Aδ) fibers that mediate acute, well-localized 'first' or fast pain. The second are unmyelinated (C) fibers that mediate poorly localized, 'second' or slow pain (Figure 1.1) and which conduct action potentials at less than 1 ms[-1].[4]

Electrophysiological studies show that Aδ fibers are divided into two subclasses. Type I Aδ fibers respond to mechanical and chemical stimuli but have a comparatively high heat threshold and are likely to mediate 'first' pain in response to pinprick and other mechanical stimuli. However, these neurons become sensitized (their threshold for stimulation will drop) if heat stimuli are sustained. Conversely, type II Aδ neurons have much lower heat thresholds but very high mechanical thresholds and are considered to mediate the 'first' acute pain response to noxious heat.[4]

Chapter 1

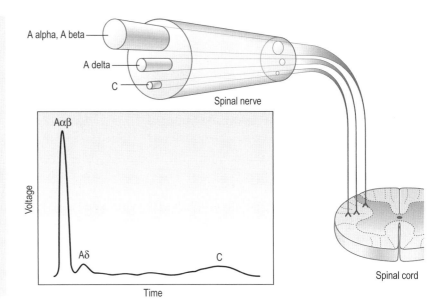

Figure 1.1

Components of peripheral primary afferent neurons that are made up of large-diameter Aβ fibers and smaller diameter Aδ and C fibers

Similarly, C fibers can be subclassified by anatomical, physiological, and biochemical criteria. A common criterion is the response profile of the afferent neuron, where those that respond

to mechanical, thermal, and chemical stimuli are referred to as polymodal nociceptors. Additionally, there are nociceptors that respond to mechanical and cold stimuli, referred to as C-MC (mechano-cold) fibers, and others that respond to chemical stimuli but are insensitive to mechanical stimuli.[5] These unmyelinated fibers are of particular interest, as these so-called 'silent nociceptors' are shown to develop mechanical sensitivity in the event of trauma and/or inflammation. While further research is required, it is probable that these C fibers become sensitized in response to inflammatory environments.[6] Box 1.1 summarizes the key points relating to primary afferent nociceptors.

Noxious stimulation of normal tissue

Nociception is unique in that individual primary afferent neurons of the pain pathway have the ability to detect a wide range of stimuli. There are qualitative and quantitative differences between neurons supplying different tissues; for example, the mechanical threshold of nociceptors may be very low (as in the cornea) or high (as in muscle).[7] Nociceptive afferent receptors are further distinct in that their receptive properties can be modulated, since nociceptors not only signal acute pain but are also responsible for persistent pain disorders that occur during injury and in which pain is produced by innocuous stimuli (allodynia) long after the injury itself has resolved. Fundamentally, peripheral nociception comprises two processes: the first is the transduction of stimuli (the triggering of a sensor potential due to a noxious stimulus) and the second, the transformation of a sensor potential into a series of action potentials.[8]

Sensory specificity of nociceptors

The sensory specificity of a nociceptor is determined by the expression of ion channels (transducers) designed to respond with a high threshold to specific features within the mechanical, thermal and chemical environment.[9] These high-threshold transducers differentiate nociceptors from $A\beta$ neurons that respond to innocuous stimuli, such as light touch, which express transducers with low thresholds.

Response to heat stimuli

Human studies show a clear difference between the perception of innocuous warmth and that of noxious heat;[4] this ability to distinguish between the two allows us to recognize, and therefore avoid, potential tissue-damaging temperatures. It is now established that ion channels of the transient receptor potential (TRP) family are responsible for the detection of thermal stimuli in peripheral nociceptors.

TRPV1 was the first of the vallinoid family of TRP channels shown to detect changes in temperature over a wide physiological range (Figure 1.2).[10] TRPV1 is a noxious heat- and capsicum-activated channel with a thermal activation threshold of ~43°C. Here sensory neurons from mice lacking TRPV1 are severely deficient in their responses to noxious heat stimuli.[11] Additionally, studies show TRPV1 as a critical part of the neuronal signaling mechanisms through which injury produces thermal hyperalgesia and pain hypersensitivity.[12] Moreover, TRPV1 channels are also acid-sensing and activated by protons (H^+) due to lowered extracellular pH during inflammation or ischemia.[13]

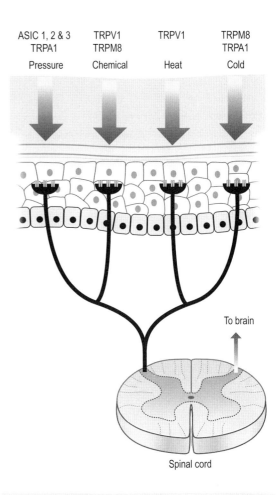

Figure 1.2
Nociceptive pain is generated by the activation of nociceptors that respond to heat, chemical, mechanical, and cold stimuli

Response to cold stimuli

TRP melastatin 8 (TRPM8) is a cold- and menthol-sensitive ion channel with an activation threshold of ~25°C and is involved in both noxious and innocuous cold sensation.[4,15,16] TRPM8 channels are found in neuronal populations, separate from TRPV1 channels, on both $A\delta$ and C fiber terminals (Figure 1.2). It has been shown that TRPM8-deficient mice nevertheless retain normal sensitivity to both noxious heat and mechanical stimuli. However, while these studies show significant deficits in both cold sensation and injury-evoked hypersensitivity,[15,16] the animals still exhibit nociceptive responses to sub-zero centigrade temperatures. This suggests the presence of at least one additional noxious cold receptor. Here, TRPA1 is suggested to detect colder stimuli, specifically within a noxious range below 15°C. However, there is uncertainty as to its precise function, with several studies producing differing results; some show normal responses in TRPA1-deficient mice[18] while others, using similar study protocols, demonstrate decreased cold sensitivity.[19] Regarding the specific role of these channels during different pathophysiological processes, several studies suggest that TRPA1 plays only a minor role in acute cold sensation, but is a key mediator in pathological conditions (tissue injury) where proinflammatory mediators of the channel are present.[4,12,20]

Response to mechanical stress

Mechanical stress resulting in direct pressure, tissue deformation, deep pressure, distension of visceral organs or the detection of touch can activate peripheral nociceptors.[21] In skin, muscle, and joints, Aδ and C fibers show increased thresholds for mechanical stimuli and thus act as nociceptors when detecting potential or actual mechanical damage. Unfortunately, as with cold-sensing channels, there is uncertainty concerning the type of channel involved in noxious mechanical transduction. Several ion channels have been proposed for this role, with acid-sensing ion channels (ASICs) and TRP channels being most extensively investigated (Figure 1.2).

ASIC channels

ASIC channels were initially associated with mechanotransduction because three members of this family (ASIC1, 2 and 3) are expressed in peripheral mechanoreceptors and nociceptors.[22,23] However, as with channels associated with cold stimuli, findings are mixed. This is likely due to separate receptor subgroup distributions in different tissues. For example, findings show that deletion of ASIC1 channel genes does not alter the function of cutaneous mechanoreceptors but does increase the mechanical sensitivity of afferents innervating the gut.[24] Likewise, several studies show that ASIC2- and ASIC3-deficient mice show only slightly decreased activity in cutaneous mechanoreceptors, but, again, increased sensitivity of colonic afferents.[24–26] Although ASIC channels play an important role in regulating receptor function, their molecular interaction at peripheral afferent terminals remains a mystery.[27] However, ASIC3 channels are found to be expressed by nociceptors innervating skeletal and cardiac muscles.[4] In these tissues, the accumulation of lactic acid and protons due to anaerobic metabolism, such as in muscle ischemia, activate ASIC3 receptors, thus generating musculoskeletal and cardiac pain.

TRP channels

Nearly all TRP subfamilies have members linked to mechanosensation in various body systems.[28] However, it is unclear whether these channels directly transduce mechanical stimuli or are an indirect part of a signaling pathway. Although TRP channels are associated with thermal sensation and the mediation of neurogenic inflammation, only two channels (TRPV4 and TRPA1) have been implicated in mechanosensation.[22] For example, TRPV4 channels are not shown to be activated by mechanical touch, but rather respond to osmolality changes due to local cell swelling[22,29] and thus indirectly affect the response of nociceptive neurons.[30] Furthermore, TRPA1 channels (associated with detecting cold stimuli) are also believed to play a part in mechanical pain sensation; again, reports are inconsistent, with just two studies showing only small changes in mechanical thresholds.[18,31] However, TRPA1 activation contributes to both normal and inflamed mechanosensory function in the gut of mice during colorectal distension in the presence of induced inflammation.[32] Thus, similar to ASIC channels, these TRP channels have a varied role, and both appear to show strongest mechanosensitive sensitivity within the gut.

In summary, the molecular basis for mechanotransduction is still far from being determined. Mechanical hypersensitivity in response to tissue or nerve injury represents a significant clinical problem in most areas of health care, not least in the area of manual therapy. There is a multitude of chronic musculoskeletal pain conditions whose response to treatment is poor. It is clear that elucidation of the biological source of touch in both normal and patho-physiological conditions is a major challenge in somatosensory and pain research.

Response to chemical stimuli

Primary afferent nociceptors also detect environmental (exogenous) irritants and endogenous (within the organism) mediators produced by physiological stress. Again, TRP channels are the predominant receptor, especially for plant-derived allergens such as capsaicin (TRPV1),[11] menthol (TRPM8),[33] and pungent elements in mustard and garlic and isothiocyanates (horseradish) (TRPA1).[4] Specifically, TRPA1 channels are stimulated by a diverse group of exogenous irritants ranging from the food ingredients described above to other toxins such as car exhausts, burning vegetation (e.g., wood fire, cigarettes), and more volatile irritants such as hydrogen peroxide. Additionally, activation of TRPA1 channels in the eyes and airways causes pain and inflammation. Animals lacking TRPA1 show a significantly reduced sensitivity to the above toxins, highlighting the sensory importance of this channel.[18,34,35]

Importantly, chemical agents are also produced endogenously as part of the inflammatory response to tissue damage and/or physiological stress. The combination of these factors is enough to sensitize nociceptors to not only chemical, but also thermal and mechanical stress. Thus, the process of chemonociception can mediate the transition between acute and persistent pain; this will be discussed further later in the chapter. The key points relating to the proposed ion channels responsible for specific nociceptive sensitivity are listed in Box 1.2.

Conduction of pain signals to the dorsal horn

The transduction of mechanical, thermal, and chemical stimuli is initiated by membrane depolarization, often referred to as either a 'generator potential' or a 'receptor

---

Box 1.2

Key points: proposed ion channels responsible for specific nociceptive sensitivity

- Heat stimuli
  - TRPV1
- Cold stimuli
  - TRPM8 (+ 0°C)
  - TRPA1 (- 0°C)
- Mechanical stress
  - ASIC1 and 2 (predominantly smooth muscle of gastrointestinal tract)
  - ASIC3 (predominantly skeletal and cardiac muscle)
  - TRPA1 (predominantly smooth muscle of gastrointestinal tract)
- Chemical stimuli
  - TRPVI (capsaicin)
  - TRPM8 (menthol)
  - TRPA1 (mustard, garlic, smoke, car exhaust)

---

potential'. If this potential is of adequate magnitude, it is transformed into an action potential. The generation of action potentials triggers a number of voltage-gated ion channels that in turn convey nociceptive signals to synapses in the dorsal horn in the spinal cord.

Voltage-gated sodium channels

Voltage-gated sodium channels (VGSC or Na_v) are proteins that span the width of neuronal cell membranes (transmembrane proteins) and mediate the inward sodium current of excitable cells. These channels are fundamental to the generation and regulation of action potentials throughout the nervous system.[36] Additionally, Na_v channels influence resting potentials of neurons and are important for setting the threshold for action potentials.[37] Changes in Na_v function or expression therefore have major effects on changes in cell excitability (Figure 1.3). While all Na$_v$ cause the rapid upstroke of action potentials, they are not entirely homogenous. For example, a toxin found in the liver of the puffer fish, tetrodotoxin (TTX), is a highly selective blocker of central nervous system (CNS) and skeletal muscle sodium currents,[38] but a weak blocker of sodium currents in cardiac muscle.[39] Here, sodium channels are classified as either TTX-sensitive (Na$_v$1.1, 1.6, and 1.7 channels) or TTX-resistant (Na$_v$ 1.8 and 1.9 channels). Here, TTX-sensitive Na$_v$1.7 channels are highly expressed in both sympathetic and small diameter C nociceptors.

Recent studies indicate that Na$_v$1.7 channels are crucial to our ability to perceive pain sensations[40] and are upregulated (increased expression on cell membrane) in inflammatory pain disorders[41] and the pathogenesis of neuropathic pain.[42] Analysis of animals lacking the Na$_v$1.7 channel in C fibers showed that all inflammatory pain responses evoked by a range of stimuli were either reduced or abolished.[43] Na$_v$1.8 channels, on the other hand, are expressed only by small-diameter C fiber neurons. Unlike other Na$_v$ channels, Na$_v$1.8 can continue generating fast action potentials and transmit nociceptive information to the CNS in cold temperatures. Thus, it is the predominant action potential generator in cold conditions.

Given the influence of Na$_v$ on the transmission of nociceptive inputs, they are the target of studies investigating subtype-specific analgesics. Concerning the selective inhibition of Na$_v$1.7, several research groups have identified a highly potent and selective Na$_v$1.7 inhibitor.[44,45] Their findings suggest these compounds may be useful as both antinociceptive and neuropathic pain agents. Thus, selective inhibition of these channels may provide a useful therapeutic option minimizing cardiac and CNS effects associated with current non-subtype-selective Na$_v$ blockers such as lidocaine and carbamazepine.[36] Interestingly, the anti-hyperalgesic effect of tricyclic antidepressants (TCAs) and selective serotonin reuptake inhibitors (SSRIs) are also due to their ability to selectively block Na$_v$1.7 channels[46] in descending pain pathways.

Voltage-gated calcium channels

Voltage-gated calcium channels (VGCCs) are also expressed along peripheral pain pathways.

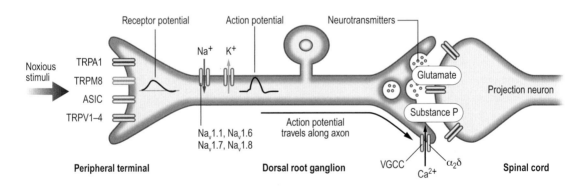

Figure 1.3

A schematic diagram of ion channels involved in nociceptive function. Peripheral terminals respond to noxious stimulation (e.g., tissue damage) through receptors and ion channels including TRP and ASIC channels. Once a defined threshold of depolarization is reached, Na$_v$ channels are activated and an action potential is generated. The action potential is transmitted along the axon to the presynaptic terminal where calcium influx through VGCCs triggers the release of neurotransmitters from the presynaptic terminals

Several VGCC subgroups play a pivotal role in neurotransmitter release and synaptic transmission. For example, T-type VGCCs are highly expressed on C fiber terminals and like Na_v are upregulated in hyperalgesic and allodynic states.[47] Interestingly, the antihyperalgesic effect of the anticonvulsant drug gabapentin is thought to act by inhibiting VGCCs, targeting specific subunits ($\alpha_2 d$ subunits) of this channel within the CNS. Animals lacking both T and N types of channel show reduced neuropathic pain behavior (e.g., anxiety) as well as a decreased likelihood of developing neuropathic pain.[48,49]

N-type VGCCs and P/Q-type VGCCs are expressed at synaptic terminals in laminae II–IV of the dorsal horn (Figure 1.3). They become active in response to incoming action potentials that in turn generate the release of calcium into the dorsal horn synapse, thus initiating the discharge of neurotransmitters (e.g., substance P, glutamate) onto spinothalamic neurons. Additionally, N-type VGCCs are uniquely inhibited by opioid receptor agonists such as morphine.[50] Moreover, mice lacking the N-type gene are, not surprisingly, shown to be less sensitive to both neuropathic and inflammatory pain, despite being otherwise normal.[51]

Peripheral sensitization and inflammatory mediators

Changes in pain sensitivity related to inflammation and nerve injury are characterized by changes in pain perception that include a reduction in pain thresholds and an increased responsiveness of the peripheral terminals of nociceptors to stimuli.[52] Enhanced sensitivity to normally noxious stimuli is classified as 'hyperalgesia' and abnormal pain sensitivity to normally non-painful stimuli is classified as 'allodynia' (Figure 1.4). Thus, peripheral sensitization is a form of stimulus-evoked functional plasticity of the nociceptive neurons.[9]

Sensitization occurs due to inflammation-associated changes in the chemical environment surrounding normally high-threshold peripheral nociceptive nerve endings.[53] First, tissue damage initiates the release of intracellular contents from damaged or inflammatory cells (including macrophages, lymphocytes, and mast cells) into the injured area. Subsequent stimulation of nociceptors further results in the release of neurotransmitters such as substance P, neurokinin A, and CGRP from local afferent nociceptive terminals. These compounds modify the excitability of adjacent sensory and sympathetic nerve endings, resulting in local vasodilatation and extravasation of plasma proteins that in turn stimulate release of additional chemical mediators by inflammatory cells.[1] Collectively, these factors, referred to as the 'inflammatory soup' (Figure 1.5), also include factors released from damaged cells, such as bradykinin, histamine, cytokines, nitric oxide, growth factors, and products of the cyclooxygenase and lipoxygenase pathways of arachidonic acid metabolism (e.g., prostaglandins).

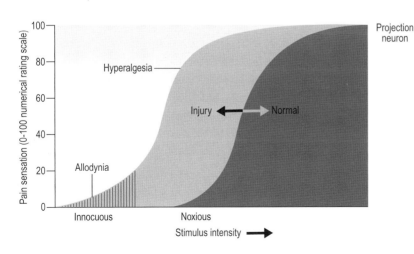

Figure 1.4

A graph showing the relationship between stimulus intensity (*x* axis) and pain sensation (*y* axis) in normal (dark) and sensitized conditions (light/lined)

Cytokines and growth factors

Cytokines are small proteins released by cells; they affect the interaction and communication between cells. Cytokines are associated with many cell populations; however, in inflammation they are produced by T cells and macrophages.[54] Additionally, during physiological and pathological processes cytokines are also produced in and released by peripheral nerve tissue. For example, following tissue injury and/or peripheral nerve injury, macrophages and Schwann cells attracted to the injured site secrete not only cytokines, but also growth factors needed for nerve regeneration.[54] In research on discogenic pain, animal studies show that growth factors are secreted from herniated nucleus pulposus and within the spinal cord.[55]

Interleukin-1β

IL-1β, a multifunctional cytokine, is released by immune cells (e.g., macrophages) as well as non-immune cells (e.g., fibroblasts) as a result of tissue injury, infection, invasion, and inflammation.[54] Furthermore, the release of IL-1β increases the production and secretion of substance P and prostaglandins (PG) in neuronal and glial cells in the spinal cord.[56] However, while IL-1β is key to a normal inflammatory response, its overproduction is also partly responsible for pathophysiological changes occurring in conditions such as rheumatoid arthritis, osteoarthritis, inflammatory bowel disease, and neuropathic pain.[57]

Interleukin-6

IL-6 plays a central role in the neuronal reaction to nerve injury,[54] with studies showing its contribution to the development of neuropathic pain following peripheral nerve injury. This is thought to be due to upregulation of IL-6, its receptor and transducer in both peripheral nociceptors and dorsal root ganglia.[58] Interestingly, IL-6 has been shown to activate pain fibers even in the absence of inflammation. Here, experimental exposure to IL-6 in peripheral nerves evokes long-lasting pain behavior indicating its direct action on nociceptive neurons.[59]

Tumor necrosis factor-α

Tumor necrosis factor (TNF-α) is a cytokine that plays a key role in peripheral pain models. Here, TNF-α is shown to (1) initiate the activation of inflammatory mediators, (2) regulate apoptotic (programmed cell death) pathways, and (3) regulate initiation and maintenance of neuropathic hyperalgesia.[54] Studies show positive correlations between levels of TNF-α expression and the development of allodynia and hyperalgesia, especially in neuropathic pain models. Importantly, nerve injury also leads to increased expression of TNF-α receptors on both damaged and adjacent non-damaged sensory neurons, resulting in an increased sensitivity in and round injury sites. Recently, the importance of TNF-α has been underlined by the success of TNF-α antagonists in the treatment of inflammatory conditions including rheumatoid arthritis, ankylosing spondylitis, and Crohn's disease.[60] This success is due mainly to the fact that TNF-α medications do not cross the blood–brain barrier and therefore act only on peripheral sites, where they are able to modify symptoms and alter disease progression. However, although risk benefit analysis is in favor of using anti-TNF-α medications, there are concerns about the potential for infections in people with rheumatoid arthritis and Crohn's disease. Additionally, anti-TNF treatments have also been shown to initiate and reactivate tuberculosis in some groups of patients.[61]

Nerve growth factor

Nerve growth factor (NGF) shares many characteristics with cytokines and is the most commonly studied growth factor relating to nociceptor sensitization.[62] While its major role lies in the area of neuronal development and survival, it also promotes neuronal sprouting (generation of additional branches) and regulates the innervation density of the peripheral sensory nervous system.[63] However, NGF is also shown to make a significant contribution to the development of mechanical and thermal hyperalgesia, with NGF levels rising significantly in inflamed tissue and injured nerves.[64] Here, NGF is released by macrophages and T lymphocytes and

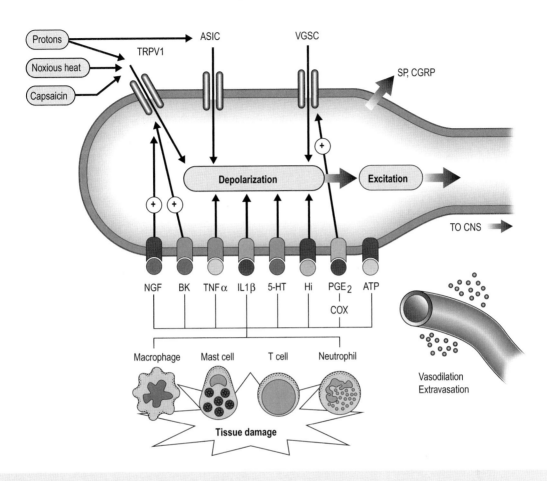

Figure 1.5

Tissue cells damaged during injury release inflammatory mediators such as prostaglandins and bradykinin into the area around nociceptors. The presence of these mediators activates immune cells such as macrophages, mast cells, and neutrophils that release further inflammatory substances. These mediators are collectively known as the 'inflammatory soup'; it includes protons (H+), purines (e.g., adenosine triphosphate, ATP), nerve growth factor (NGF), bradykinin (BK), tumor necrosis factor (TNF-α), interleukins (e.g., IL-1β), serotonin (5-HT), histamine (Hi), and prostaglandins (e.g., PGE2). Prostaglandins are formed by cyclooxygenase (COX) enzyme

has a cytokine-type action on inflammatory cells. Importantly, NGF is a powerful degranulator of mast cells (Figure 1.6) that contribute to hyperalgesia through the release of histamine and bradykinin.[1] Tyrosine kinase receptors are the predominant NGF receptor. These are expressed in about 50% of peripheral nociceptors, where their activation leads to the sensitization of TRPV1 receptors $Na_v1.8$ channels and the release of substance P, thus explaining its role in amplification of hyperalgesia.[60]

Cyclo-oxygenase, prostaglandins, and bradykinin

Prostaglandin E2 (PGE2) is a pivotal mediator of inflammatory pain sensitization and is produced in response to peripherally damaged and/or inflamed tissues. During tissue injury, arachidonic acid is released from cell membranes and is transformed into the prostaglandins precursor PGH2 by the action of constitutively expressed cyclooxygenase

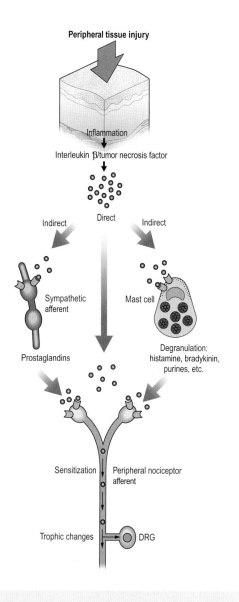

Peripheral tissue injury

Inflammation

Interleukin β/tumor necrosis factor

Indirect   Direct   Indirect

Sympathetic afferent

Mast cell

Prostaglandins

Degranulation: histamine, bradykinin, purines, etc.

Sensitization   Peripheral nociceptor afferent

Trophic changes   DRG

Figure 1.6

The role of nerve growth factor (NGF) in peripheral sensitization. NGF has (1) a direct effect on primary afferent nociceptors by activating tyrosine kinase A receptors (TrKA) and (2) indirect effects on both mast cells (stimulating the release of inflammatory mediators including bradykinin and histamine) and sympathetic efferents (activating the release of prostaglandins), all of which activate receptors on peripheral nociceptors

1 (COX1) or inducible cyclooxygenase 2 (COX2). PGH2 is then converted to PGE2 that then acts on nociceptor G protein-coupled receptors (GPCRs). The activation of GPCRs triggers the release of intracellular second messengers within the nociceptive neuron (discussed in the following section).[65] The release of bradykinin during the inflammatory process stimulates further synthesis and release of PGE2. An increase in PGE2 concentration is strongly associated with inflammation-induced hyperalgesia, with studies demonstrating that PGE2 injection evokes hyperalgesia.

The primary analgesic effect of nonsteroidal anti-inflammatory drugs (NSAIDs) is the inhibition of COX and the subsequent reduction of peripheral PGE2. Previously, it was understood that COX1 was a constitutive enzyme, distributed throughout the body with a 'housekeeping' role related to cell homeostasis, most commonly associated with the gastrointestinal tract, whereas COX2 was an enzyme upregulated in response to inflammatory stimuli.[67] Thus, while COX inhibits the action of PGE2, the use of COX1 inhibitors also results in side effects such as gastric ulceration. Fortunately, the introduction of COX2 selective antagonists has been shown to be more specific to inflammation. However, there are also cautions to be observed with COX2 medications, since its inhibition has been shown to be associated with increased risk of cardiovascular events (myocardial infarction, stroke).[67]

Intracellular secondary messenger pathways

Activation of GPCRs and ionotropic (ligand-gated ion channels) receptors such as ASICs and TRP channels directly and/or indirectly activate intracellular second messenger pathways that augment or inhibit nociceptive processing.[68] Second messengers activated by GPCRs include cyclic adenosine monophosphate (cAMP), cyclic guanosine monophosphate (cGMP), inositol triphosphate (IP_3) and diacylglycerol (DAG). Ionotropic receptors also activate second messenger systems by increasing calcium influx (Figure 1.7),[68] which then mediate numerous biological processes that lead to generation and maintenance of pain.

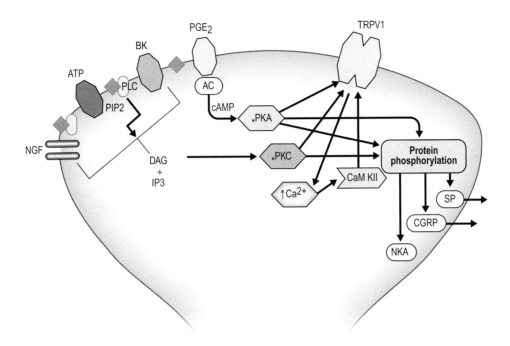

Figure 1.7

A schematic representation of intracellular cAMP-PKA and IP3/DAG-PKC pathways that (1) modulate the activation of TRPV1 channels and (2) increase expression of substance P (SP), calcitonin gene-related peptide (CGRP), and neurokinin A (NKA). Concerning the IP3/DAG pathway, activated ATP and bradykinin (BK) receptors stimulate phospholipase C (PLC) to split phosphatidylinositol 4–5 bisphosphate (PIP2) into IP3 and DAG. DAG and IP3 then activate PKC pathways that lead to the increased activation of TRPV1 receptors and intracellular protein phosphorylation that in turn increase the release of neurotransmitters such as substance P and Neurokinin A

The cAMP protein kinase A pathway

An increased level of intracellular cAMP is shown to be an important measure of nociceptive sensitivity.[69] Increases in cAMP-activated protein kinase A (PKA) in turn activate processes such as altered mRNA transcription and calcium mobilization that increase pain sensitivity (Figure 1.7). It is important to understand that while increases in cAMP cause inflammation-driven hyperalgesia, the activation of PKA is required to maintain it.[2] Activated intracellular cAMP also causes the phosphorylation and subsequent opening of TTX-resistant Na channels (e.g., $Na_v1.8$) from inside the neuron. These actions further enhance nociceptor excitability and thus lower pain thresholds.

The IP3/DAG protein kinase C pathway

The activation of GPCRs also activates DAG and IP3 (Figure 1.7). DAG then stimulates another protein kinase, protein kinase C (PKC), which, with IP3, promotes intracellular calcium mobilization.[68] Continued activation of PKC has also been found to evoke TRPV1 sensitization from inside the activated neuron through protein phosphorylation, and also to contribute to heat hyperalgesia.[70] Interestingly, PKC also mediates mechanical hyperalgesia when associated with peripheral neuropathy. Here, studies show that mechanical allodynia generated by chronic alcohol consumption is dramatically reduced by injection of PKC inhibitor at the site of nociceptive testing.[71]

Intracellular activation of TRPV1 receptors and neurogenic inflammation

Cumulative evidence now shows that nociceptive sensitization by inflammatory mediators is primarily due to the potentiation of TRPV1 channel activity.[72] TRPV1 sensitization by proalgesic agents is due either to direct activation of the channel or to its potentiation (increase in degree of activity). In addition to activation of TRPV1 via extracellular inflammatory agents, intracellular pathways within C fiber terminals also modulate TRPV1 channels. Here, direct activation of GPCRs by bradykinin, NFG, and PGE2 triggers various intracellular mechanisms through the phosphorylation of intracellular protein kinases.[73] It is the activation of these kinases that not only modulates TRPV1, but also acts to increase the release of substance P, neurokinin A, and CGRP from the C fiber terminal (Figure 1.7). Release of these substances further facilitates the increase in vascular permeability, vasodilation, and the release of a complex assortment of proinflammatory and proalgesic factors. Importantly, these mediators stimulate adjacent sensory nerve endings that further enhance their own sensitivity to temperature and touch.

Sympathetically maintained pain

The sympathetic nervous system (SNS) is best known as an efferent neuroeffector system modulating visceral, cardiovascular, bronchial, metabolic, and sudomotor function. Although the SNS is shown to play an essential role in global responses to noxious stimuli as observed with fight or flight, it also has a peripheral role. Here, NGF influences peripheral 'sprouting' of sympathetic nerves and subsequent 'coupling' of sensory and SNS neurons that cause increases in spontaneous (without stimulus) firing.[2] Patients with SNS-dependent pain complain of diffuse burning pain and hyperalgesia following nerve injury.

Sympathetic coupling

Several forms of coupling between SNS and adjacent neurons are proposed. First, ephaptic coupling describes electrical activity cross-talk that occurs not via the release of neurotransmitters but through the direct flow of current to an adjacent nociceptive neuron.[74] However, while this hypothesis may explain forms of hyperalgesia experienced by the patient, it offers no explanation for the SNS dependency of the pain state or the spread of symptoms beyond the injured tissue. Second, there is mounting evidence showing that damaged nociceptive neurons increase their expression of adrenergic receptors[75]. Blockade of α-adrenergic receptor function leads to significant pain relief in patients with chronic regional pain syndrome, a disorder showing severe pain typically in the extremities.[76] Additionally, patients with sympathetically maintained pain also describe pain relief on receiving a sympathetic ganglion block. Third, the release of NGF from injured peripheral tissue stimulates SNS neurons that in turn form 'basket-like' outgrowths (sprouting) at the dorsal root ganglion that further drives ganglion activity.

Proinflammatory mediators and joint pain

The cytokines and growth factors described above induce and maintain many types of arthritis.[77,78] Degenerative disorders such as osteoarthritis (OA) occur owing to locally activated inflammation, while systemic disorders, including rheumatoid arthritis, are activated by autoimmune stimuli. However, both local and systemic immune pathologies show similar levels of proinflammatory mediators such as TNF-α, several interleukins, NGF, and prostaglandins.

People with arthritis typically experience ongoing pain in the absence of deliberate stimulation, especially with movements within the non-painful normal range. In such cases, the patient experiences mechanical hyperalgesia. Equally, if normally non-painful heat or cold stimuli induce pain, the patient experiences thermal hyperalgesia.[77] Therefore, proinflammatory mediators not only have a direct impact on the joint disease process, but also affect the nervous system, where they act to initiate and mediate pain elicited from the neurons themselves. Importantly, pathological changes in nerve fibers in the long term in joint pathology may also trigger more centrally mediated pain disorders via central sensitization (Chapter 2).[79]

Silent nociceptors

There is one more, rarely described class of nociceptor categorized by unique properties. 'Sleeping' or 'silent' nociceptors are typically unresponsive or inactive under most circumstances and are unresponsive to noxious mechanical stimulation except in extreme ranges of intensity. However, this class of nociceptor becomes active following inflammation and sensitization by NGF. Typically, they have been identified within joint capsules and in the wall of the gastrointestinal tract.[80,81] Following sensitization, they become responsive and discharge vigorously even within the normal physiological range of ordinary movement. Furthermore, activation of silent nociceptors creates new and extra nociceptive input that significantly contributes to mechanical allodynia and hyperalgesia associated with inflammation in arthritis and in visceral pain disorders such as interstitial cystitis and inflammatory bowel disease.[1]

Treatment approaches

Drug treatment

Given the large range and number of inflammatory (sensitizing) mediators acting in parallel, alleviation of their effects is challenging. At present, treatment blocking PGE2 synthesis via the inhibition of COX1 and COX2 is the standard approach for most nonsteroidal anti-inflammatory (NSAIDs) analgesics. Treatment approaches targeting other proinflammatory mediators exist, including anti-NGF agents. A recent systematic review found that in the treatment of osteoarthritis (OA) of hip/knee, anti-NGF agents, either alone or in combination with NSAIDs, were more efficacious for the treatment of pain when compared to NSAIDs alone. However, more adverse effects, including increasingly progressive OA and increased likelihood of joint replacement, were found with the combination treatment than with either treatment used on its own.[78] These adverse effects are most likely due to the fact that NGF regulates a number of metabolic processes that affect organ function, wound healing, neoplastic disease, and immunosuppression. Thus, although NGF

antagonists decreased pain in people with OA, their effect on other metabolic processes lead to increased joint cartilage degeneration due to both overuse and changes in wound healing mechanisms. Nevertheless, promising findings were observed in a double-blind controlled clinical trial in people with chronic low back pain (LBP), with subjects reporting improvements rated as 'good' to 'very good' at six weeks using anti-NGF treatment when compared to placebo.[82,83] However, as the adverse effects observed in OA subject groups appear to be similar across all treatments, further development is on regulatory hold.

Anti-TNFα agents have also been investigated in a variety of different chronic pain conditions. Most studies investigate the effect of these drugs in subjects with autoimmune disorders such as ankylosing spondylitis, rheumatoid arthritis, and Crohn's disease.[84,85] However, despite the proven therapeutic value of these agents, there have been reports of potentially serious adverse effects, including an increased risk of infection, malignancies, and worsening of conditions such as multiple sclerosis and congestive heart failure.[86] Encouragingly, however, a recent Cochrane review showed not only evidence that anti TNF-α agents improve clinical symptoms of ankylosing spondylitis, including reductions in both pain and physical function, but equally, they found no evidence of increases in serious adverse effects.[87]

Exercise

Exercise has been shown to be a valuable intervention, with enormous benefits, including reductions in morbidity in cardiovascular disease, obstructive pulmonary disease, and age-related chronic disorders.[88] While the effects of exercise on improved physical fitness and enhancement of cardiovascular and pulmonary perfusion are well-established, its effect on levels of inflammatory mediators is less clear. Recently, several interesting findings have emerged showing decreases in proinflammatory neurotransmitters and increases in anti-inflammatory mediators in both healthy patients and patients suffering a variety of pain-related conditions.[88–91] Here, findings also suggest that regular exercise of moderate intensity increases circulating levels of IL-6 that in turn induce an anti-inflammatory response by triggering the release of inhibitory IL-1ra and IL-10 from local endothelial cells, while also inhibiting the production of TNF-α.[92] Studies also show that moderate cycling[91] and aquatic exercise[93] improve the inflammatory status of fibromyalgia patients as well as healthy but usually sedentary women.[90]

Manual therapy

It is proposed that manual therapy can influence the effect of inflammatory mediators on peripheral nociceptors. Studies have investigated the effects of joint manipulation and soft tissue techniques on both inflammatory mediators such as substance P and blood levels of endogenous analgesic peptides such as β-endorphins. For example, healthy subjects treated with spinal manipulation showed downregulation of substance P compared to subjects receiving sham manipulation.[94] Similarly, soft-tissue techniques are shown to decrease levels of substance P; however, these findings are also correlated to an increase in sleep hours and decreases in anxiety and depression.[95] Thus, it is not known whether such techniques have a direct or indirect effect on peripheral levels of inflammatory mediators. As such, further investigation in these areas would help to explain the significance of variables affecting not only the perception of pain but also peripheral inflammatory mediators driving pain.

Alternatively, studies using osteopathic manipulative treatment show altered blood levels of several pain biomarkers, including serotonin, cannabinoids, and inflammatory cytokines. Here, people with chronic low back pain show greater changes in biomarker levels, especially directly after treatment.[96] However, as with many studies of this nature, while there are significant correlations between treatment and changes in inflammatory biomarkers, underlying mechanisms behind these changes remain unidentified. In another study, researchers compared baseline and post osteopathic manipulative treatment (12 weeks) levels of several proinflammatory cytokines.[97] Interestingly, although results showed significant correlations between concentrations of IL-1β and IL6 in people presenting with severe somatic dysfunction, TNF-α was the only inflammatory marker to show reductions over the 12-week treatment period. These conflicting results clearly show that there is a need for further research, including investigations to address more specific pain conditions, as, for example, the expression of inflammatory mediators in the presence of facet joint dysfunction may be unlike that in people presenting with disc-related low back pain.

Summary

Peripheral pain mechanisms are significantly altered both during and after inflammation and/or nerve damage. Inflammatory mediators initiate action potentials along nociceptive neurons by acting on receptors, ion channels, and immune cells that generate and maintain nociceptor stimulation and ultimately sensitization. Intracellular mechanisms further contribute to peripheral sensitization where, for example, the phosphorylation of protein kinases not only enhances the activity of TRPV1 channels but also the expression and release of inflammatory peptides such as substance P and CGRP. Together, these extra- and intracellular nociceptive processes result in increased primary afferent input to the spinal cord, which, in turn, leads to alterations in nociceptive processing in the dorsal horn (Chapter 2). Importantly, recent studies show that drug treatment, exercise, and manual therapy can all help to reduce levels of inflammatory markers. However, it remains unclear as to what mechanisms underlie reductions in some but not all inflammatory mediators in different chronic pain conditions. Thus future studies must focus their objectives toward more specific causes of musculoskeletal pain conditions as opposed to nonspecific anatomical pain presentations.

References

1. Hudspeth M, Siddall P, Munglani R. Physiology of pain. In: Hemmings H, Hopkins P, editors. Foundations of anesthesia basic sciences for clinical practice. 2nd ed. Philadelphia: Elsevier; 2006. p. 267–85.

2. Farquhar Smith P. Peripheral mechanisms. In: Hughes J, editor. Pain management. Edinburgh: Elsevier Health Sciences; 2008. p. 48–65.

3. MacCallum D. Peripheral nervous system. University of Michigan Medical School; 2014.

4. Basbaum AI, Bautista DM, Scherrer G, Julius D. Cellular and molecular mechanisms of pain. Cell. 2009;139(2):267–84.

5. Gold MS, Gebhart GF. Nociceptor sensitization in pain pathogenesis. Nature Medicine. 2010;16(11):1248–57.

6. Schmidt R, Schmelz M, Forster C, Ringkamp M, Torebjork E, Handwerker H. Novel classes of responsive and unresponsive C nociceptors in human skin. Journal of Neuroscience. 1995;15(1/1):333–41.

7. Schaible HG. Peripheral and central mechanisms of pain generation. Handbook of Experimental Pharmacology. 2007(177):3–28.

8. Schaible H-G. Emerging concepts of pain therapy based on neuronal mechanisms. In: Schaible H-G, editor. Pain control. Handbook of Experimental Pharmacology. 227: Springer Berlin Heidelberg; 2015. p. 1–14.

9. Woolf CJ, Ma Q. Nociceptors – noxious stimulus detectors. Neuron. 2007;55(3):353–64.

10. Patapoutian A, Peier AM, Story GM, Viswanath V. ThermoTRP channels and beyond: mechanisms of temperature sensation. Nature Reviews Neuroscience. 2003;4(7):529–39.

11. Caterina MJ, Leffler A, Malmberg AB, Martin WJ, Trafton J, Petersen-Zeitz KR, et al. Impaired nociception and pain sensation in mice lacking the capsaicin receptor. Science (New York, NY). 2000;288(5464):306–13.

12. Julius D. TRP channels and pain. Annual Review of Cell and Developmental Biology. 2013;29:355–84.

13. Rosenbaum T, Simon S. TRPV1 receptors and signal transduction. In: Liedtke W, Heller S, editors. TRP ion channel function in sensory transduction and cellular signaling cascades. Boca Raton, FL: CRC Press; 2007.

14. Liu L, Simon SA. Capsaicin, acid and heat-evoked currents in rat trigeminal ganglion neurons: relationship to functional VR1 receptors. Physiology and Behavior. 2000;69(3):363–78.

15. Bautista DM, Siemens J, Glazer JM, Tsuruda PR, Basbaum AI, Stucky CL, et al. The menthol receptor TRPM8 is the principal detector of environmental cold. Nature. 2007;448(7150):204–8.

16. Dhaka A, Murray AN, Mathur J, Earley TJ, Petrus MJ, Patapoutian A. TRPM8 is required for cold sensation in mice. Neuron. 2007;54(3):371–8.

17. McCoy DD, Knowlton WM, McKemy DD. Scraping through the ice: uncovering the role of TRPM8 in cold transduction. 2011;300(6):R1278–87.

18. Bautista DM, Jordt SE, Nikai T, Tsuruda PR, Read AJ, Poblete J, et al. TRPA1 mediates the inflammatory actions of environmental irritants and proalgesic agents. Cell. 2006;124(6):1269–82.

19. Story GM, Peier AM, Reeve AJ, Eid SR, Mosbacher J, Hricik TR, et al. ANKTM1, a TRP-like channel expressed in nociceptive neurons, is activated by cold temperatures. Cell. 2003;112(6):819–29.

20. Del Camino D, Murphy S, Heiry M, Barrett LB, Earley TJ, Cook CA, et al. TRPA1 contributes to cold hypersensitivity. Journal of Neuroscience. 2010;30(45):15165–74.

21. Julius D, Basbaum AI. Molecular mechanisms of nociception. Nature. 2001;413(6852):203–10.

22. Delmas P, Hao J, Rodat-Despoix L. Molecular mechanisms of mechanotransduction in mammalian sensory neurons. Nature Reviews Neuroscience. 2011;12(3):139–53.

23. Hughes PA, Brierley SM, Young RL, Blackshaw LA. Localization and comparative analysis of acid-sensing ion channel (ASIC1, 2, and 3) mRNA expression in mouse colonic sensory neurons within thoracolumbar dorsal root ganglia. Journal of Comparative Neurology. 2007;500(5):863–75.

24. Page AJ, Brierley SM, Martin CM, Martinez-Salgado C, Wemmie JA, Brennan TJ, et al. The ion channel ASIC1 contributes to visceral but not cutaneous mechanoreceptor function. Gastroenterology. 2004;127(6):1739–47.

25. Price MP, Lewin GR, McIlwrath SL, Cheng C, Xie J, Heppenstall PA, et al. The mammalian sodium channel BNC1 is required for normal touch sensation. Nature. 2000;407(6807):1007–11.

26. Price MP, McIlwrath SL, Xie J, Cheng C, Qiao J, Tarr DE, et al. The DRASIC cation channel contributes to the detection of cutaneous touch and acid stimuli in mice. Neuron. 2001;32(6):1071–83.

27. Omerbašić D, Schuhmacher L-N, Bernal Sierra Y-A, Smith ESJ, Lewin GR. ASICs and mammalian mechanoreceptor function. Neuropharmacology. 2015;94:80–6.

28. Christensen AP, Corey DP. TRP channels in mechanosensation: direct or indirect activation? Nature Reviews Neuroscience. 2007;8(7):510–21.

29. Zhu C. Mechanochemistry: a molecular biomechanics view of mechanosensing. Annals of Biomedical Engineering. 2014;42(2):388–404.

30. Alessandri-Haber N, Dina OA, Yeh JJ, Parada CA, Reichling DB, Levine JD. Transient receptor potential vanilloid 4 is essential in chemotherapy-induced neuropathic pain in the rat. Journal of Neuroscience. 2004;24(18):4444–52.

31. Petrus M, Peier AM, Bandell M, Hwang SW, Huynh T, Olney N, et al. A role of TRPA1 in mechanical hyperalgesia is revealed by pharmacological inhibition. Molecular Pain. 2007;3:40.

32. Brierley SM, Hughes PA, Page AJ, Kwan KY, Martin CM, O'Donnell TA, et al. The ion channel TRPA1 is required for normal mechanosensation and is modulated by algesic stimuli. Gastroenterology. 2009;137(6):2084–95.e3.

33. Peier AM, Moqrich A, Hergarden AC, Reeve AJ, Andersson DA, Story GM, et al. A TRP channel that senses cold stimuli and menthol. Cell. 2002;108(5):705–15.

34. Bandell M, Story GM, Hwang SW, Viswanath V, Eid SR, Petrus MJ, et al. Noxious cold ion channel TRPA1 is activated by pungent compounds and bradykinin. Neuron. 2004;41(6):849–57.

35. Akopian AN, Ruparel NB, Patwardhan A, Hargreaves KM. Cannabinoids desensitize capsaicin and mustard oil responses in sensory neurons via TRPA1 activation. Journal of Neuroscience. 2008;28(5):1064–75.

36. Theile JW, Cummins TR. Recent developments regarding voltage-gated sodium channel blockers for the treatment of inherited and acquired neuropathic pain syndromes. Frontiers in Pharmacology. 2011;2:54.

37. Rush AM, Cummins TR, Waxman SG. Multiple sodium channels and their roles in electrogenesis within dorsal root ganglion neurons. Journal of Physiology. 2007;579(1):1–14.

38. Ritchie JM, Rogart RB. The binding of saxitoxin and tetrodotoxin to excitable tissue. Reviews of Physiology, Biochemistry and Pharmacology. 1977;79:1–50.

39. Cummins TR, Sheets PL, Waxman SG. The roles of sodium channels in nociception: implications for mechanisms of pain. Pain. 2007;131(3):243–57.

40. Goldberg YP, MacFarlane J, MacDonald ML, Thompson J, Dube MP, Mattice M, et al. Loss-of-function mutations in the Nav1.7 gene underlie congenital indifference to pain in multiple human populations. Clinical Genetics. 2007;71(4):311–19.

41. Estacion M, Dib-Hajj SD, Benke PJ, Te Morsche RH, Eastman EM, Macala LJ, et al. NaV1.7 gain-of-function mutations as a continuum: A1632E displays physiological changes associated with erythromelalgia and paroxysmal extreme pain disorder mutations and produces symptoms of both disorders. Journal of neuroscience. 2008;28(43):11079–88.

42. Dib-Hajj SD, Black JA, Waxman SG. Voltage-gated sodium channels: therapeutic targets for pain. Pain Medicine (Malden, Mass). 2009;10(7):1260–9.

43. Nassar MA, Stirling LC, Forlani G, Baker MD, Matthews EA, Dickenson AH, et al. Nociceptor-specific gene deletion reveals a major role for Nav1.7 (PN1) in acute and inflammatory pain. Proceedings of the National Academy of Sciences of the United States of America. 2004;101(34):12706–11.

44. Sun S, Jia Q, Zenova AY, Chafeev M, Zhang Z, Lin S, et al. The discovery of benzenesulfonamide-based potent and selective inhibitors of voltage-gated sodium channel Nav1.7. Bioorganic and Medicinal Chemistry Letters. 2014;24(18):4397–401.

45. Ho GD, Tulshian D, Bercovici A, Tan Z, Hanisak J, Brumfield S, et al. Discovery of pyrrolo-benzo-1,4-diazines as potent Nav1.7 sodium channel blockers. Bioorganic and Medicinal Chemistry Letters. 2014;24(17):4110–13.

46. Dick IE, Brochu RM, Purohit Y, Kaczorowski GJ, Martin WJ, Priest BT. Sodium channel blockade may contribute to the analgesic efficacy of antidepressants. Journal of Pain. 2007;8(4):315–24.

47. Luo ZD, Chaplan SR, Higuera ES, Sorkin LS, Stauderman KA, Williams ME, et al. Upregulation of dorsal root ganglion (alpha)2(delta) calcium channel subunit and its correlation with allodynia in spinal nerve-injured rats. Journal of Neuroscience. 2001;21(6):1868–75.

48. Hansson P. [Peripheral neuropathic pain more researched than central]. Lakartidningen. 2008;105(39):2700–5.

49. Choi S, Na HS, Kim J, Lee J, Lee S, Kim D, et al. Attenuated pain responses in mice lacking Ca(V)3.2 T-type channels. Genes, Brain, and Behavior. 2007;6(5):425–31.

50. Altier C, Zamponi GW. Targeting Ca2+ channels to treat pain: T-type versus N-type. Trends in Pharmacological Sciences. 2004;25(9):465–70.

51. Saegusa H, Kurihara T, Zong S, Kazuno A, Matsuda Y, Nonaka T, et al. Suppression of inflammatory and neuropathic pain symptoms in mice lacking the N-type Ca2+ channel. EMBO Journal. 2001;20(10):2349–56.

52. Schaible H-G. Peripheral and central mechanisms of pain generation. In: Stein C, editor. Analgesia. Berlin, Heidelberg: Springer Berlin Heidelberg; 2007. p. 3–28.

53. McMahon SB, Bevan S. Inflammatory mediators and modulators of pain. In: Koltzenburg M, editor. Wall and Melzack's textbook of pain. E-dition: Churchill Livingstone (Elsevier Health Sciences); 2005. p. 49–72.

54. Zhang J-M, An J. Cytokines, inflammation and pain. International Anesthesiology Clinics. 2007;45(2):27–37.

55. DeLeo JA, Colburn RW, Nichols M, Malhotra A. Interleukin-6-mediated hyperalgesia/allodynia and increased spinal IL-6 expression in a rat mononeuropathy model. Journal of Interferon and Cytokine Research. 1996;16(9):695–700.

56. Jeanjean AP, Moussaoui SM, Maloteaux JM, Laduron PM. Interleukin-1 beta induces long-term increase of axonally transported opiate receptors and substance P. Neuroscience. 1995;68(1):151–7.

57. Ren K, Torres R. Role of interleukin-1β during pain and inflammation. Brain Research Reviews. 2009;60(1):57–64.

58. De Jongh RF, Vissers KC, Meert TF, Booij LH, De Deyne CS, Heylen RJ. The role of interleukin-6 in nociception and pain. Anesthesia and Analgesia. 2003;96(4):1096–103, table of contents.

59. Eliav E, Benoliel R, Herzberg U, Kalladka M, Tal M. The role of IL-6 and IL-1beta in painful perineural inflammatory neuritis. Brain, Behavior, and Immunity. 2009;23(4):474–84.

60. Marchand F, Perretti M, McMahon SB. Role of the immune system in chronic pain. Nature Reviews Neuroscience. 2005;6(7):521–32.

61. Antoni C, Braun J. Side effects of anti-TNF therapy: current knowledge. Clinical and Experimental Rheumatology. 2002;20(6 Suppl 28):S152–7.

62. Jankowski M, Koerber H. Neurotrophic factors and nociceptor sensitization. In: Kruger L, Light A, editors. Translational pain research: from mouse to man. Boca Raton, FL: CRC Press; 2010.

63. Diamond J, Holmes M, Coughlin M. Endogenous NGF and nerve impulses regulate the collateral sprouting of sensory axons in the skin of the adult rat. Journal of Neuroscience. 1992;12(4):1454–66.

64. Moalem G, Tracey DJ. Immune and inflammatory mechanisms in neuropathic pain. Brain Research Reviews. 2006;51(2):240–64.

65. Hata AN, Breyer RM. Pharmacology and signaling of prostaglandin receptors: multiple roles in inflammation and immune modulation. Pharmacology and Therapeutics. 2004;103(2):147–66.

66. Wang H, Ehnert C, Brenner GJ, Woolf CJ. Bradykinin and peripheral sensitization. Biological Chemistry. 2006;387(1):11–14.

67. Bingham S, Beswick PJ, Blum DE, Gray NM, Chessell IP. The role of the cylooxygenase pathway in nociception and pain. Seminars in Cell and Developmental Biology. 2006;17(5):544–54.

68. Sluka K, Skyba D, Hoeger Bement M, Audette K, Radhakrishnan R. Second messenger pathways in pain. In: Zhuo M, editor. Molecular pain. New York: Springer; 2007. p. 219–34.

69. Taiwo YO, Levine JD. Further confirmation of the role of adenyl cyclase and of cAMP-dependent protein kinase in primary afferent hyperalgesia. Neuroscience. 1991;44(1):131–5.

70. Cortright DN, Szallasi A. Biochemical pharmacology of the vanilloid receptor TRPV1. An update. European Journal of Biochemistry/FEBS. 2004;271(10):1814–19.

71. Dina OA, Barletta J, Chen X, Mutero A, Martin A, Messing RO, et al. Key role for the epsilon isoform of protein kinase C in painful alcoholic neuropathy in the rat. Journal of Neuroscience. 2000;20(22):8614–19.

72. Planells-Cases R, Garcia-Sanz N, Morenilla-Palao C, Ferrer-Montiel A. Functional aspects and mechanisms of TRPV1 involvement in neurogenic inflammation that leads to thermal hyperalgesia. Pflugers Archiv: European Journal of Physiology. 2005;451(1):151–9.

73. Bhave G, Gereau RWt. Posttranslational mechanisms of peripheral sensitization. Journal of Neurobiology. 2004;61(1):88–106.

74. McMahon SB. Mechanisms of sympathetic pain. British Medical Bulletin. 1991;47(3):584–600.

75. Campbell JN, Meyer RA. Mechanisms of neuropathic pain. Neuron. 2006;52(1):77–92.

76. Raja SN, Treede RD. Testing the link between sympathetic efferent and sensory afferent fibers in neuropathic pain. Anesthesiology. 2012;117(1):173–7.

77. Schaible HG. Nociceptive neurons detect cytokines in arthritis. Arthritis Research and Therapy. 2014;16(5):470.

78. Seidel MF, Wise BL, Lane NE. Nerve growth factor: an update on the science and therapy. Osteoarthritis and Cartilage/OARS, Osteoarthritis Research Society. 2013;21(9):1223–8.

79. Phillips K, Clauw DJ. Central pain mechanisms in the rheumatic diseases: future directions. Arthritis and Rheumatism. 2013;65(2):291–302.

80. Gebhart G. Visceral pain – peripheral sensitisation. Gut. 2000;47(Suppl 4):iv54-iv5.

81. Cavanaugh JM, Lu Y, Chen C, Kallakuri S. Pain generation in lumbar and cervical facet joints. Journal of Bone and Joint Surgery. American volume. 2006;88(Suppl 2):63–7.

82. Katz N, Borenstein DG, Birbara C, Bramson C, Nemeth MA, Smith MD, et al. Efficacy and safety of tanezumab in the treatment of chronic low back pain. Pain. 2011;152(10):2248–58.

83. Kivitz AJ, Gimbel JS, Bramson C, Nemeth MA, Keller DS, Brown MT, et al. Efficacy and safety of tanezumab versus naproxen in the treatment of chronic low back pain. Pain. 2013;154(7):1009–21.

84. Chaabo K, Kirkham B. Rheumatoid arthritis – anti-TNF. International Immunopharmacology. 2015;27(2):180–4.

85. Dretzke J, Edlin R, Round J, Connock M, Hulme C, Czeczot J, et al. A systematic review and economic evaluation of the use of tumour necrosis factor-alpha (TNF-alpha) inhibitors, adalimumab and infliximab, for Crohn's disease. Health Technology Assessment (Winchester, England). 2011;15(6):1–244.

86. Connor V. Anti-TNF therapies: a comprehensive analysis of adverse effects associated with immunosuppression. Rheumatology International. 2011;31(3):327–37.

87. Maxwell L, Zochling J, Boonen A, et al. TNF-alpha inhibitors for ankylosing spondylitis. Cochrane Database of Systematic Reviews. 2015(4).

88. Di Raimondo D, Tuttolomondo A, Buttà C, Casuccio A, Giarrusso L, Miceli G, et al. Metabolic and anti-inflammatory effects of a home-based programme of aerobic physical exercise. International Journal of Clinical Practice. 2013;67(12):1247–53.

89. Ortega E, Collazos ME, Maynar M, Barriga C, De la Fuente M. Stimulation of the phagocytic function of neutrophils in sedentary men after acute moderate exercise. European Journal of Applied Physiology and Occupational Physiology. 1993;66(1):60–4.

90. Giraldo E, Garcia JJ, Hinchado MD, Ortega E. Exercise intensity-dependent changes in the inflammatory response in sedentary women: role of neuroendocrine parameters in the neutrophil phagocytic process and the pro-/anti-inflammatory cytokine balance. Neuroimmunomodulation. 2009;16(4):237–44.

91. Bote ME, Garcia JJ, Hinchado MD, Ortega E. Fibromyalgia: anti-inflammatory and stress responses after acute moderate exercise. PLoS ONE. 2013;8(9):e74524.

92. Petersen AM, Pedersen BK. The role of IL-6 in mediating the anti-inflammatory effects of exercise. Journal of Physiology and Pharmacology. 2006;57(Suppl 10):43–51.

93. Bote ME, Garcia JJ, Hinchado MD, Ortega E. An exploratory study of the effect of regular aquatic exercise on the function of neutrophils from women with fibromyalgia: role of IL-8 and noradrenaline. Brain, Behavior, and Immunity. 2014;39:107–12.

94. Teodorczyk-Injeyan JA, Injeyan HS, Ruegg R. Spinal manipulative therapy reduces inflammatory cytokines but not substance P production in normal subjects. Journal of Manipulative and Physiological Therapeutics. 2006;29(1):14–21.

95. Field T, Diego M, Cullen C, Hernandez-Reif M, Sunshine W, Douglas S. Fibromyalgia pain and substance P decrease and sleep improves after massage therapy. Journal of Clinical Rheumatology. 2002;8(2):72–6.

96. Degenhardt BF, Darmani NA, Johnson JC, Towns LC, Rhodes DC, Trinh C, et al. Role of osteopathic manipulative treatment in altering pain biomarkers: a pilot study. Journal of the American Osteopathic Association. 2007;107(9):387–400.

97. Licciardone JC, Kearns CM, Hodge LM, Bergamini MV. Associations of cytokine concentrations with key osteopathic lesions and clinical outcomes in patients with nonspecific chronic low back pain: results from the OSTEOPATHIC Trial. Journal of the American Osteopathic Association. 2012;112(9):596–605.

Introduction

The spinal cord is the lowest level of the central nociceptive system.[1] Here, second order neurons convert peripheral afferent signals from multiple sites into encoded messages that are sent to many parts of the central nervous system (CNS). Any type of injury to tissues (such as disease, trauma, or inflammation) activates high-threshold nociceptors that in turn transmit action potentials to the dorsal horn of the spinal cord. The dorsal horn is the major receiving zone for primary afferent neurons that communicate information from sensory receptors in the skin, joints, viscera, and muscles to the CNS. Here, the excitability of nociceptive spinal neurons can change due to peripheral inputs in painful conditions. Additionally, nociceptive processing in the spinal cord is also modified by local interneurons as well as descending facilitatory and inhibitory influences from supraspinal regions. Thus, plasticity or modification of synaptic activity in the dorsal horn due to prolonged nociceptive input is fundamental to the generation and maintenance of pain and increased sensitivity.

Although peripheral sensitization is something of a local phenomenon, central sensitization refers to altered neuronal process in all areas of the central nervous system.[2] The term 'central sensitization' refers to the increase in responsiveness (sensitivity) to peripheral inputs coming into the spinal cord. However, from a diagnostic perspective this can be confusing to the clinician as central sensitization includes altered nociceptive processing in the spinal cord, different areas of the brain, and descending pain modulatory pathways. Thus, difficulties arise when attempting to determine which central pain pathways are responsible for driving symptoms of increased responsiveness to peripheral inputs. Given that central sensitization is often present in many musculoskeletal conditions that include chronic low back pain, whiplash, osteoarthritis, and fibromyalgia, the clinical presentation becomes more complicated due an increase in unrelated or atypical symptoms, and hence a more difficult clinical reasoning process.[3]

This chapter will first describe normal nociceptive processes within the spinal cord. Thereafter, central sensitization is described as three successive processes that are dependent not only on duration and intensity of incoming peripheral inputs but also individual phenotypic predisposition to increased pain responses. It is intended that information in this chapter be used as an adjunct for subsequent chapters that describe the many considerations and issues faced when managing people with chronic pain.

Normal nociception

Primary afferent inputs to the dorsal horn

In response to painful stimuli, action potentials are conducted along sensory fibers to corresponding cell bodies in the dorsal root ganglion. Primary afferent neurons terminate in the dorsal horn with a specific distribution pattern based on their response function, their peripheral targets (cutaneous, visceral afferents), conduction velocity (size and myelination), response properties (intensity of stimulus needed for activation), and neurochemical phenotype (e.g., individual differences in peptide expression).[4] Generally, cutaneous nociceptive and thermoreceptive Aδ and C fibers terminate in laminae I and II, although some Aδ fibers reach deeper laminae. More specifically, studies also show that thermoreceptive C fibers terminate in lamina I[4] whereas mechanoreceptive neurons terminate in lamina II.[5] Alternatively, large myelinated low-threshold mechanoreceptive afferents (Aβ fibers) have recently been shown to terminate between lamina II and lamina V (Figure 2.1). Nociceptive fibers are divided into two neurochemical groups: those that contain neuropeptides such as substance P and those that do not.[4] These two groups terminate at different sites within the superficial dorsal horn lamina. Generally speaking, non-peptidergic C fibers innervate the epidermis and terminate in laminae I and II (Figure 2.1) while peptidergic fibers innervating tissue deeper to the skin terminate at lamina II only.[4,6]

Differences in distribution of somatic and visceral central terminals

It was originally thought that the C fibers innervating muscle and those innervating viscera both terminated at lamina II. However, it has since been shown that those innervating cutaneous structures project to

lamina II,[7] while also terminating in discreet areas of laminae I, II, IV, and V. Conversely, unmyelinated C fibers innervating abdominal viscera spread profusely in the spinal cord where they bifurcate, and run both rostrally and caudally in the dorsal columns and in Lissauer's tract. From here, they give rise to many collateral branches that ramify to several different locations and segments in the spinal cord, including laminae I, II, V, and X, while also crossing to contralateral laminae (Figure 2.2).[8] Generally speaking, cutaneous fibers show the most dense and defined projections, while visceral afferents have the most wide-ranging and diffuse projections.[9] Nociceptive fibers innervating muscle

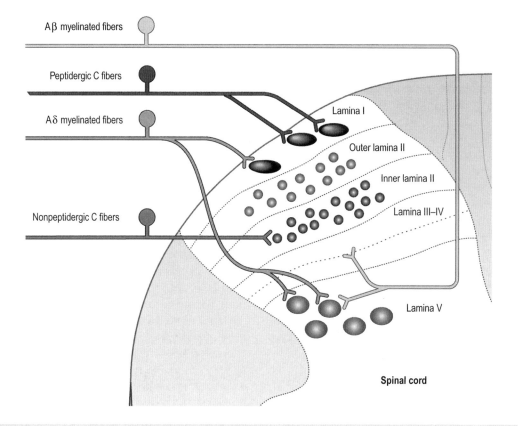

Figure 2.1
Nociceptive afferent fibers terminate in the superficial dorsal horn. Central terminals of peptidergic fibers (substance P, CGRP) terminate in lamina I and the outer area of lamina II. Non-peptidergic fibers (P2X2, isolectin IB4) terminate in deeper part of lamina II. Thinly myelinated Aδ fibers terminate in lamina I and deeper laminae. Large myelinated fibers (Aβ fibers) terminate at laminae IV–VI

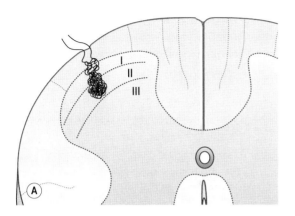 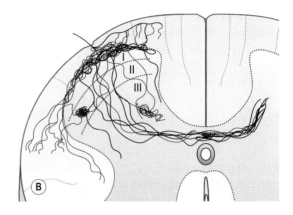

Figure 2.2
Difference in distribution of central terminals between visceral and somatic unmyelinated primary afferent fibers[8]

have projections that lie in between these extremes. Interestingly, it is thought that these differences in central projection arrangements contribute to the difficulty in localizing muscle and visceral pain (Table 2.1).

Sensory transmission in the dorsal horn

Nociceptive-specific cells are located in superficial laminae and synapse with Aδ and C fibers and

Table 2.1
General differences in cutaneous, muscle and visceral pain characteristics dependent on density of nociception and distribution of terminals in the spinal cord

	Character	Discrimination
Cutaneous pain	• Sharp/stabbing	• Easily localized
Muscle pain	• Ache/cramp	• Difficult to localize
Visceral pain	• Colicky pain • Autonomic responses • Affective responses	• Very poorly defined and perceived around the midline and often referred to somatic structures

only fire action potentials when painful stimuli are detected in the periphery. Other dorsal horn cells receive inputs only from proprioceptive Aβ fibers and respond only to light touch and vibration. A third type of neuronal cell, termed a wide dynamic range neuron (WDR), receives inputs from all three types of sensory fiber and thus responds to the full spectrum of stimulation, ranging from light touch to mechanical, thermal, and chemical noxious stimuli. These WDRs may be projection neurons or interneurons receiving signals from both the periphery and other parts of the spinal cord. Thus, they are able to capture information from external and internal (locally at the spinal cord and from other regions of the CNS) environments.[10] WDRs also demonstrate 'wind-up', a short-lasting form of synaptic plasticity in which repetitive stimulation of the same intensity produces an increase in their evoked response with each stimulus.[11] This effect when applied to human subjects is known as temporal summation (see p. 34).

The role of interneurons

Most neurons in laminae I–III have axons that remain in the spinal cord and ramify locally within the same segment, and are thus defined as interneurons.[4] These neurons are involved in the modulation (modification) and transmission of sensory information.[12] Interneurons are divided into excitatory (glutamatergic) and inhibitory (GABA/glycine) classes. While no reliable immunocytochemical markers exist for cell bodies of glutamatergic neurons, findings from animal studies show GABA is present in 25%, 30%, and 40% of neurons in laminae I, II, and III respectively.[4] However, while interneurons in lamina II have been extensively studied, findings generally show poor correlations between neuron morphology and their function. Additionally, our knowledge of the organization of interneurons in laminae I and III is even more limited.

Interneurons and projection wide dynamic range neurons

Interestingly, when acting as a projection neuron to the brain, WDRs receive signals from both excitatory (C fiber activated)[12] and inhibitory (Aβ fiber activated) interneurons.[13] Recent studies show that excitatory C fiber wind-up and Aβ fiber inhibition of interneurons exist in tandem. These studies support the convergence of excitation and inhibition onto WDRs. Importantly, differences in firing behavior between interneurons may contribute to the balance between the excitatory influence (C fibers) and inhibitory influence (Aβ fibers) of afferent inputs and subsequent evoked responses in WDR projection neurons.[14]

Projection (second-order) neurons

Projection neurons are defined as neurons whose axons extend from a neuronal cell body within the CNS to one or more of its distant regions.[15] Concerning nociception, projection neurons are concentrated in laminae I and II and scattered throughout laminae III–VI.[4] Most projection neurons cross the midline of the spinal cord and travel in the contralateral white matter to brainstem and midbrain nuclei along the spinothalamic tract. The main supraspinal targets of these projection neurons include the:

- ventrolateral medulla (endogenous pain modulation)
- nucleus of solitary tract (cardiorespiratory responses to nociception)

- lateral parabrachial area (autonomic fear responses to nociception)
- periaqueductal gray (endogenous pain modulation)
- thalamus (relay and processing of signals to other brain regions).

Descending inputs

Descending pathways from higher center regions also project to the dorsal horn. Two types of descending pathways exist: a serotonergic system originating from the nucleus raphe magnus and noradrenergic pathways from the locus coeruleus and other pontine areas. These two pathways are responsible for modulating pain. Both serotonergic and noradrenergic pathways terminate throughout the dorsal horn, and while some form synapses, most of their action is mediated through volume transmission.[9] Volume transmission is defined as the diffusion of neurotransmitters through CNS extracellular fluid causing the activation of extrasynaptic receptors. This results in a longer activation time course than transmissions via a single synapse. A further descending pathway involved in pain modulation consists of GABAergic axons from the ventromedial medulla which ramifies within the dorsal horn and synapses with lamina II interneurons. Descending pain modulation is described in more detail in Chapter 3 and key features of synaptic transmission of nociceptive inputs in the dorsal horn are summarized in Box 2.1.

Presynaptic neurotransmitters and receptors

Glutamate is the primary excitatory neurotransmitter in the CNS and is released from the terminal endings of primary afferents and dorsal horn interneurons which activate receptors on projection neurons. GABA and glycine are the major inhibitory neurotransmitters released by both interneurons and descending pathways. Interneurons also release excitatory substance P, calcitonin gene-related peptide (CGRP), and cholecystokinin, especially in laminae I and II, where they further increase postsynaptic activity on projection neurons.[16] Concerning inhibition, opioid peptides (enkephalins and endorphins) are also released in the dorsal horn via descending pathways owing to activation in the midbrain of the periaqueductal gray that also plays a role in presynaptic inhibition of primary afferents (Figure 2.3).[17]

Postsynaptic neurotransmitters and receptors

Transmission of action potentials are either fast (e.g., action of glutamate and ATP at ionic receptors) or slower (neuropeptides at protein-coupled receptors). Glutamate is released from central terminals of primary afferents and activates ligand-operated ionotropic S-alpha-amino-3-hydroxy-5-methyl-4-isoxazolepropionic acid receptors (AMPA), N-mythyl-D-aspartate receptors (NMDA), kainate receptors, and G-protein coupled receptors.[18] Additionally, substance P, also released from primary afferent central terminals, further activates postsynaptic neurokinin 1 (NK1) receptors (Figure 2.4).

AMPA receptors

AMPA receptors, when activated, permit the selective entry of sodium ions (Na+) under normal physiological conditions. This activation results in 'fast pain' transmission along brain-directed projection neurons, otherwise known as short latency excitatory postsynaptic action potentials (EPSPs).[19] AMPA receptors are distributed throughout the CNS,

especially in the spinal cord, as well as in different brain regions such as the hippocampus and cerebellum.[20] Importantly, prolonged release of glutamate or simultaneous activation of NK1 receptors by substance P results in increased and sustained activation of AMPA and NK1 receptors (Figure 2.4). This is now shown to be crucial in the development of abnormal responses to further stimuli. In fact, studies show that glutamate-mediated excitatory synaptic transmission efficiency is dependent on both the number and function of AMPA receptors at glutamatergic synapses.[21]

Neurokinin 1 receptors

80% of NK1 receptors in the dorsal horn are expressed in lamina I; however, they are also expressed in laminae III and IV.[22] Because of these concentrations, NK1 receptors have received much attention as their expression is restricted to dorsal horn neurons that are activated by noxious stimuli.[23] The effects of substance P on NK1 receptors are reduced by NK1 receptor antagonists, while destruction of lamina I neurons expressing NK1 receptors in animal studies also show substantial reductions in hyperalgesia.[22]

NMDA receptors

NMDA receptors are glutamate-gated cation channels that are permeable to Na+ and calcium ions (Ca^{2+}) and is both voltage and ligand gated. NMDA receptors are not critical for basic synaptic transmission, but instead regulate functional and structural plasticity of individual synapses and neurons. Whereas AMPA and kainate receptors are responsible for fast transmission, NMDA receptors are much slower. Normally, glutamate molecules released from the presynaptic terminal are efficiently removed from the synaptic space by glutamate transporters and such are only briefly available for receptor binding. While NMDA receptors have a high affinity for glutamate, individual synaptic inputs during baseline activity are not sufficient to initiate Ca^{2+} influx. This is because at normal resting potential, NMDA receptors are silent where magnesium (Mg^{2+}) ions bind tightly to the receptor preventing the influx of Ca^{2+} ion.[24] Once NMDA receptors are activated the Mg^{2+} leaves the channel (Figure 2.5). This amount of

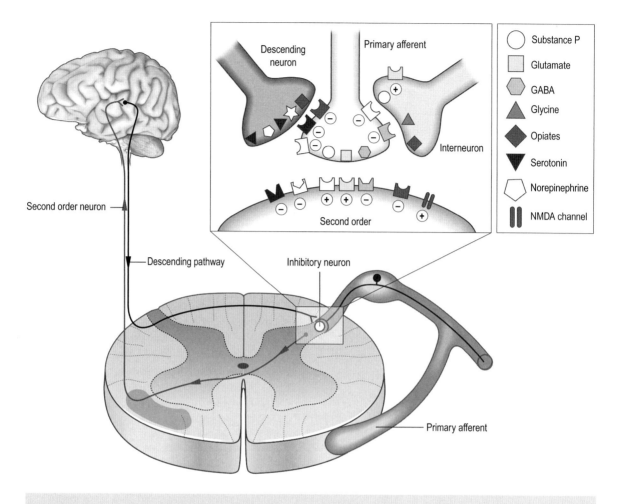

Figure 2.3

This figure shows (1) incoming primary afferent neurons, interneurons, and descending neurons, and (2) associated excitatory and inhibitory neurotransmitters involved in dorsal horn pain modulation

depolarization only occurs when glutamate and substance P are co-released after intense primary afferent activation that acts on AMPA and NK1 receptors.[19] Subsequent activation of NMDA receptors causes large and continued depolarization and subsequent intracellular Ca^{2+} mobilization in the postsynaptic (projection) neuron. It is this process at NMDA receptors at pre- and postsynaptic locations that initiates long-term changes observed in chronic pain states.

NMDA receptor activation is shown to have a significant role in pain arising from both superficial and deep muscles and from joints.[25] Indeed, animal studies show that exercise-induced pain in sedentary mice is strongly associated with increased activation of supraspinal NMDA receptors.[26] Interestingly, these receptors are also sensitized by unaccustomed exercise that causes them to respond more strongly to minor muscle use. Additionally, NMDA receptors located in medullary regions are involved in descending pain modulation, and it is thought that 'ON' cells (facilitation cells) located in the rostral ventral medulla become activated and thus initiate descending facilitatory inputs that enhance dorsal horn synaptic activity[27]

(Chapter 3). Box 2.2 summarizes some key points concerning NMDA receptors and musculoskeletal pain.

Central sensitization and synaptic plasticity

As stated in the introduction, central sensitization is defined as an amplification of responsiveness in which increased activity in pain facilitatory pathways and/or decreases in pain inhibitory pathways lead to alterations of both 'bottom-up' (periphery to brain) and 'top-down' (brain to periphery) pain mechanisms. Thus, central sensitization plays a significant role in the pathophysiology of many musculoskeletal pain conditions. Given these centrally mediated mechanisms, it is uncertain whether physical therapies are reliably effective in such conditions, and whether manual therapists always recognize signs and symptoms of this kind of pathophysiology. Helpfully, several authors describe ways in which central sensitization symptoms in patients presenting with musculoskeletal pain can be recognized during the processes of history taking and clinical examination, and importantly, via self-reporting measures aimed at quantifying symptoms of central sensitization such as hyperalgesia, allodynia, and its global effect on the individual.[28] Tools include the Central Sensitization Inventory,[29] the Allodynia Symptom Checklist,[30] and other, more specific, neuropathic pain questionnaires.[31] This information, as it becomes more available in the future, will allow quicker recognition and more effective management of patients with centrally mediated pain.

The remainder of this section describes pathophysiological mechanisms and, for ease of understanding, is divided into three successive processes that are dependent not only on the duration and intensity of incoming peripheral inputs, but also on individual genomic predisposition to increased pain responses. It is these mechanisms that contribute to the following characteristics, shown in Boxes 2.3 and 2.4.

Postsynaptic activity in second-order neurons

Activation of NMDA receptors is an essential step in both initiating and maintaining activity-dependent central sensitization. This has been shown by the prevention and reversal of hyperexcitability in nociceptive neurons using NMDA receptor antagonists.[26] Increases in intracellular Ca^{2+} beyond a certain threshold appears to be key to the initiation of central sensitization. This occurs not only through the activation of NMDA, but also AMPA receptors. NMDA receptor

---

Box 2.2

Key points: NMDA receptors and musculoskeletal pain

- Shown to play a critical role in pain arising from subcutaneous and deep muscle and joint tissue

- NMDA receptor antagonists (ketamine); effective in the clinical treatment of deep tissue pain

- Maintenance of proinflammatory muscle pain is also associated with ongoing activation of supraspinal NMDA receptors in the medulla

---

Box 2.3

Key points: pain history characteristics of central sensitization

- Disproportionate/unpredictable patterns of pain in response to nonspecific aggravating factors

- Pain – disproportionate to the nature of injury

- Pain – unremitting/constant

- Widespread, non-anatomical distribution of pain

- History of failed interventions

- Unresponsive to nonsteroidal anti-inflammatory drugs (NSAIDs)

- More responsive to centrally acting drugs

- Associated psychological factors

- Night pain/disturbed sleep

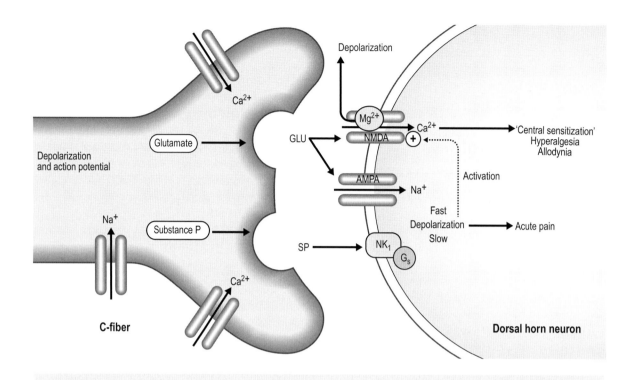

Figure 2.4

Normal nociceptive transduction in the spinal cord. Incoming primary afferent inputs activate presynaptic excitatory neurotransmitters that cross the synapse activating S-alpha-amino-3-hydroxy-5-methyl-4-isoxazolepropionic acid receptors (AMPA) and neurokinin 1 (NK1) channels causing short-latency action potentials in the postsynaptic projection neuron. Note, N-methyl-D-aspartate (NMDA) channels are silent during normal nociceptive input

activation and subsequent influx of Ca^{2+} ions initiate a cascade of secondary events within the projection neuron. Influx of Ca^{2+} activates several pathways involving second messengers similar to those at distal peripheral terminals (Chapter 1), including inositol triphosphate (IP_3), cyclic guanosine monophosphate (cGMP), protein kinase C (PKC) and nitric oxide (NO). While NO does not appear to be important in acute nociception, it is, however, involved in the initiation and maintenance of chronic pain states. This is because NO activation requires the influx of Ca^{2+} through NMDA channels. NO also diffuses out of the postsynaptic neuron to effect incoming presynaptic nerve fibers and local astrocytes acting as a neurotransmitter.32 NO acts on presynaptic C fiber terminals by enhancing the release of substance P and CGRP which contributes to the development of

secondary hyperalgesia (centrally mediated hyperalgesia in tissue adjacent to the injury zone). Moreover, it is proposed that spinal NO also contributes glutamatergic mechanisms of descending facilitation by interfering with GABAergic and glycinergic effects on projection neurons.33 Continued influx of Ca^{2+} also leads to alterations in gene expression and protein synthesis, causing longer term changes in neuronal excitability. These sensitizing mechanisms are discussed in the next section.

Central sensitization – synapse activity-dependent (wind-up)

Wind-up is a form of activity-dependent plasticity that occurs only in dorsal horn postsynaptic neurons that are specifically activated by a presynaptic stimulus (input-specific activation of postsynaptic neurons).[34] As the term suggests, 'wind-up' is characterized by a progressive increase in action potential output from dorsal horn neurons during a succession of repeated low-frequency nociceptor stimuli of the same intensity.[35] The release of excitatory neurotransmitters from primary afferent terminals elicits slow synaptic potentials where their summation results in a cumulative depolarization, leading to the removal of the Mg^{2+} blockade of NMDA receptors. As NMDA receptors become more sensitive to glutamate, each action potential progressively increases in response to each stimulus. A behavioral comparison may be produced by repeated noxious mechanical stimuli, known as temporal summation, where pain increases with each successive stimulus, even though the stimulus intensity does not change.[35,36]

Central sensitization – intracellular calcium store activation-dependent

Nociceptive activity caused either by successive synchronous inputs such as heat stimulation to the skin or by multiple (asynchronous) stimulation due to frank trauma evokes facilitated transmission in dorsal horn neurons.[35] These repeated inputs increase responses in the activated pathway (homosynaptic potentiation) and novel inputs in adjacent non-stimulated afferents (heterosynaptic potentiation). The release of many excitatory neurotransmitters, including substance P, glutamate, and brain-derived neurotrophic factor (BDNF), from nociceptive terminals activates a multitude of postsynaptic intracellular signaling pathways initially involving the activation of NMDA, AMPA, NK1 and GPCR, metabotropic glutamate receptors (mGlu), and tyrosine kinase receptors (TrkB) (Figure 2.5).

Inside the postsynaptic neuron, two mechanisms are shown to contribute to and maintain increased synaptic efficiency. First, alterations in postsynaptic receptor activity occur due to intracellular processing and the trafficking of 'modified' NMDA and AMPA receptors to the synaptic membrane (Figure 2.5). An increased release of intracellular Ca^{2+} activates intracellular protein kinases (PKA, PKC) that in turn phosphorylate NMDA and AMPA channels.[37] This process brings about increased channel open-times, quicker removal of the Mg^{2+} channel blockade, and the modification and trafficking of newly synthesized receptors to the synaptic membrane. Together these actions lead to prolonged postsynaptic hyperexcitability. Second, Ca^{2+} also activates calmodulin-dependent protein kinase (CaMK) II that not only phosphorylates AMPA receptors, but also traffics new, more efficient AMPA receptors that open at lower activation thresholds.[37]

In addition to the removal of the Mg^{2+} block in NMDA receptors, intracellular PKC reduces local segmental inhibition by reducing the effects of GABA and glycine and the effect of descending inhibition directed by the periaqueductal gray (PAG) in the midbrain[37] onto projection neurons in the dorsal horn. Thus, disinhibition, in whatever form, increases the likelihood of activation by excitatory inputs that incidentally also include non-nociceptive A fibers. Additionally, together with PKA, PKC contributes to the activation of extracellular signal-regulated kinases (ERK) that in turn regulate and decrease inward currents through potassium channels, further contributing to postsynaptic hyperexcitability (see Figure 2.5).[38]

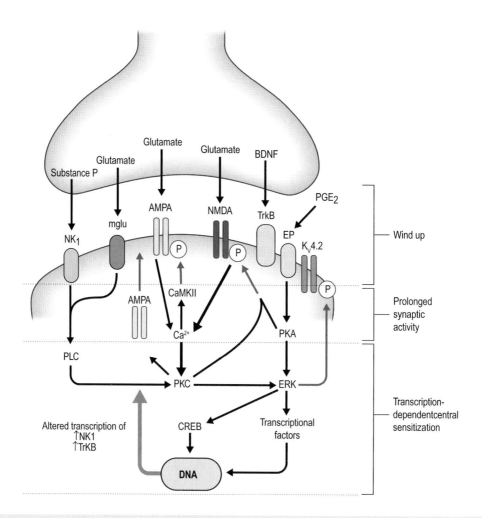

Figure 2.5

Central sensitization at the dorsal horn. Glutamate binds to postsynaptic ion channels (S-alpha-amino-3-hydroxy-5-methyl-4-isoxazolepropionic acid receptors (AMPA); N-methyl-D-aspartate (NMDA)) and metabotropic glutamate receptors (mGlu). Substance P binds to neurokinin 1 (NK1) receptors while brain-derived neurotrophic factor (BDNF) binds with tyrosine kinase receptors (TrkB). Additionally, prostaglandins (PGE2) bind to EP receptors. Activation of these receptors trigger an increase in intracellular $Ca2+$ concentrations, which in turn activate protein kinases (PKA, PKC). These kinases phosphorylate AMPA and NMDA receptors and recruit new AMPA receptors to the synapse surface. Lastly, extracellular signal-related kinase (ERK) phosphorylates potassium voltage gated channels, further enhancing the sensitization process.

Long-term potentiation

Long-term potentiation (LTP) defines a long-lasting and activity-dependent increase in synaptic activity and a mechanism that leads to more permanent amplification of nociceptive inputs in the spinal cord.[39] LTP has been studied most predominantly in the hippocampus and cortical areas of the brain in the form of homosynaptic potentiation. However, while LTP has been found to occur in the spinal cord, alterations in activity-dependent central sensitization come in the form of heterosynaptic potentiation in which activated synapses initiate activity in adjacent non-activated synapses, something that never occurs in cortical LTP.[37]

Central sensitization – altered gene transcription-dependent

As described above, the activation of NMDA, AMPA, NK1, and mGlu receptors by glutamate, substance P, and BDNF initiates the activation of postsynaptic PKC, PKA, and ERK. Other than affecting K^+ channels, ERK can also enter the neuronal nucleus, where it helps to phosphorylate cAMP-response element binding protein (CREB). CREB and other transcription factors can alter the expression of genes, including NK1 and TrkB, that produce long-term strengthening of the synapse hyperexcitability (Figure 2.5). Importantly, activity-dependent transcriptional changes in the spinal cord are accompanied by similar changes in the primary afferent neurons. Studies show that induced peripheral inflammation produces increased release of substance P and BDNF, both of which are ligands for TrkB and NK1 receptors.[35] Additionally, with prolonged noxious stimuli, there follows phenotypic switching where, for example, large dorsal horn ganglion neurons (A fibers) express substance P and BDNF. Thus, supposed non-nociceptive afferents gain the capability to induce central sensitization where repeated light-touch can trigger progressive tactile pain hypersensitivity as tested with temporal summation.[40]

The neuroimmune system: the role of glial cells

Glial cells represent by far the most abundant cells in the spinal cord and are observed throughout the entire nervous system. In particular, microglia and astrocytes are shown to undergo structural and functional change during injury and have been shown thereby to contribute significantly to the excitation of dorsal horn neurons as well as the onset and maintenance of central sensitization (Figure 2.6).

Microglia

Microglia are the immune system's representatives in the CNS, where they act as macrophages. They are homogeneously distributed within the gray matter and act within hours of peripheral injury, accumulating in the superficial dorsal horn around the termination zone of injured peripheral nerve fibers.[41] Additionally, microglia aggregate around cell bodies of ventral horn motor neurons whose peripheral nerve fibers are also damaged. These stimulated glia release inflammatory cytokines that further augment spinal neuron excitation. The role of microglia as modulators of pain has received much attention in recent years. Previously, they were considered to be inactive during non-injured conditions. They have been shown, however, to actively sense the local environment with their ramified processes.[42] It is important to note that microglia become activated after nerve injury, but not after inflammatory tissue injury; thus, the activation of the afferent fiber in any injury condition is not the trigger for microglial activation.[41] Under normal conditions, glial cell proliferation is rarely observed. While nerve injury triggers significant morphological changes (from ramified to amoeboid), it is the biochemical changes after nerve injury that induce pain. These biochemical changes include the release of inflammatory mediators (cytokines, glutamate) and a substantial upregulation of receptors on microglia, chief of which are the ATP P2X-type purinogenic receptors in the ipsilateral spinal cord.[43] Animal studies show that by administering an intraspinal P2X receptor blocker, tactile allodynia after nerve injury is suppressed. Further research shows that ATP-evoked activation of P2X receptors further stimulates the release of BDNF, which in turn acts upon TrkB receptors in lamina I projection neurons (Figure 2.5).[44] Altered microglia function also causes dysregulation of ion channels in astrocytes, thus facilitating changes in astrocyte activity.[45]

Astrocytes

Astrocytes have received less attention concerning their contribution to pain processing in the spinal cord, despite evidence showing activation during peripheral nerve injury.[46] A full description of astrocyte function is beyond the scope of this chapter. However, their function influences:

- extracellular ion homeostasis
- neurotransmitter reuptake and release

- control of synaptic strength
- control of the blood–brain barrier.

In other words, when in a resting state, astrocytes exert a constant maintenance function.[47] When externally stimulated, however, astrocytes switch phenotype, resulting in morphological changes such as enlargement of their astrocytic processes, an increase in glial fibrillary acidic protein (GFAP), and a reduction in glutamate reuptake.[48] Animal studies have shown an ipsilateral increase in astrocytic activation during nerve injury, with a subsequent increase in the expression of GFAP that correlated with levels of paw hypersensitivity.[48,49] Once stimulated, astrocytes release inflammatory mediators such as glutamate, NO, and PGE2.[50] Unlike microglia, astrocytes become activated under peripheral inflammatory conditions (Figure 2.6), and spinal astrocytic activation has been shown following colonic inflammation.[51] Interestingly, astrocytic activation has also been observed in chemotherapeutic and morphine tolerance animal models, suggesting a wide range of triggers contributing to central sensitization.

Schwann cells

There is also evidence showing the contribution of Schwann cells to chronic pain, both peripherally and in the brain. Schwann cells form the myelin sheath around Aβ and Aδ fibers as well as Remak bundles that wrap around groups of unmyelinated C fibers. However, after injury, Schwann cells, like other glial cells, undergo phenotypic modulation that causes them to proliferate, migrate, and secrete mediators

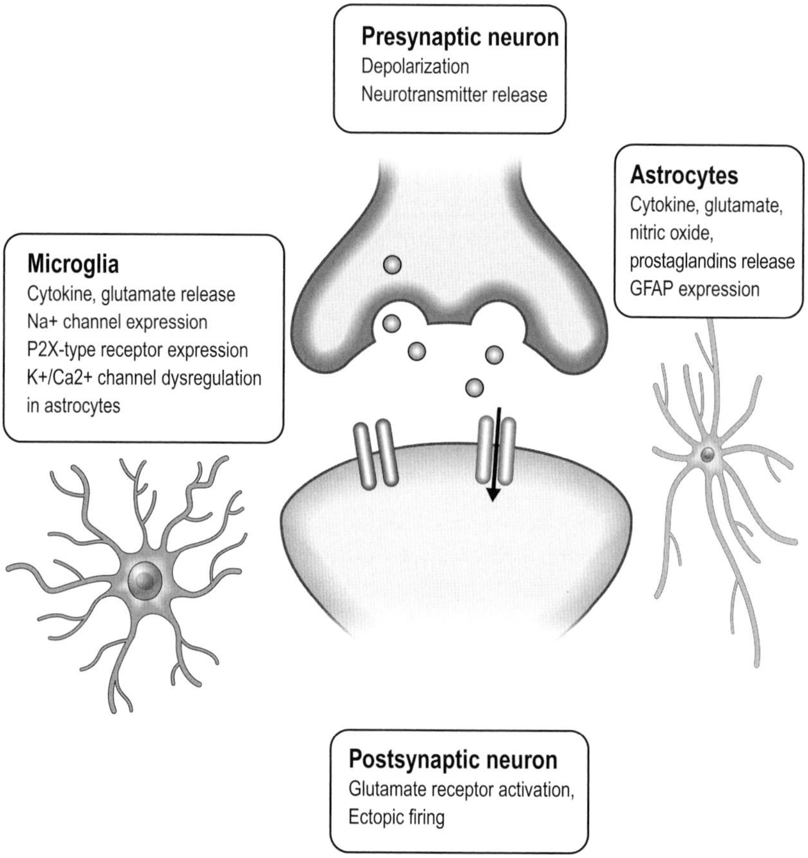

Figure 2.6
A schematic representation of spinal microglial and astrocyte function during noxious conditions. Microglia receive neuronal signals that in noxious conditions act like macrophages and release inflammatory mediators that further augment dorsal horn excitation. Astrocytes show a similar function, but in addition to spinal activation are also stimulated in peripheral inflammatory conditions

Presynaptic neuron
Depolarization
Neurotransmitter release

Astrocytes
Cytokine, glutamate, nitric oxide, prostaglandins release
GFAP expression

Microglia
Cytokine, glutamate release
Na+ channel expression
P2X-type receptor expression
K+/Ca2+ channel dysregulation in astrocytes

Postsynaptic neuron
Glutamate receptor activation, Ectopic firing

that control Wallerian degeneration (axonal degeneration distal to nerve injury site) and regeneration. Schwann cells also express pro-inflammatory cytokines such as IL-10 and TNFα.[52]

Central sensitization in humans

The term 'central sensitization' as applied to humans is a broad one, and difficult to apply in a mechanistic sense. 'Central' can apply to:

- ipsilateral sensitization associated with local nociceptive input
- segmental sensitization contralateral to local nociceptive inputs
- spreading sensitization to segments adjacent to local nociceptive inputs
- generalized widespread sensitization.

The development of chronic pain progresses and spreads over time in 10–20% of people who initially present with local pain conditions.[53,54] For example, a number of patients presenting with low back pain (25%)[55] and whiplash disorders (17%)[56] go on to develop chronic widespread pain (CWP). While the mechanisms underlying CWP are unclear, recent patient data suggest both social and psychological conditions as strong predisposing factors.[57] Additionally, genetic and familial factors have recently been shown to significantly predict the development of CWP, especially in conditions such as fibromyalgia.[58] Studies examining patients with recent-onset CWP have found further risk factors, including age, family, longer duration of pain, and self-reported anxiety and depression.[59–60]

Widespread manifestations of central sensitization

Pain duration, the number of pain locations, and pain intensity are important indicators of spreading sensitization.[61] For example, people presenting with neck and shoulder pain also show mechanical hyperalgesia in lower body regions,[62] while those presenting with chronic tension headaches and osteoarthritis also present with extrasegmental hyperalgesia.[63,64] Similar

observations have also been reported in people with painful osteoarthritis of the knee, rheumatoid arthritis, and visceral conditions such as endometriosis and irritable bowel syndrome.[65,66] Interestingly, several studies show that if persistent pain (e.g., whiplash, knee/hip osteoarthritis) is reduced using nerve blocks or successful knee replacement, widespread hyperalgesia is also reduced.[67–69] Thus, by minimizing the source of nociception, widespread sensitization may be modulated, at least in the short term. Given these encouraging results, clinical trials involving long-term follow-up interventions aimed at reducing the primary source of pain are necessary. However, it should be noted that levels of primary nociceptive input may vary between central sensitization-type conditions. Evidence now suggests that some conditions are more 'centrally driven' than others. For example, knee osteoarthritis shows an obvious source of primary nociceptive input, whereas many functional pain disorders (e.g., functional abdominal pain, irritable bowel syndrome, fibromyalgia) show little or no primary nociceptive input.

Measurement of central sensitization

Pain sensitization in which nociceptive neurons are activated by nociceptive input manifests as pain hypersensitivity and is now shown to contribute to clinical pain. Clifford Woolf, in his seminal work, found that long-lasting increases in the excitability of spinal cord neurons manifests as a reduction in pain threshold (allodynia), an increase in responsiveness to noxious stimuli (hyperalgesia) (Figure 2.7), and an increase of the receptive field enabling nociceptive input from adjacent (and beyond) non-injured tissue to produce pain (secondary hyperalgesia).[70] Additionally, prolonged excitability of spinal cord neurons also manifests in temporal summation, which refers to the mechanism in which repetitive noxious stimulation of the same intensity results in an increase in pain in humans.[71]

While pain hypersensitivity may be reported locally or generally in the presence of central sensitization, quantitative sensory testing (QST) provides a more sophisticated method to assess sensory symptoms associated with sensitization-type pain conditions. QST allows sensitive detection of alterations

Chapter 2

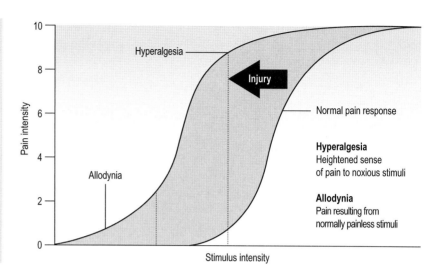

Figure 2.7
A pain intensity–stimulus intensity graph showing the 'sensitization' shift to the left where the stimulus intensity reduces and the pain intensity increases

as well as patterns of hyperalgesia and allodynia that may be attributed to sensitization of the peripheral or central nociceptive systems. QST involves a number of stimulus modalities (thermal, mechanical, chemical, electrical), assessment methods (psychometric, electrophysiological, imaging), and target structures (skin, muscle, viscera).[61] However, problems arise in the case of local pain; hyperalgesia cannot be compared contralaterally due to central manifestations associated with widespread pain. Additionally, both allodynia and hyperalgesia also manifest as a result of peripheral nociceptor sensitization.[72]

Temporal summation and after-sensation

As stated previously in this chapter, wind-up type pain is an important and strong central mechanism in dorsal horn neurons. The initial part of the wind-up process in animals translates into temporal summation in humans:[61] if a stable noxious stimulus of equal strength is repeated 1–3 times per second, pain will become more intense (Figure 2.8).[73]

While sophisticated electrical, mechanical and thermal modalities are used for research purposes, testing in clinical settings may be performed using simple devices such as tapping the skin with a nylon filament or with a pin. Patients also experience pain sensations after noxious stimuli have stopped (aftersensation),

a feature which has also been proposed as diagnostic of central sensitization. Interestingly, temporal summation in people with chronic pain is inhibited by NMDA receptor antagonists in conditions such as fibromyalgia[74] and neuropathic pain.[75]

Spatial summation

Spatial summation occurs when excitatory inputs from several different presynaptic neurons cause action potentials in a postsynaptic neuron. The manifestation of excitatory spatial summation is due to the sensitization of dorsal horn neurons and is key to initiation and maintenance of general sensitization.[76,77] Spatial summation is assessed by stimulating two different areas using mechanical or thermal stimuli, and has been observed in many pain conditions including fibromyalgia and osteoarthritis.[69,77]

Referred pain

Referred pain resulting from deep somatic or visceral structures is very often accompanied by secondary hyperalgesia and trophic changes in more superficial structures.[78] These referred pain areas are initiated and maintained as a result of central sensitization in pain conditions such as chronic low back pain[79] and irritable bowel syndrome.[80] Indeed, secondary hyperalgesia is affirmed by pain threshold decreases and spatial summation from muscles in visceral pain conditions.[78]

This phenomenon occurs as a result of the barrage of visceral afferent input on viscerosomatic convergent (WDR) neurons in the dorsal horn. This barrage of visceral afferent input further activates reflex arcs towards not just somatic structures, but also back to visceral structures innervated by the same segments.[81] Similar to studies investigating temporal summation, researchers have found that pharmacological intervention in dorsal horn pathways reduces areas of referred pain. For example, it has been shown that ketamine (NMDA channel blocker)[82] and gabapentin (Ca^{2+} channel blocker)[83] reduce temporal summation of pressure and electrical stimulation respectively.

Descending pain modulation

There is increasing evidence that altered descending pain modulation plays a significant role in maintaining central sensitization. This topic is described in detail in Chapter 3, but we can state here that less efficient descending pain modulation, with its effects on dorsal horn pain processes, has been observed, and stated as a general phenomenon, in many chronic pain disorders.

Key points concerning clinical pain syndromes associated with central sensitization are listed in Box 2.5.

Treatment approaches

Manual therapy

Manual therapy (MT) is aimed at exerting peripheral effects, for example, decreasing muscle tension and increasing joint range of motion, in order to relieve musculoskeletal pain.[84] However, various chronic pain disorders such as fibromyalgia, irritable bowel syndrome, and chronic low back pain are associated with altered spinal and cortical pain processing of

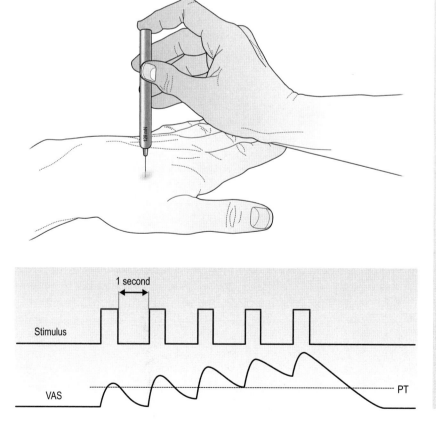

Figure 2.8
Temporal summation and aftersensation pain scores are assessed with a visual analog scale (VAS) in response to repetitive stimulations of identical intensity, in this case applied as pinpricks to the lower arm or volar aspect of the hand. PT – pain threshold

Box 2.5

Key points: clinical pain syndromes associated with central sensitization

- Osteoarthritis: well understood peripheral pathology where pain is shown to be augmented by a central component

- Temporomandibular joint (TMJ) disorders: pathophysiology – not well understood. Generalized pain sensitivity suggestive of central sensitization

- Musculoskeletal disorders (e.g., whiplash, shoulder impingement syndrome): characterized by the spread of pain sensitivity to deep uninjured tissue, indicating central sensitization maintained by low-level peripheral inputs

- Headache: both migraine and chronic tension headache show high temporal summation ratios, commonly associated with central sensitization

- Fibromyalgia: major role for central sensitization, but thought to be induced by abnormal peripheral muscle afferent input

- Neuropathic pain: NMDA receptor synaptic plasticity may contribute to enhanced neural activity which are normalized by centrally acting antidepressants

noxious stimuli suggestive of central sensitization.[2,85,86] Thus, central sensitization is considered a major factor in the maintenance of chronic pain. However, despite growing evidence and support for the effectiveness of MT on somatic pain disorders, the mechanisms by which it functions are not fully understood. Additionally, diagnoses are based on clusters of signs and symptoms that while aiming to direct clinical diagnosis and management, struggle to predict clinical outcomes. Thus an understanding of the mechanisms underlying MT with central sensitization-driven pain disorders may help to recognize individuals who are more likely to respond positively to MT. Encouragingly, findings from human and animal

studies show that joint mobilization exerts temporal activation of antinociceptive pathways. Human studies show that joint mobilization produces both local and widespread hypoalgesic effects.[87,88] Animal studies go further by showing these effects to be mediated by descending pathways, and that spinal blockade of serotonin receptors (neurotransmitters associated with descending pathways) prevented hypoalgesia while spinal blockade of opioid and GABA receptors had no effect on joint manipulation-induced hypoalgesia.[89] However, these and MT effects are shown to be short-lived and thus limited as long-term treatment strategies without repeated treatments. Conversely, MT may also function as a source of nociceptive input to the central nervous system and thus maintain the central sensitization processes.[84] For this reason, physical therapists must understand central pain processes, as peripheral treatments may cause more harm than good.

Exercise therapy

Exercise activates endogenous analgesia in healthy people, in whom increased pain thresholds are observed following exercise, especially aerobic exercise such as cycling and static contractions of local muscle groups. This is due to the release of endogenous opioids and the activation of supraspinal inhibitory mechanisms thought to be due to increases in heart rate and blood pressure. Research in this area indicates that cardiovascular responses are associated with alterations in pain perception, with blood pressure activating arterial baroreceptors, leading to interactions of adjacent pain inhibitory and vasomotor brainstem nuclei.[90] Exercise also triggers many other peripheral and central processes involving the pituitary (e.g., beta-endorphin and growth hormone) and hypothalamus that may also enable analgesic effects. However, a review of these mechanisms is beyond the scope of this chapter; and they are well described by Godfrey et al. and Bender et al., to whom the reader is referred.[91,92]

Conversely, some people with chronic pain conditions such as fibromyalgia and whiplash respond poorly, often complaining of increased rather than decreased pain, especially after exercise.[93] Pain management programs including exercise are therefore often prone to early dropouts. Importantly, it is suggested that when chronic pain patients exercise already painful muscles, this causes new and further nociceptive input, resulting in flare-ups following the exercise. However, Lannersten and Kosek further show that when patients with pain conditions in specific body regions exercise the non-painful parts of the body, exercise analgesia is activated.[93] Significantly, they also show that people with fibromyalgia fail to activate endogenous analgesia during all exercise, suggesting that centrally driven pain mechanisms may be responsible. Such central mechanisms are more driven by the brain, which produces pain and other warning signs even when no tissue damage occurs. Further information regarding this area of exercise therapy is reviewed in Chapter 3.

Pharmacological therapy

Pharmacological approaches to central sensitization in people with chronic pain are wide ranging and complex. This chapter presents a brief overview of the evidence; however, an in-depth review of pharmacotherapy is beyond the scope of this chapter and the therapies are well-described elsewhere, most recently by Nijs et al.[84]

Nonsteroidal anti-inflammatory drugs

Nonsteroidal anti-inflammatory drugs (NSAIDs) have long been considered unsuitable for the treatment of central sensitization, mainly because of their anti-inflammatory action on peripheral nociceptors. However, although direct effects on central mechanisms are uncertain, the peripheral effects of NSAIDs act to reduce peripheral activity and thus attenuate nociceptor-mediated hyperalgesia.[94] More recently, the inhibitory effect of NSAIDs on cyclooxygenases and the formation of prostaglandins (PGE2) have also been observed at central sites.[95] Several studies in this area of pain research show that NSAIDs also inhibit the action of PEG2 in the dorsal horn by acting on pre- and postsynaptic membranes (Figure 2.5). Here, PEG2 receptors facilitate the spinal release of glutamate and

glycine, and thus inhibition of these receptors reduces postsynaptic activity in the dorsal horn.

Serotonin and norepinephrine/noradrenaline-reuptake inhibitors

Serotonin and norepinephrine/noradrenaline-reuptake inhibitors (SSRIs, SNRIs) activate serotonergic and noradrenergic descending pain modulatory pathways. Originally developed for the treatment of depression, these antidepressants block the reuptake of serotonin and norepinephrine and in the spinal cord they partly activate opioid-containing interneurons that in turn inhibit dorsal horn synaptic nociceptive activity.[84] A Cochrane review showed that an SNRI such as duloxetine provides a small incremental benefit in reducing pain while also improving quality of life in chronic pain conditions such as fibromyalgia. However, this review further highlights the negative effects of such medication, showing high dropout rates due to adverse events such as nausea, dry mouth, and headache.[96]

Opioids

Opioids are powerful analgesics used to treat both acute and chronic pain. They target a wide variety of opioid receptors (μ, δ and κ types) with μ-opioid receptors the most often targeted by drugs such as codeine, morphine, buprenorphine, hydromorphone, and fentanyl. Endogenous opioid-containing neurons are found throughout pain pathways of the central nervous system including superficial and deep laminae of the dorsal horn, spinal cord interneurons, and supraspinal regions such as the thalamus, limbic system, cerebral cortex, and descending pain modulatory pathways.[84] Activation of δ-opioid receptors has a pain inhibitory effect that in the dorsal horn includes presynaptic inhibition of incoming primary afferent inputs as well as postsynaptic inhibition of projection neurons. However, opioids have also been found to induce hyperalgesia and central sensitization, often increasing pain severity in people with chronic pain.[97] In this case, opioids elicit pronociceptive pathways that include increased activation of NMDA receptors, the release of intracellular protein kinases, apoptosis of dorsal horn neurons, and increased descending pain facilitation.[98]

NMDA receptor blockers

As described in this chapter, NMDA receptors play a key role in the development and maintenance of central sensitization. It has been shown that blockade of NMDA receptors may help to reduce increase and spread of hyperalgesia and allodynia caused by central sensitization.[99] However, these drugs have a narrow therapeutic window and there is little difference between toxic and therapeutic doses. This is due to the widespread distribution of NMDA receptors throughout the central nervous system and their differing functions, including memory, cognition, and anxiety.[100,101] Thus, despite the effectiveness of these agents in reducing levels of hyperalgesia and allodynia, they are associated with many unavoidable and often intolerable side effects. The aim of recent pharmacological strategies is therefore to combine current analgesics with non-toxic doses of NMDA-receptor antagonists to enhance their analgesic effect.[84]

Calcium channel alpha-2-delta ligands

Originally designed as anticonvulsants and analogs of the inhibitory neurotransmitter GABA, calcium channel alpha-2-delta (Ca $\alpha_2\delta$) ligands gabapentin and more recently pregabalin in fact show no obvious effects on GABA receptors.[102] Instead these agents bind selectively to Ca $\alpha_2\delta$, a subunit of voltage-gated calcium channels. These subunits are shown to sustain increased release of pain neurotransmitters between incoming primary afferent fibers and second order neurons.[103] Gabapentin and pregabalin, in particular, bind to the subunits, reducing the release of glutamate, and substance P by reducing the influx of calcium during depolarization.[104]

Summary

Central sensitization provides an evidence-based explanation for people suffering unexplained chronic musculoskeletal pain and is found to some degree in many pain conditions. We now know that in central sensitization conditions, pain arises as a result of changes in the properties of neurons in the CNS, where it is sufficient to reduce pain thresholds and increase the severity and duration of responses to noxious input. Thus, pain is not only initiated by peripheral inputs but is also maintained and augmented by central neuronal plasticity. Clifford Woolf, in his seminal work on central sensitization, showed that this plasticity profoundly alters sensitivity to such an extent that it must be considered as a major contributor to most chronic pain disorders. We also know that central sensitization can be both measured and to some degree treated. Concerning non-pharmacological treatments, findings from both animal and human studies provide strong evidence showing positive changes in spinal neurophysiological function immediately after some forms of manual therapy. However, most of these studies provide weak but encouraging evidence and are limited mostly to spinal manipulation. Future studies must investigate different types of manual therapy techniques, their location, duration, and numbers of treatments needed for long-term pain relief.

References

1. Schaible HG. Peripheral and central mechanisms of pain generation. Handbook of Experimental Pharmacology. 2007(177):3–28.

2. Woolf CJ. Central sensitization: implications for the diagnosis and treatment of pain. Pain. 2011;152(3 Suppl):S2–15.

3. Nijs J, Van Houdenhove B. From acute musculoskeletal pain to chronic widespread pain and fibromyalgia: application of pain neurophysiology in manual therapy practice. Manual Therapy. 2009;14(1):3–12.

4. Todd AJ. Neuronal circuitry for pain processing in the dorsal horn. Nature Reviews Neuroscience. 2010;11(12):823–36.

5. Seal RP, Wang X, Guan Y, Raja SN, Woodbury CJ, Basbaum AI, et al. Injury-induced mechanical hypersensitivity requires C-low threshold mechanoreceptors. Nature. 2009;462(7273):651–5.

6. Bennett DL, Dmietrieva N, Priestley JV, Clary D, McMahon SB. trkA, CGRP and IB4 expression in retrogradely labelled cutaneous and visceral primary sensory neurones in the rat. Neuroscience Letters. 1996;206(1):33–6.

7. Ling L-J, Honda T, Shimada Y, Ozaki N, Shiraishi Y, Sugiura Y. Central projection of unmyelinated (C) primary afferent fibers from gastrocnemius muscle in the guinea pig. Journal of Comparative Neurology. 2003;461(2):140–50.

8. Sugiura Y, Terui N, Hosoya Y. Difference in distribution of central terminals between visceral and somatic unmyelinated (C) primary afferent fibers. Journal of Neurophysiology. 1989;62(4):834–40.

9. Todd A, Koerber H. Neuronanatomical substrates of spinal nociception In: McMahon S, Koltzenberg M, Tracey I, editors. Textbook of pain. 6th ed. Edinburgh: Elsevier; 2012. p. 73–90.

10. Le Bars D, Cadden SW. What is a wide-dynamic-range cell? In: Gardner E et al., editors. The senses: a comprehensive reference. New York: Academic Press; 2008. 5.25. p. 331–8.

11. Guan Y, Raja SN. Wide-dynamic-range neurons are heterogeneous in windup responsiveness to changes in stimulus intensity and isoflurane anesthesia level in mice. Journal of Neuroscience Research. 2010;88(10):2272–83.

12. Yasaka T, Tiong SY, Hughes DI, Riddell JS, Todd AJ. Populations of inhibitory and excitatory interneurons in lamina II of the adult rat spinal dorsal horn revealed by a combined electrophysiological and anatomical approach. Pain. 2010;151(2):475–88.

13. Ratte S, Hong S, De Schutter E, Prescott SA. Impact of neuronal properties on network coding: roles of spike initiation dynamics and robust synchrony transfer. Neuron. 2013;78(5):758–72.

14. Zhang TC, Janik JJ, Grill WM. Modeling effects of spinal cord stimulation on wide-dynamic range dorsal horn neurons: influence of stimulation frequency and GABAergic inhibition. Journal of Neurophysiology. 2014;112(3):552–67.

15. Nusbaum M. Modulatory projection neurons. In: Binder M, Hirokawa N, Windhorst U, editors. Encyclopedia of neuroscience. Berlin Heidelberg: Springer; 2009. p. 2385–8.

16. Sasek CA, Seybold VS, Elde RP. The immunohistochemical localization of nine peptides in the sacral parasympathetic nucleus and the dorsal gray commissure in rat spinal cord. Neuroscience. 1984;12(3):855–73.

17. Budai D, Fields HL. Endogenous opioid peptides acting at mu-opioid receptors in the dorsal horn contribute to midbrain modulation of spinal nociceptive neurons. Journal of Neurophysiology. 1998;79(2):677–87.

18. Traynelis SF, Wollmuth LP, McBain CJ, Menniti FS, Vance KM, Ogden KK, et al. Glutamate receptor ion channels: structure, regulation, and function. Pharmacological Reviews. 2010;62(3):405–96.

19. Hudspeth M, Siddall P, Munglani R. Physiology of pain. In: Hemmings H, Hopkins P, editors. Foundations of anesthesia basic sciences for clinical practice. 2nd ed. Philadelphia: Elsevier; 2006. p. 267–85.

20. Wang Y, Wu J, Wu Z, Lin Q, Yue Y, Fang L. Regulation of AMPA receptors in spinal nociception. Molecular Pain. 2010;6:5.

21. Gu JG, Heft MW. P2X receptor-mediated purinergic sensory pathways to the spinal cord dorsal horn. Purinergic Signalling. 2004;1(1):11–16.

22. Todd AJ, McGill MM, Shehab SA. Neurokinin 1 receptor expression by neurons in laminae I, III and IV of the rat spinal dorsal horn that project to the brainstem. European Journal of Neuroscience. 2000;12(2):689–700.

23. Salter MW, Henry JL. Responses of functionally identified neurones in the dorsal horn of the cat spinal cord to substance P, neurokinin A and physalaemin. Neuroscience. 1991;43(2–3):601–10.

24. Blanke M, van Dongen A. Activation mechanisms of the NMDA receptor. In: Van Dongen A, editor. Biology of the NMDA receptor. Boca Raton, FL: CRC Press; 2009.

25. Henriksson KG, Sorensen J. The promise of N-methyl-D-aspartate receptor antagonists in fibromyalgia. Rheumatic Diseases Clinics of North America. 2002;28(2):343–51.

26. Sluka KA, Danielson J, Rasmussen L, DaSilva LF. Exercise-induced pain requires NMDA receptor activation in the medullary raphe nuclei. Medicine and Science in Sports and Exercise. 2012;44(3):420–7.

27. Zhuo M, Gebhart GF. Biphasic modulation of spinal nociceptive transmission from the medullary raphe nuclei in the rat. Journal of Neurophysiology. 1997;78(2):746–58.

28. Nijs J, Paul van Wilgen C, Van Oosterwijck J, van Ittersum M, Meeus M. How to explain central sensitization to patients with 'unexplained' chronic musculoskeletal pain: practice guidelines. Manual Therapy. 2011;16(5):413–8.

29. Mayer TG, Neblett R, Cohen H, Howard KJ, Choi YH, Williams MJ, et al. The development and psychometric validation of the central sensitization inventory. Pain Practice. 2012;12(4):276–85.

30. Lipton RB, Bigal ME, Ashina S, Burstein R, Silberstein S, Reed ML, et al. Cutaneous allodynia in the migraine population. Annals of Neurology. 2008;63(2):148–58.

31. Rog DJ, Nurmikko TJ, Friede T, Young CA. Validation and reliability of the Neuropathic Pain Scale (NPS) in multiple sclerosis. Clinical Journal of Pain. 2007;23(6):473–81.

32. Cury Y, Picolo G, Gutierrez VP, Ferreira SH. Pain and analgesia: the dual effect of nitric oxide in the nociceptive system. Nitric Oxide: Biology and Chemistry. 2011;25(3):243–54.

33. Millan MJ. Descending control of pain. Progress in Neurobiology. 2002;66(6):355–474.

34. Mulkey RM, Malenka RC. Mechanisms underlying induction of homosynaptic long-term depression in area CA1 of the hippocampus. Neuron. 1992;9(5):967–75.

35. Ji RR, Kohno T, Moore KA, Woolf CJ. Central sensitization and LTP: do pain and memory share similar mechanisms? Trends in Neurosciences. 2003;26(12):696–705.

36. Staud R, Cannon RC, Mauderli AP, Robinson ME, Price DD, Vierck CJ, Jr. Temporal summation of pain from mechanical stimulation of muscle tissue in normal controls and subjects with fibromyalgia syndrome. Pain. 2003;102(1–2):87–95.

37. Latremoliere A, Woolf CJ. Central sensitization: a generator of pain hypersensitivity by central neural plasticity. Journal of Pain. 2009;10(9):895–926.

38. Schrader LA, Birnbaum SG, Nadin BM, Ren Y, Bui D, Anderson AE, et al. ERK/ MAPK regulates the Kv4.2 potassium channel by direct phosphorylation of the pore-forming subunit. American Journal of Physiology Cell Physiology. 2006;290(3):C852–61.

39. Yang F, Guo J, Sun WL, Liu FY, Cai J, Xing GG, et al. The induction of long-term potentiation in spinal dorsal horn after peripheral nociceptive stimulation and contribution of spinal TRPV1 in rats. Neuroscience. 2014;269:59–66.

40. Noguchi K, Kawai Y, Fukuoka T, Senba E, Miki K. Substance P induced by peripheral nerve injury in primary afferent sensory neurons and its effect on dorsal column nucleus neurons. Journal of Neuroscience. 1995;15(11):7633–43.

41. Basbaum AI, Bautista DM, Scherrer G, Julius D. Cellular and molecular mechanisms of pain. Cell. 2009;139(2):267–84.

42. Nimmerjahn A, Kirchhoff F, Helmchen F. Resting microglial cells are highly dynamic surveillants of brain parenchyma in vivo. Science (New York, NY). 2005;308(5726):1314–8.

43. Tsuda M, Shigemoto-Mogami Y, Koizumi S, Mizokoshi A, Kohsaka S, Salter MW, et al. P2X4 receptors induced in spinal microglia gate tactile allodynia after nerve injury. Nature. 2003;424(6950):778–83.

44. Coull JA, Beggs S, Boudreau D, Boivin D, Tsuda M, Inoue K, et al. BDNF from microglia causes the shift in neuronal anion gradient underlying neuropathic pain. Nature. 2005;438(7070):1017–21.

45. Palygin O, Lalo U, Verkhratsky A, Pankratov Y. Ionotropic NMDA and P2X1/5 receptors mediate synaptically induced Ca2+ signalling in cortical astrocytes. Cell Calcium. 2010;48(4):225–31.

46. Coyle DE. Partial peripheral nerve injury leads to activation of astroglia and microglia which parallels the development of allodynic behavior. Glia. 1998;23(1):75–83.

47. Ji RR, Berta T, Nedergaard M. Glia and pain: is chronic pain a gliopathy? Pain. 2013;154(Suppl 1):S10–28.

48. Garrison CJ, Dougherty PM, Kajander KC, Carlton SM. Staining of glial fibrillary acidic protein (GFAP) in lumbar spinal cord increases following a sciatic nerve constriction injury. Brain Research. 1991;565(1):1–7.

49. Kane CJ, Sims TJ, Gilmore SA. Astrocytes in the aged rat spinal cord fail to increase GFAP mRNA following sciatic nerve axotomy. Brain Research. 1997;759(1):163–5.

50. Bal-Price A, Moneer Z, Brown GC. Nitric oxide induces rapid, calcium-dependent release of vesicular glutamate and ATP from cultured rat astrocytes. Glia. 2002;40(3):312–23.

51. Sun YN, Luo JY, Rao ZR, Lan L, Duan L. GFAP and Fos immunoreactivity in lumbo-sacral spinal cord and medulla oblongata after chronic colonic inflammation in rats. World Journal of Gastroenterology. 2005;11(31):4827–32.

52. Wagner R, Myers RR. Schwann cells produce tumor necrosis factor alpha: expression in injured and non-injured nerves. Neuroscience. 1996;73(3):625–9.

53. Lee J, Ellis B, Price C, Baranowski AP. Chronic widespread pain, including fibromyalgia: a pathway for care developed by the British Pain Society. British Journal of Anaesthesia. 2014;112(1):16–24.

54. Papageorgiou A, Silman A, Macfarlane G. Chronic widespread pain in the population: a seven year follow up study. Annals of the Rheumatic Diseases. 2002;61(12):1071–4.

55. Viniol A, Jegan N, Leonhardt C, Brugger M, Strauch K, Barth J, et al. Differences between patients with chronic widespread pain and local chronic low back pain in primary care – a comparative cross-sectional analysis. BMC Musculoskeletal Disorders. 2013;14:351.

56. Holm LW, Carroll LJ, Cassidy JD, Skillgate E, Ahlbom A. Widespread pain following whiplash-associated disorders: incidence, course, and risk factors. Journal of Rheumatology. 2007;34(1):193–200.

57. Mundal I, Grawe RW, Bjorngaard JH, Linaker OM, Fors EA. Psychosocial factors and risk of chronic widespread pain: an 11-year follow-up study – the HUNT Study. Pain. 2014;155(8):1555–61.

58. Kindler LL, Jones KD, Perrin N, Bennett RM. Risk factors predicting the development of widespread pain from chronic back or neck pain. Journal of Pain. 2010;11(12):1320–8.

59. de Heer EW, Gerrits MMJG, Beekman ATF, Dekker J, van Marwijk HWJ, de Waal MWM, et al. The Association of Depression and Anxiety with Pain: A Study from NESDA. PLoS ONE. 2014;9(10):e106907.

60. Rohrbeck J, Jordan K, Croft P. The frequency and characteristics of chronic widespread pain in general practice: a case–control study. British Journal of General Practice. 2007;57(535):109–15.

61. Arendt-Nielsen L. Central sensitization in humans: assessment and pharmacology. Handbook of Experimental Pharmacology. 2015;227:79–102.

62. Scott D, Jull G, Sterling M. Widespread sensory hypersensitivity is a feature of chronic whiplash-associated disorder but not chronic idiopathic neck pain. Clinical Journal of Pain. 2005;21(2):175–81.

63. King CD, Sibille KT, Goodin BR, Cruz-Almeida Y, Glover TL, Bartley E, et al. Experimental pain sensitivity differs as a function of clinical pain severity in symptomatic knee osteoarthritis. Osteoarthritis and Cartilage/OARS, Osteoarthritis Research Society. 2013;21(9):1243–52.

64. Fernandez-de-las-Penas C, Caminero AB, Madeleine P, Guillem-Mesado A, Ge HY, Arendt-Nielsen L, et al. Multiple active myofascial trigger points and pressure pain sensitivity maps in the temporalis muscle are related in women with chronic tension type headache. Clinical Journal of Pain. 2009;25(6):506–12.

65. Laursen BS, Bajaj P, Olesen AS, Delmar C, Arendt-Nielsen L. Health related quality of life and quantitative pain measurement in females with chronic non-malignant pain. European Journal of Pain. 2005;9(3):267–75.

66. Kato K, Sullivan PF, Evengard B, Pedersen NL. Chronic widespread pain and its comorbidities: a population-based study. Archives of Internal Medicine. 2006;166(15):1649–54.

67. Schneider GM, Smith AD, Hooper A, Stratford P, Schneider KJ, Westaway MD, et al. Minimizing the source of nociception and its concurrent effect on sensory hypersensitivity: an exploratory study in chronic whiplash patients. BMC Musculoskeletal Disorders. 2010;11:29.

68. Aranda-Villalobos P, Fernandez-de-Las-Penas C, Navarro-Espigares JL, Hernandez-Torres E, Villalobos M, Arendt-Nielsen L, et al. Normalization of widespread pressure pain hypersensitivity after total hip replacement in patients with hip osteoarthritis is associated with clinical and functional improvements. Arthritis and Rheumatism. 2013;65(5):1262–70.

69. Graven-Nielsen T, Wodehouse T, Langford RM, Arendt-Nielsen L, Kidd BL. Normalization of widespread hyperesthesia and facilitated spatial summation of deep-tissue pain in knee osteoarthritis patients after knee replacement. Arthritis and Rheumatism. 2012;64(9):2907–16.

70. Woolf CJ. Evidence for a central component of post-injury pain hypersensitivity. Nature. 1983;306(5944):686–8.

71. Gracely RH, Grant MA, Giesecke T. Evoked pain measures in fibromyalgia. Best Practice and Research Clinical Rheumatology. 2003;17(4):593–609.

72. Truini A, Biasiotta A, Di Stefano G, La Cesa S, Leone C, Cartoni C, et al. Peripheral nociceptor sensitization mediates allodynia in patients with distal symmetric polyneuropathy. Journal of Neurology. 2013;260(3):761–6.

73. Arendt-Nielsen L, Brennum J, Sindrup S, Bak P. Electrophysiological and psychophysical quantification of temporal summation in the human nociceptive system. European Journal of Applied Physiology. 1994;68(3):266–73.

74. Graven-Nielsen T, Aspegren Kendall S, Henriksson KG, Bengtsson M, Sorensen J, Johnson A, et al. Ketamine reduces muscle pain, temporal summation, and referred pain in fibromyalgia patients. Pain. 2000;85(3):483–91.

75. Felsby S, Nielsen J, Arendt-Nielsen L, Jensen TS. NMDA receptor blockade in chronic neuropathic pain: a comparison of ketamine and magnesium chloride. Pain. 1996;64(2):283–91.

76. Bouhassira D, Gall O, Chitour D, Le Bars D. Dorsal horn convergent neurones: negative feedback triggered by spatial summation of nociceptive afferents. Pain. 1995;62(2):195–200.

77. Staud R, Koo E, Robinson ME, Price DD. Spatial summation of mechanically evoked muscle pain and painful aftersensations in normal subjects and fibromyalgia patients. Pain. 2007;130(1–2):177–87.

78. Giamberardino MA. Referred muscle pain/hyperalgesia and central sensitization. Journal of Rehabilitation Medicine. 2003;41(Suppl):85–8.

79. Chen CK, Nizar AJ. Myofascial pain syndrome in chronic back pain patients. Korean Journal of Pain. 2011;24(2):100–4.

80. Sikandar S, Dickenson AH. Visceral pain – the ins and outs, the ups and downs. Current Opinion in Supportive and Palliative Care. 2012;6(1):17–26.

81. Giamberardino MA, Valente R, de Bigontina P, Vecchiet L. Artificial ureteral calculosis in rats: behavioral characterization of visceral pain episodes and their relationship with referred lumbar muscle hyperalgesia. Pain. 1995;61(3):459–69.

82. Graven-Nielsen T, Aspegren Kendall S, Henriksson KG, Bengtsson M, Sörensen J, Johnson A, et al. Ketamine reduces muscle pain, temporal summation, and referred pain in fibromyalgia patients. Pain. 2000;85(3):483–91.

83. Arendt-Nielsen L, Frokjaer JB, Staahl C, Graven-Nielsen T, Huggins JP, Smart TS, et al. Effects of gabapentin on experimental somatic pain and temporal summation. Regional Anesthesia and Pain Medicine. 2007;32(5):382–8.

84. Nijs J, Malfliet A, Ickmans K, Baert I, Meeus M. Treatment of central sensitization in patients with 'unexplained' chronic pain: an update. Expert Opinion on Pharmacotherapy. 2014;15(12):1671–83.

85. Giesecke T, Gracely RH, Grant MA, Nachemson A, Petzke F, Williams DA, et al. Evidence of augmented central pain processing in idiopathic chronic low back pain. Arthritis and Rheumatism. 2004;50(2):613–23.

86. Moshiree B, Zhou Q, Price DD, Verne GN. Central sensitization in visceral pain disorders. Gut. 2006;55(7):905–8.

87. Sluka KA, Skyba DA, Radhakrishnan R, Leeper BJ, Wright A. Joint mobilization reduces hyperalgesia associated with chronic muscle and joint inflammation in rats. Journal of Pain. 2006;7(8):602–7.

88. Moss P, Sluka K, Wright A. The initial effects of knee joint mobilization on osteoarthritic hyperalgesia. Manual Therapy. 2007;12(2):109–18.

89. Skyba DA, Radhakrishnan R, Rohlwing JJ, Wright A, Sluka KA. Joint manipulation reduces hyperalgesia by activation of monoamine receptors but not opioid or GABA receptors in the spinal cord. Pain. 2003;106(1–2):159–68.

90. Umeda M, Newcomb LW, Ellingson LD, Koltyn KF. Examination of the dose-response relationship between pain perception and blood pressure elevations induced by isometric exercise in men and women. Biological Psychology. 2010;85(1):90–6.

91. Godfrey RJ, Madgwick Z, Whyte GP. The exercise-induced growth hormone response in athletes. Sports Medicine (Auckland, NZ). 2003;33(8):599–613.

92. Bender T, Nagy G, Barna I, Tefner I, Kadas E, Geher P. The effect of physical therapy on beta-endorphin levels. European Journal of Applied Physiology. 2007;100(4):371–82.

93. Nijs J, Kosek E, Van Oosterwijck J, Meeus M. Dysfunctional endogenous analgesia during exercise in patients with chronic pain: to exercise or not to exercise? Pain Physician. 2012;15(3 Suppl):Es205–13.

94. Petersen KL, Brennum J, Dahl JB. Experimental evaluation of the analgesic effect of ibuprofen on primary and secondary hyperalgesia. Pain. 1997;70(2–3):167–74.

95. Burian M, Geisslinger G. COX-dependent mechanisms involved in the antinociceptive action of NSAIDs at central and peripheral sites. Pharmacology and Therapeutics. 2005;107(2):139–54.

96. Hauser W, Urrutia G, Tort S, Uceyler N, Walitt B. Serotonin and noradrenaline reuptake inhibitors (SNRIs) for fibromyalgia syndrome. Cochrane Database of Systematic Reviews. 2013(1):Cd010292.

97. Ruscheweyh R, Sandkuhler J. Opioids and central sensitization: II. Induction and reversal of hyperalgesia. European Journal of Pain. 2005;9(2):149–52.

98. Silverman SM. Opioid induced hyperalgesia: clinical implications for the pain practitioner. Pain Physician. 2009;12(3):679–84.

99. Sang CN. NMDA-receptor antagonists in neuropathic pain: experimental methods to clinical trials. Journal of Pain and Symptom Management. 2000;19(1 Supplement 1):21–5.

100. Hoeller AA, Costa APR, Bicca MA, Matheus FC, Lach G, Spiga F, et al. The role of hippocampal NMDA receptors in long-term emotional responses following muscarinic receptor activation. PLoS ONE. 2016;11(1):e0147293.

101. Rowland LM, Astur RS, Jung RE, Bustillo JR, Lauriello J, Yeo RA. Selective cognitive impairments associated with NMDA receptor blockade in humans. Neuropsychopharmacology. 2005;30(3):633–9.

102. Cheng J-K, Lee S-Z, Yang J-R, Wang C-H, Liao Y-Y, Chen C-C, et al. Does gabapentin act as an agonist at native GABAB receptors? Journal of Biomedical Science. 2004;11(3):346–55.

103. Patel R, Dickenson AH. Mechanisms of the gabapentinoids and α2 δ-1 calcium channel subunit in neuropathic pain. Pharmacology Research and Perspectives. 2016;4(2):e00205.

104. Tuchman M, Barrett JA, Donevan S, Hedberg TG, Taylor CP. Central sensitization and CaVα2δ ligands in chronic pain syndromes: pathologic processes and pharmacologic effect. Journal of Pain. 2010;11(12):1241–9.

Introduction

Until the introduction of noninvasive human brain imaging methods, our understanding of the role of the brain and associated supraspinal structures was limited to findings from animal anatomical and electrophysiological studies.[1] Functional imaging in humans has now made it possible to identify the main supraspinal components of the human nociceptive system, adding to our understanding of the role of the cortex and its different regions in pain perception and modulation. Concerning cerebral cortex function, two nociceptive systems, known as the lateral and medial pain pathways, work in parallel to provide a physical concept that in part helps to explain pain in humans.[2] Additionally, subcortical pain modulatory pathways have been identified in animals that show projections involving the hypothalamus, periaqueductal gray (PAG), rostroventral medulla (RVM), and other nuclei in the midbrain and brainstem.[3–5] Interaction between these brain areas shapes our experience of pain, with our interpretation of peripheral nociceptive input being influenced by emotion, memories, pathological, genetic, and cognitive factors.

Various models exist regarding the effect of manual therapy on both spinal and supraspinal pain mechanisms. For example, animal studies show the benefit of manual therapy to the lower extremities following noxious injections. Here, functional brain imaging show decreases in activation in supraspinal regions responsible for pain processing following light touch to the hind paw after introduction of capsaicin.[6] Findings in human studies also show possible supraspinal responses to manual therapy, with associated autonomic[7] and opioid responses[8] and subjective pain relief. Additionally, psychological variables such as placebo and expectation may also be considered a supraspinal response to peripheral interventions.

This chapter will first describe supraspinal pain mechanisms in sequence from the spinal cord to the thalamus, somatosensory, limbic, and motor cortices followed by descending pain mechanisms. It is intended that information in this chapter be used as an adjunct for subsequent chapters that describe the many considerations and issues faced when managing people with chronic pain.

Projection neurons

After the direct or indirect interactions of neurons in the dorsal horn (DH), axons of second order neurons form afferent bundles that transmit nociceptive impulses to structures in the brainstem, diencephalon (posterior part of forebrain), including the thalamus, PAG, parabrachial regions, the reticular formation of the medulla, the amygdala complex, and the hypothalamus.[9] Anatomically, ascending sensory neurons associated with nociceptive transmission form two pathways: the anterolateral system and the dorsal columns. The anterolateral system includes predominantly the spinothalamic, spinomesencephalic, and spinoreticular tracts that transmit pain and temperature, crude or poorly localized touch, pressure, and some nociception respectively,[10] and are described briefly in the following sections, Table 3.1, and shown in Figure 3.1.

The spinothalamic tract

The spinothalamic tract (STT) mediates sensations of pain, temperature, and light touch. The cell bodies originate predominately in spinal cord (SC) laminae I and V, but are also found in laminae II, IV, VI, VII, VIII, and X.[11] The axons of these projection neurons cross the midline of the SC and ascend to the brainstem and thalamus through the anterolateral quadrant of the SC. Based on their DH origin, STT fibers follow specific pathways that terminate at the different areas of the thalamus, where they project to specific cortical regions. STT fibers projecting to the lateral thalamus have receptive fields on specific areas of contralateral skin and are thus suited to function in the signaling of sensory-discriminative components

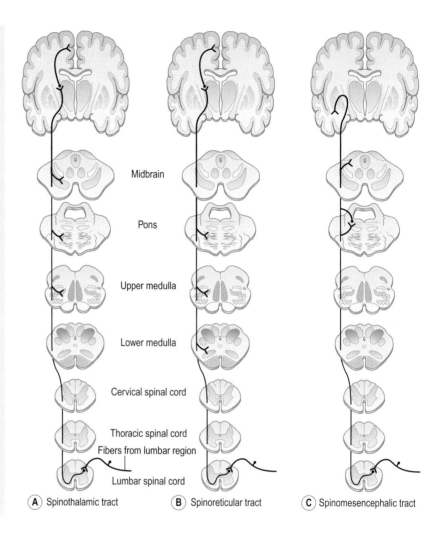

Figure 3.1

A schematic diagram showing the pathways of (A) the spinothalamic tracts, (B) the spinoreticular tracts, and (C) the spinomesencephalic tracts

Midbrain

Pons

Upper medulla

Lower medulla

Cervical spinal cord

Thoracic spinal cord

Fibers from lumbar region

Lumbar spinal cord

(A) Spinothalamic tract   (B) Spinoreticular tract   (C) Spinomesencephalic tract

of pain such as intensity and character. Alternatively, STT fibers that project to the medial thalamus have large receptive fields that often include the entire surface of the body and face.[12] STT neurons with large receptive fields are more related to motivational and affective features of pain as opposed to sensory discrimination.[9] Interestingly, STT fibers that project to the medial thalamus also receive input from visceral structures, suggesting one other explanation for the diffuse nature of visceral pain.[13]

The spinomesencephalic tract

Cell bodies of the spinomesencephalic tract (SMT) originate from wide dynamic range neurons and neurons in laminae I and IV–VI. SMT fibers travel up from the spinal cord to the midbrain, terminating at various midbrain nuclei including the PAG,[9] where they are shown to activate descending analgesic pathways.[9] SMT fibers are also thought to play a role in emotional components of pain as they also terminate at the parabrachial nucleus that in turn sends projections to the amygdala, an integral part of the limbic system.[10] In contrast to the STT, SMT neurons respond to both noxious and innocuous stimuli and are shown to have complex widespread receptive fields in separated areas of the body, including muscles, joints, cornea, dura, and all limbs.[14]

Table 3.1: Comparisons of ascending pathways for pain transmission

Tract	Spinothalamic tract	Spinomesence-phalic tract	Spinoreticular tract	Dorsal columns
Origin	Laminae I, IV, V	Laminae I, IV–VI	Laminae VII, VIII	Gracilis and cuneatus nuclei in the medulla
Somatotopic organization	Yes	No	No	Yes
Body representation	Contralateral	Bilateral	Bilateral	Contralateral
Subcortical targets	None	Periaqueductal gray, parabrachial nucleus, raphe nuclei	Hypothalamus, autonomic centers, reticular formation	None
Thalamic nucleus	Ventral posterolateral nucleus (VPL)	None	Intralaminar nuclei	VPL nucleus
Cortical location	Primary somatosensory cortex	None	Cingulate and insular cortex	Primary somatosensory cortex
Role	Discriminatory pain (intensity, location, quality)	Descending pain modulation, pain-related emotional processing	Affective and arousal components of pain	Discriminatory visceral pain
Pain function	Pain and temperature	Control of pain sensation	Sensation of poorly localized pain	Poorly localized visceral pain

The spinoreticular tract

The spinoreticular tract (SRT) has been shown to originate mostly in laminae VII and VIII in the ventral horn and is similar to the STT. However, the path of the SRT is interrupted several times by synapses where it gives off branches to the reticular formation in both the pons and the medulla oblongata.[15] Here, they are directed to the precerebellar nucleus in the lateral reticular formation, which is involved in motor control. SRT projections are also directed to the medial reticular formation involved more with nociception. Additionally, research shows scattered SRT neurons originating in lamina I.[9] These neurons send projections to catecholamine cell groups in reticular areas that respond specially to noxious stimuli. Thus, the primary functions of SRT neurons appear to include the influence of autonomic centers, endogenous pain modulation, and motivational and affective responses.

The dorsal columns

While the dorsal columns (DCs) have been viewed as a pathway involving positional sense and two-point discrimination, there is also compelling evidence showing an important role of the DCs in the transmission of visceral nociceptive information.[16] In addition to responding to chemical and mechanical irritation of the gastrointestinal tract, mechanical stimulation of the perineum, sacral region, and uterus also activates nociceptive transmission in the DCs.[17] Furthermore, behavioral and electrophysiological experimental methods show that DC lesions lead to reduced activity of thalamic and gracile neurons by visceral stimuli.[16] These observations have been substantiated, with several clinical studies showing that small lesions interrupting fibers of the DCs relieve pain and decrease analgesic requirements in patients with cancer arising in visceral organs.[18,19]

The thalamus

The thalamus is the last nociceptive center below the cortex and is involved in sensory discriminative and affective motivational components of pain. In general, each group of thalamic nuclei concerned with pain transmission has a distinct function for a specific pain component.

The lateral nociceptive thalamus

The lateral nociceptive thalamus includes areas of the ventral posterolateral nucleus (VPL) that receive nociceptive information from the body, while the ventral posteromedial nucleus (VPM) receives nociceptive information from the face, both being received via the STT (Figure 3.2).[15] Given that the bulk of STT neurons from both musculoskeletal and visceral systems terminate in both nuclei, neurons respond predominantly to heat and noxious mechanical stimuli but respond weakly to innocuous cutaneous mechanical stimuli.[20,21] Concerning cutaneous inputs, neurons in the VPL nucleus are also somatotopic and have restricted receptive fields and precisely code the intensity of noxious stimuli.[22] The ventral posterior inferior nucleus (VPI) also receives nociceptive signals from the STT; however, unlike the VPL and VPM that send

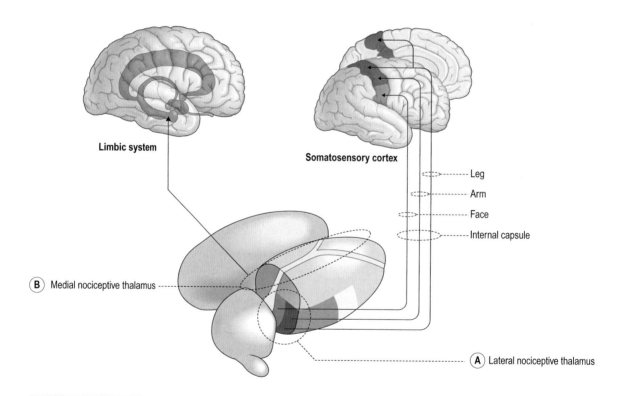

Limbic system

Somatosensory cortex

- - - - - Leg
- - - - - Arm
- - - - - Face
- - - - - Internal capsule

(B) Medial nociceptive thalamus - - - - - - -

(A) Lateral nociceptive thalamus

Figure 3.2
This shows (A) the lateral nociceptive nucleus that receives nociceptive information from the spinothalamic tract (STT). This includes the ventral posterolateral nucleus (VPL) that receives nociceptive information from the body and the ventral posteromedial nucleus (VPM) that receives information from the face. These nuclei send ascending projections to the primary and secondary somatosensory cortices. (B) The medial nociceptive thalamus receives nociceptive information from both the spinoreticular (SRT) and spinomesencephalic (SMT) tracts. This nucleus sends ascending projections to the limbic system.

projections to S1, the VPI sends projections to the secondary somatosensory cortex (S2) (pages 47-48) and the insular cortex (page 49).[23]

The medial nociceptive thalamus

The medial nociceptive thalamus comprises two nuclei situated in a thin sheet of myelinated fiber bundles contained in a Y-shaped lamina that dissect the body of the thalamus (Figure 3.2). The medial nociceptive thalami receive nociceptive information mostly via the SMT and SRT.[9] The ventromedial nuclei have large bilateral receptive fields and respond to noxious mechanical and thermal stimuli from any part of the body, suggesting they do not play a significant role in discrimination but do, however, distinguish intensity.[24] Neurons in this nucleus do not respond to innocuous stimuli and project to limbic system areas of the neocortex including the insula. Here, they play an important role in motivational and affective responses and/or the coordination of motor responses to pain.[22]

The thalamus and pain modulatory responses

Evidence now shows the thalamus to have an important contribution to hyperalgesic responses associated with peripheral injury. Animal studies show that following limb inflammation or peripheral nerve injury, VPL and VPM neurons exhibit lower thresholds and increased responses from peripherally evoked stimuli.[22,25] Additionally, other thalamic nuclei such as the nucleus submedius have also been shown to be involved in descending pain inhibition. Activation of the nucleus submedius stimulates projections to the ventrolateral orbital cortex (VLO), a region of the prefrontal cortex (PFC). Activation of this brain region leads to subsequent activation of the PAG–brainstem descending inhibitory system (pages 53-54).

Thalamic pain

A stroke anywhere along the spinothalamic pathway and its cortical projections can result in central post-stroke pain (CPSP).[26] It is now known that VPL lesions are most likely to cause pain than lesions elsewhere. In supratentorial lesions, most pain is observed in the extremities and there are likely to be sensory deficits of sharpness and cold (peripherally mediated Aδ fibers), while patients with infratentorial lesions report mostly facial pain and deficits of warmth and hot pain (peripherally mediated C fibers).[26,27] Thus, patients describe their pain as either burning-scalding or burning-freezing, depending on the site of the lesion. Additionally, CPSP often appears after post-stroke care is finished, and thus is often misdiagnosed, resulting in significant delays before treatment begins.[28] Unfortunately,

---

Box 3.1

Key points: thalamus

- Not purely a relay center but also involved in processing nociceptive information
- Involved in transmission of both sensory-discriminative and motivation mechanisms of pain
- Thalamic neurons show decreased thresholds in the presence of peripheral inflammation
- Involved in descending modulation via direct connections to the PAG
- Lesions in the VP nuclei cause thalamic pain

Box 3.2

Key points: the somatosensory cortex

- Key roles of S1
  - pain localization
  - pain sensation intensity
  - small receptive fields
- Key roles of S2
  - large bilateral receptive fields
  - possible role in learning and memory of painful events via connections with limbic system

diagnosis may be further complicated by cognitive and speech difficulties due to the stroke in addition to comorbid depression, anxiety, and sleep disturbance. Thankfully, the incidence of CPSP in stroke patients is relatively small, and while many patients experience abnormal sensory signs (42%), CPSP is found in under 10% of cases.[29]

The lateral pain system

Somatosensory cortex and pain processing

Current knowledge shows that the lateral pain system is chiefly involved processing sensory-discriminative features of pain.[30] Sensory-discriminative components of pain relate to at least three features: stimulus localization, intensity discrimination, and quality discrimination. The ability to perceive the locality and severity of pain is used daily in clinical practice when patients are asked about where their pain is felt and requested to rate its severity. Localization is clearly defined for the skin but more difficult for deeper tissues such as joints and muscles, and especially difficult for visceral structures.

The primary somatosensory cortex

The role of the primary somatosensory cortex (S1) in pain perception has long been disputed. Historically, findings differ between human and animal studies. In early human studies, lesions of the S1 have shown to produce either hypoalgesia or hyperalgesia, or to have no effect on pain perception,[31] whereas findings from animal studies clearly indicate the participation of S1 in pain processing. Several studies show that S1 responds to noxious activity in both anesthetized and awake animals where the activity of these neurons correlates with both duration and intensity of applied stimuli.[32–34] However, in later human studies, patients with epileptic foci involving the S1 cortex experience painful seizures,[35] slow temporal summation, and post noxious stimulus activity in the S1 cortex.[36]

Overall, the S1 is involved in the sensory-discriminative function of pain perception, especially in the localization of painful stimuli on the body surface. Thus, S1 activation correlates with intensity of pain sensation[31] but not with levels of pain unpleasantness, which is associated with anterior cingulate cortex activation.[37] However, attention and anticipation of sensory features of pain are shown to produce increases in S1 activity and increases in stimulus perception.[31] Thus, while S1 has a critical role in sensory-discriminative features of pain, cognitive factors can alter perceived intensity and thus modulate S1 activity.[38]

The secondary somatosensory cortex

Like S1, the secondary somatosensory cortex (S2) receives nociceptive projections from lateral thalamic nuclei. However, unlike S1, the S2 receives fibers mostly from the ventral posterolateral inferior nucleus.[39] Whereas nociceptive neurons in S1 are unilateral and correlate with locality and intensity of pain sensation, nociceptive neurons in S2 encode pain intensity poorly, have large bilateral receptive fields, and respond to stimuli presented on both sides of the body. Functional imaging also shows a somatotopic map (like the somatosensory homunculus in S1) in S2, but the neural areas for each body part are not as precise; thus, direct stimulation of S2 (in patients undergoing surgery) leads to vague non-localized pain.[40] Additionally, S2 projects neurons to limbic system structures via the insular cortex, where it is believed to be involved in recognition, learning, and memory of painful events.[31] Given these multisensory properties, the precise role(s) of S2 remain undetermined. For example, imaging work of the S2 shows that fMRI activation does not differ across different levels of painful and non-painful stimuli, thus supporting the theory that S2 is the target for independent pathways for the integration of painful and non-painful stimuli necessary for higher order processing.[41]

The medial pain system

The limbic system and pain processing

Limbic system structures are activated during noxious stimulation. Signals from the intramedullary lamina of the thalamus project to the limbic system structures, the periaqueductal gray, the amygdala, and the cingulate and insular cortices via the medial pain system (Figure 3.1).[42] Current evidence shows that the medial pain system is primarily involved in the processing of affective and motivational features of pain.[30] These components of pain are essential and involve the negative emotional reaction ('I don't like it'), arousal and selective attention ('it preoccupies me'), and the motivation to terminate the stimulus causing pain ('stop it').[43]

The cingulate cortex

The cingulate cortex is a major part of the limbic system and is associated with emotional-motivational components of pain. However, the cingulate cortex is an anatomically and functionally heterogeneous area. It is generally divided into the anterior cingulate cortex (ACC) and the posterior cingulate cortex (PCC). The ACC receives little afferent input from other cortical areas but does receive extensive projections from the dorsomedial thalamic nucleus, and generally connects with various regions of the descending pain modulation system.[30] The PCC, however, has extensive inputs from frontal, parietal, temporal, and occipital lobes and is thought to be involved in visuospatial orientation toward both innocuous and noxious somatosensory stimuli[42]. While these two regions of the cingulate cortex are well connected, there are striking differences in connections to the amygdala, where it has extensive reciprocal connections with the ACC but very little with the PCC.[44] Because of the amygdala's role in the storage of emotional memory, its connections with the ACC serve to communicate ongoing with past emotional experiences toward emotional and affective responses to incoming noxious inputs. Interestingly, functional imaging data show evidence that the rostral ACC (rACC) is a critical area for placebo analgesia.[45] This is likely due to connections between the rACC, the amygdala and other subcortical structures such as the hippocampus[46] and descending pain inhibitory pathways that are shown to be activated by placebo analgesia.[3]

Animal studies investigating cell recordings in the ACC show that nociceptive neurons are not organised somatotopically, and like the S2 area of the somatosensory cortex have a large receptive field that in some cases includes the entire body.[47] Additionally, the ACC has been shown to be associated with both somatic and visceral pain. Somatically, electrical stimulation of the ACC can activate nociceptive reflexes,[48] while in visceral pain models similar stimulation to the rACC in rats enhances visceromotor responses to colorectal distension.[49] Additionally, the ACC is also shown to be involved in both attention and escape from pain as well as the anticipation that leads to avoidance of noxious stimuli.[50,51] Furthermore, cognitive color-word tests are shown to increase activation of inhibitory regions of the cingulate cortex that include the perigenual ACC, an inhibitory region rich in opioid receptors and the PAG. These results highlight the role of the cingulate in affective-motivational factors of pain.

Single-neuron recordings from ACCs of patients undergoing cingulotomy during treatment for psychiatric disease show selective responses to painful thermal and mechanical stimuli.[52] As stated above, receptive fields were large and mostly bilateral where in all cases no cells responded to innocuous mechanical or thermal stimuli. Moreover, clinical reports show that patients with cingulotomies still feel pain but describe the pain as less distressing or bothersome.[53] Interestingly, these results are supported by findings in which the use of hypnosis shows a reduction in the unpleasantness of painful stimuli without changing perceived pain intensity. Imaging in such cases shows activation changes in the ACC but not in other brain regions.[37]

Key points relating to the cingulate cortex are summarized in Box 3.3 and nociceptive afferent inputs to the brain via spinal ascending pathways including the spinothalamic, spinomesencephalic and spinoreticular tracts are illustrated in Figure 3.3.

The insular cortex

The insular cortex is activated during noxious somatosensory stimulation. Afferent nociceptive information is mostly transmitted to the insular cortex from the somatosensory cortex and the thalamus (VPI), where it is processed with the aid of additional information related to working memory due to reciprocal connections of the insula with the PFC, ACC, amygdala, hippocampus and S2 (Figure 3.4).[54] Lesion studies in human subjects show that damage to the insula reduces pain effect and behavioral actions. Patients display a lack of withdrawal from painful stimuli anywhere on the body.[55] Similarly, animal studies further show that nociceptive responses in the insula, S2 and the ACC, have large bilateral receptive fields and respond to multimodal stimulation, in particular noxious stimulation to the viscera.[56,57] Additionally, functional imaging studies consistently show pain-related activation of the insula.[54,58,59] Thus, the insula is well positioned to utilize cognitive information to modulate connected brain regions involved in the

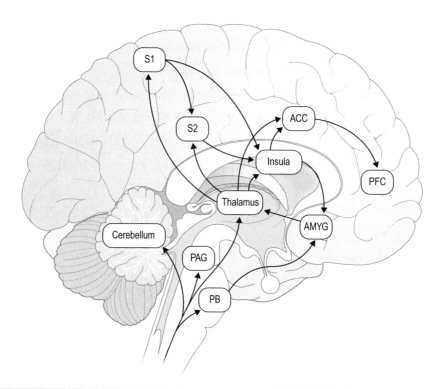

Figure 3.3

Nociceptive afferent inputs project to the brain via spinal ascending pathways including the spinothalamic, spinomesencephalic, and spinoreticular tracts. Nociceptive inputs entering the thalamus are then projected to the primary and secondary somatosensory cortices (S1/S2) along the lateral pain pathway, whereas medial pain pathways project from the thalamus to the anterior cingulate (ACC), insular, and prefrontal (PFC) cortices. PAG – periaqueductal gray; PB – parabrachial nucleus

processing of sensory-discriminative, affective and cognitive-evaluative mechanisms of pain.

The insula consists of anatomically and functionally different areas. Studies suggest that the posterior areas of the insula are related to interoceptive awareness to auditory, visual, and somatosensory function whereas anterior areas are associated with limbic, olfactory, gustatory, and viscero-autonomic function.[31] In relation to pain modulation, the rostral agranular insular cortex (RAIC) is shown to be important in the modulation of nociception in both humans and rats (Figure 3.4)[60]. The RAIC receives sensory information from the ventral posterior nuclei of the thalamus and sends efferent fibers to the amygdala, hypothalamus, PAG, and RVM. These and other widespread reciprocal connections with the ACC and orbitofrontal cortex suggest that the RAIC is involved with multiple features of pain behavior. Indeed, studies show that projections to the RAIC from medial thalamic nuclei are associated with motivational/affective mechanisms of pain, while projections from the RAIC to midbrain-limbic (mesolimbic) circuits

are likely to contribute to sensorimotor integration of nociceptive processing.[61] Furthermore, given that the RAIC sends neurons to the brainstem, it probably contributes to descending inhibitory control. Box 3.4 summarizes key points relating to the insular cortex.

The amygdala

As part of the limbic system, the amygdala is involved in emotional evaluation of sensory stimuli, emotional learning, and memory and is associated with affective disorders such as anxiety and depression.[62] The amygdala, like other areas of the pain system, shows high levels of neuronal plasticity, including long-term potentiation, that result in altered behavior and fear conditioning.[63,64] The amygdala is made up of several distinct nuclei: the lateral nucleus (LA) receives processed affective, cognitive, and sensory information from the thalamus and somatosensory and limbic cortical areas (Figure 3.5), which then project information to the central nucleus (CeA), which acts as the amygdala's output nucleus.[62]

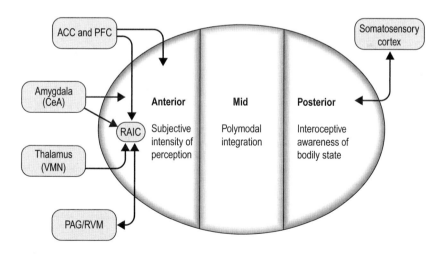

Figure 3.4

A schematic diagram showing the insula and its major connections involved in pain processing. (1) The posterior insula and the sensory-motor cortex; (2) the anterior insula and the thalamus, ACC, PFC, and amygdala. (3) The RAIC has reciprocal connections with a multitude of limbic system areas, namely the thalamus, amygdala, ACC, PFC, PAG, and RVM. ACC – anterior cingulate cortex; PFC – prefrontal cortex; RAIC – rostral agranular insular cortex; PAG – periaqueductal gray; RVM – rostral ventromedial medulla

Chapter 3

Nociceptive inputs to the CeA

Two main pathways convey nociceptive information to the central nucleus of the amygdala (CeA). First, via the LA, the CeA receives highly integrated polymodal inputs from the thalamus and somatosensory and limbic cortical areas related mainly to fear and anxiety.[64] The second major pathway to the CeA is more direct and consists of less integrated 'raw' nociceptive inputs directly from the spinal cord via the parabrachial nucleus located in the pons (Figure 3.5). The parabrachial nucleus receives and integrates information from all cutaneous, deep, and visceral tissues which through highly organized and specific connections sends nociceptive information to the CeA.[65] Animal studies show that noxious stimulation to musculoskeletal tissues such as the knee joint[66] and visceral tissues (colon)[67] activate CeA neurons. However, while CeA neurons respond to noxious tissue stimulation over wide receptive fields, the CeA does not have a major role in sensory-discriminative aspects of pain, rather, it is involved in emotional-affective pain mechanisms.

The influence of the CeA on nociceptive centers

The CeA also projects to other areas of the amygdala that influence affective and cognitive aspects of pain. The CeA integrates nociceptive information with previously acquired affective and cognitive memory through connections with other amygdaloid regions.[68] Additionally, the CeA projects opioidergic neurons to centers related to descending nociceptive control such as the PAG[69] and the dorsal reticular nucleus, associated with diffuse noxious inhibitory control (DNIC) (see p. 55). The CeA also projects directly to other structures that influence the modulation of nociception such as the substantia nigra (dopamine), locus coeruleus (norepinephrine/noradrenaline) and the raphe nucleus (serotonin).[64]

The amygdala and chronic pain

The role of the amygdala, in particular the CeA, has been investigated in animal studies using persistent somatic, visceral, and intra-articular and neuropathic pain models.[64] Generally, these studies do not show changes in reaction to spontaneous pain behaviors; however, chronic pain conditions do lead to increased neuronal activity and synaptic transmission in the CeA. Animal studies also show that the administration of CeA GABA agonists[70] as well as NMDA and mGlu receptor antagonists[71] results in decreases in pain-related behaviors.

The ventrolateral orbital cortex

As stated on page 46, the VLO region of the prefrontal cortex receives somatosensory inputs and is activated by both cutaneous and visceral noxious stimuli in normal and pain-sensitive states.[72] Studies in which morphine is injected into the VLO of animals show an increase in pain thresholds (tail flick) as well as analgesia in neuropathic pain states.[73] These antinociceptive effects are reversed by the administration of naloxone (mu-opioid receptor antagonist). Furthermore, electrophysiological studies show that nucleus submedius of the thalamus and VLO neurons respond specifically to noxious stimuli received from widespread receptive fields from skin, muscle, and viscera.[74] The VLO is predominantly involved in affective-motivational aspects of pain as shown in studies in both animals and humans. However, the VLO also projects neurons to the PAG, a region implicated in descending pain modulation.[75] Here, electrolytic lesions in the PAG and VLO eliminate inhibitory effects provoked by stimulation of the nucleus submedius.[75,76] Although there has been very little human study, surgical lesions

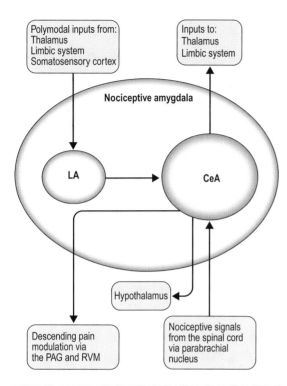

Figure 3.5

A schematic diagram showing ascending nociceptive inputs to the amygdala's central nucleus (CeA) from the spinal cord via the parabrachial nucleus in the brainstem. The CeA also receives modified nociceptive inputs from both limbic and somatosensory cortices and the thalamus via the lateral nucleus of the amygdala (LA). The CeA also sends inputs to (1) the PAG and RVM and thus having a role in descending pain modulation and (2) the hypothalamus where it influences autonomic and neuroendocrine components of pain

of the orbital cortex in patients have been shown to provide relief from chronic pain.[77,78]

The motor cortex

Functions of the motor cortex are primarily related to sensorimotor integration, control of voluntary movements and processing of motor-related information.[79] Evidence of motor cortex involvement in pain modulation has come about due to studies investigating motor cortex stimulation (MCS), showing that motor cortex stimulation increases nociceptive thresholds in both humans and animals.[80,81] Animal studies show that transdural stimulation of the motor cortex induces inhibition of thalamic sensory neurons and disinhibition of PAG neurons (activation of descending inhibitory neurons inducing antinociception). Earlier studies also show the inhibitory effects of MCS on neuropathic pain due to sciatic nerve injury by activation of the limbic and descending pain inhibitory systems described in the previous section.[82] Here, immunolabeling also shows decreases in CNS glutamate expression, a facilitatory neurotransmitter found extensively in pain pathways.

Encouragingly, human studies show MCS as a treatment for refractory peripheral neuropathic pain conditions such as trigeminal neuralgia, amputation, and brachial plexus lesions. MCS also has an analgesic effect on sensory discriminative aspects of pain with reductions in pain intensity rather than affective aspects of pain where sickness (affective) profile scores varied significantly depending on ongoing medical management.[80] However, treatment with repetitive MCS in conjunction with a battery of psychological function measures shows that fibromyalgia patients report not only significantly reduced levels of pain but also improved quality of life.[83] Moreover, MCS is also longer lasting for affective (fatigue, morning tiredness, and walking) than for sensory pain for up to 2 weeks. These results suggest that MCS also 'interferes' with emotional input of pain perception.

Imaging studies also support the above research. For example, MCS is associated with increases in cerebral blood flow in both prefrontal and cingulate cortices. However, concerning therapeutic value, post-stimulation periods are further associated with increases in blood flow within cortical (ACC, orbitofrontal cortex) and subcortical (thalamus, putamen, PAG and pons) regions.[84] Additionally, biochemical processes involved in the effect of MCS are due to increased GABAergic and opioid activity along inhibitory pathways.[85,86] Thus, it is thought that MCS, could, in part help to re-establish defective intracortical inhibitory processes.

Chapter 3

Descending pain modulation

Descending pain modulatory systems send brain-processed pain outputs to the DH that can either inhibit or facilitate sensory inputs coming from the periphery and/or ongoing DH synaptic processes. Importantly, descending inhibitory outputs block spinal transmission at the DH which leads to reduced pain perception despite ongoing peripheral inputs. These inhibitory mechanisms have evolutionary value in that they allow organisms to ignore pain in critical situations such as fight-or-flight and they are also considered to be the basis for placebo-induced analgesia.[87] Descending control arises from several supraspinal sites; however, the most studied is the PAG-RVM system mentioned in previous sections.

The PAG-RVM system

The PAG was the first brain region to have been shown to activate endogenous pain inhibitory outputs. Early studies using microinjections of opioids or electrical stimulation to the PAG showed strong antinociceptive effects in both animals and humans that are reversible by the introduction of naloxone.[88,89] The PAG receives inputs from cortical sites and has reciprocal connections with the amygdala as well as connections with ascending spinomesencephalic tracts. Additionally, human imaging studies have shown that the rACC probably facilitates expectation and placebo activation of the PAG.[90] Furthermore, activation of PAG neurons stimulates the RVM situated in the brainstem, which then may inhibit or facilitate depending on inputs from the PAG.[91]

The RVM receives neuronal inputs from the PAG and is suggested to be the final common relay station in the descending inhibition of nociception from supraspinal brain regions.[3] Additionally, the RVM also receives neurons from the thalamus, the parabrachial nucleus (involved in medial pain pathways via the thalamus to limbic structures) and the noradrenergic locus coeruleus. Inputs from these supraspinal regions on the RVM allow it to exert a bidirectional pain modulatory effect on the PAG, both facilitating and inhibiting pain.[88]

The RVM and ON and OFF cells

Important developments in our understanding of descending pain modulation have emerged from the studies of Fields and colleagues in which the activity of neurons in the RVM were compared with behavior in animals provoked by noxious stimuli (tail-flick response to heat).[92] They identified two distinct populations of RVM neurons: (1) a population of neurons (on-cells) that increase firing in response to noxious stimuli prior to the initiation of a nociceptive withdrawal reflex (tail flick) and (2), another population of neurons (off-cells) that 'ceased' firing immediately prior to the tail flick. The same authors subsequently showed that opiate microinjections into the nucleus raphe magnus within the RVM inhibited on-cells while also causing excitation of off-cells sufficient to produce analgesia.[93] Importantly, the PAG-RVM system receives inputs from higher cortical centers and thus provides a mechanism whereby homeostatic or experiential priorities due to fear, illness, and psychological stress may increase or decrease nociceptive inputs.[91]

Interestingly, descending control of nociception from the PAG-RVM system has also been shown to preferentially suppress nociceptive inputs mediated by peripheral C fibers, but preserving sensory-discriminatory information conveyed by more rapidly conducting A fibers.[91] C fibers predominantly terminate in the superficial DH while A fibers terminate mostly in the deep DH. Thus, while the activity of the deep DH cells may be influenced by descending pathways, most descending influence is likely to be secondary to modulation in the superficial DH via dendrites or relayed superficial interneurons.[94] Figure 3.6 shows integral connections between supraspinal regions involved in endogenous pain modulation.

Neurotransmitters modulating descending pain modulation

Early studies show that activation of descending tracts from the RVM stimulates release of serotonin in spinal DH, either from terminals of descending projections or from spinal interneurons.[88] However,

Figure 3.6

A schematic diagram showing cortical regions involved in endogenous pain modulation. SI – primary somatosensory cortex; S2 – secondary somatosensory cortex; ACC – anterior cingulate cortex; VLO – ventrolateral orbital cortex; PAG – periaqueductal gray, RVM – rostral ventral medulla

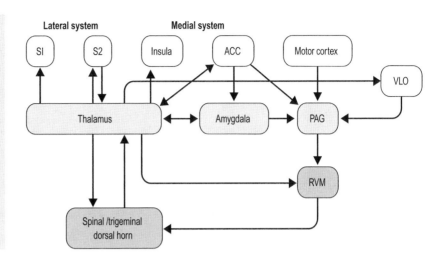

later studies show very few RVM neurons to be serotonergic (<20%), with most of those identified being either glycinergic or GABAergic.[95] However, electrophysiological studies show that descending serotonergic fibers from the RVM facilitate pain in inflammatory and neuropathic pain states and GABAergic and glycinergic inputs to the spinal cord mediate general antinociception.[3]

Another important component of descending pain modulation are noradrenergic projections, chiefly from the locus coeruleus and other pontine nuclei, that communicate with the PAG and RVM.[96] Many studies show that stimulation of these nuclei in addition to the PAG and/or RVM produce pain inhibition, blocked by α2-adrenergic receptor antagonists.[97] However, like serotonin, the effect of norepinephrine/noradrenaline depends which specific receptors are activated. Thus, just as α2-adrenergic receptor agonists (e.g., clonidine) show strong inhibitory effects on noxious stimuli-activated pain, activation of α1-adrenergic receptors produces pain facilitatory effects.[98] Importantly, the descending noradrenergic system has been shown to be enhanced during nerve injury.[3] This increase in noradrenergic activity during nerve injury or inflammation provides a mechanistic model for the clinical success of serotonin/norepinephrine reuptake inhibitors (e.g., duloxetine) in conditions such as diabetic neuropathy and fibromyalgia.[99,100]

Diffuse noxious inhibitory control (DNIC)

Diffuse noxious inhibitory control (DNIC) refers to the phenomenon that pain in one body region can inhibit pain in another body region.[101] DNIC involves a spino-medullary-spinal loop in which projection neurons ascend from the spinal cord to the subnucleus reticularis dorsalis (SRD) in the caudal medulla and descend through the dorsal funiculi, affecting only wide dynamic range (WDR) neurons in lamina V of the dorsal horn and trigeminal nociceptive neurons.[101,102] WDR neurons, as reviewed in Chapter 2, are important conversion sites for both excitatory and inhibitory inputs arising from many types tissue. Interestingly other types of cell in the DH such as C and AΔ neurons are not affected by this type of control.[101]

DNIC effects are activated through a complex feedback loop involving supraspinal structures as, unlike segmental inhibitions, these effects are not observed in either animals or humans where the spinal cord has been sectioned at cervical segments.[101] Although supraspinal structures are suggested to be involved in this form of descending inhibition, lesions of the PAG, RVM, and thalamus do not reduce or modify DNIC and thus are not presumed to modify the activity of WDR neurons.[103] In contrast, experimental lesions in the SRD and the presence of Wallenberg syndrome (brainstem stroke) significantly reduced DNIC,[104] thus, the SRD is considered a

Chapter 3

key relay station in the DNIC loop. Importantly, more recent data shows that the SRD is influenced by cortical regions such as the ACC and the PFC, thus explaining why psychological factors affect DNIC responses.[105]

Measurement of endogenous pain modulation

Many observational studies show that chronic pain conditions occur due in part to the loss of DNIC. Loss in DNIC has been shown to lead to either reduced endogenous pain inhibition or worse, an increase in endogenous pain facilitation. Cumulating evidence now suggests that by measuring levels of DNIC, one can determine to what extent supraspinal pain processing influences chronic pain states. Studies of DNIC-like effects in humans report subjective experiences similar to the behavioral responses found in animals. However, given that the origin of neurophysiological effects is uncertain, the term conditioned pain modulation (CPM) is recommended.[106]

CPM studies in humans repeatedly show dysfunctional pain modulation in conditions such as fibromyalgia, painful arthritis, and irritable bowel syndrome.[107] The technique involves simultaneously applying painful stimuli at distant body regions and assessing how much a (conditioning stimulus) reduces pain evoked by another (test) stimulus.[108] The most reliable forms of test stimuli for are pressure and thermal pain while cold water immersion is the most reliable as the conditioning pain (Figure 3.7).[109] Generally, in case-control studies, healthy control groups show a decreased sensitivity to test stimuli in the presence of or immediately after a conditioning stimulus, whereas, people with chronic pain conditions show, absent or in many cases increased sensitivity to pain.

Treatment approaches

As discussed in Chapter 2, it is often difficult to successfully treat people with chronic pain. Despite much effort, chronic, unexplained pain remains a significant challenge both clinically and in research. Although evidence suggests that conditions such as fibromyalgia, chronic low back pain, and headache are driven by central mechanisms, efforts to disentangle these pathways remain relatively unanswered. This is due to 'central sensitization', a term that encompasses a multitude of different processes such as increased temporal summation and pain facilitation at the dorsal horn, altered sensory and affective processing in the brain,

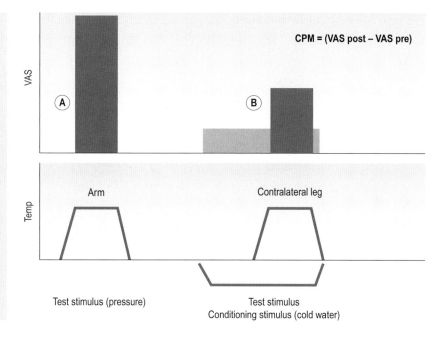

Figure 3.7
A diagram showing a typical protocol for measuring CPM. This graph shows (A) a VAS score for a test stimulus applied to the arm and (B) a second test stimulus given during a simultaneous conditioning stimulus applied at the contralateral lower limb. The level of CPM is given as the second VAS score minus the first VAS score. A negative score indicates an inhibitory effect of the second conditioning stimulus

CPM = (VAS post − VAS pre)

VAS

A

B

Temp

Arm

Contralateral leg

Test stimulus (pressure)

Test stimulus
Conditioning stimulus (cold water)

and malfunctioning descending inhibitory pathways. The majority of treatment approaches towards central sensitization are reviewed in Chapter 2; however, therapeutic interventions related to physical therapies shown to have effects on brain and descending pain modulatory pathways are described below.

Cognitive behavioral therapy

Many studies show strong associations between maladaptive thoughts about pain and a number of pain conditions.[110] Here, several psychological variables including catastrophizing, increased pain vigilance, and depression are shown to negatively influence chronic pain conditions. There have been many meta-analyses evaluating the effect of cognitive behavioral therapy (CBT) on chronic pain. For example, a Cochrane review found that CBT, which focuses on helping people to change any aspects of their behavior that worsen or maintain pain, disability, distress, and catastrophic thinking, was the most commonly used psychological treatment.[111] The authors found that although CBT is effective in altering mood and catastrophizing when compared to usual treatment or waiting list subjects, it only has small effects on pain-related disability and weak effects in reducing pain intensity. Nevertheless, experts agree that CBT is beneficial in increasing self-control over understanding and the effect of pain on the individual, a self-management strategy essential for improving health-related quality of life.[112] It is thought that CBT helps to reduce or deactivate brain-coordinated facilitatory pathways and thus decrease the amount of CNS hyperexcitability.

Acceptance-based therapies

Recently, there has been a growing interest in acceptance-based therapies in which the aims are related to acceptance rather than the control of pain.[113] One such therapy is mindfulness-based stress reduction (MBSR), which teaches formal types of practice including meditation, yoga, and the daily exercise of mindfulness; it involves training the mind or inducing a state of consciousness that 'disidentifies' from the moment-to-moment experience of pain.[114] The aim of MBSR is to alleviate pain and improve emotional well-being through moment-to-moment non-judgmental awareness (e.g.,

yoga, walking, and meditation). Randomized controlled studies (RCTs) suggest these techniques are helpful in reducing both pain severity and pain-related comorbidities such as anxiety and depression.[115,116]

Another more recently developed acceptance-based intervention is acceptance and commitment therapy (ACT). ACT aims to address ineffective control strategies by staying in contact with negative emotions such as avoidance and hypervigilance.[113] The aim is to understand why a particular behavior is maintained and thus is more focused on behavioral change. For example, this perspective suggests that chronic pain is an experiential avoidance disorder that attempts to avoid thoughts, feelings, memories, and physical sensations that create suffering.[117] Similar to MBSR, ACT data show that regardless of chronic pain condition, ACT participants report reduced pain interference, and better pain-related mood.[118] Meta-analyses suggest that MBSR and ACT both show small to medium effects on physical and mental health in people with chronic pain.[113] However, given the importance of acceptance and mindfulness in chronic pain conditions, the search for other similar but more effective treatments should continue.

Exercise therapy

Although exercise therapy is reviewed in Chapter 2, it has equal relevance to more cognitive-targeted approaches. Exercise therapy is described as a form of neuroscience education that aims to be continued over long-term rehabilitation programs.[112] Nijs and colleagues suggest a time-dependent approach, for five minutes regardless of pain, over a more symptom-dependent approach in which exercise stops once it hurts. Here, they argue that symptom-dependent approaches facilitate the brain to produce abnormal (hypersensitive) warning signs of pain while time-dependent exercise approaches may deactivate brain-coordinated, descending facilitatory pain pathways. Although our understanding of brain circuitry involved in exercise analgesia is incomplete, a recent animal study showed significant correlations between increased withdrawal thresholds and reduced expression of mu-opioid receptors (MORs) in the RVM of animals with sciatic neuropathy.[119]

Pain facilitatory 'on-cells' in the RVM reportedly express MORs, and thus a reduction or desensitization of these receptors will decrease 'on-cell' activity.

However, such studies do not address cognitive-emotional factors found in human subjects with chronic pain. This issue is underlined by the fact that healthy people and some with persistent musculoskeletal pain, including low back and shoulder pain, show exercise-induced analgesia, while other patients with other pain conditions, such as fibromyalgia and chronic whiplash, do not.[112] Importantly, however, recent human brain imaging data show that fibromyalgia patients do show post-exercise reductions in pain sensitivity after a short session of acute intense cycling versus those participating in quiet rest.[120] Furthermore, imaging data in the exercise group also show increased activity in the dorsolateral PFC, a brain region known to be involved in endogenous pain modulation. These results go some way to confirming the ideas of Nijs and colleagues concerning shorter, more intense exercise strategies.

Pain neuroscience education

Understanding of central mechanisms involved in the contribution and maintenance of chronic pain conditions is important for all stakeholders in management and care of people with chronic pain. Thus, it is important not only for practitioners working in multidisciplinary pain management but for all those working throughout primary and secondary care settings. Prior to the treatment of chronic pain it is essential that patients are educated about mechanisms associated with centrally driven pain. Studies show that pain education is independently therapeutic, with

evidence pointing towards changes in pain beliefs and improving health status in fibromyalgia and chronic low back pain.[112] This education is particularly valuable in helping patients grasp the concept that pain is maintained by hypersensitivity of the CNS rather than by local tissue damage where their pain is experienced. Throughout this publication, it is shown that misconceived beliefs and understanding, such as pain hypervigilance, anxiety, and catastrophizing, all add significantly to the contribution and/or continuation of central sensitization. Nijs and colleagues rightly suggest that written information about pain physiology should be provided at the first pain education setting as homework so that in the second session misunderstandings can be discussed and corrected.[121] Pain education programs with other active treatments are also shown to improve levels of endogenous pain inhibition at three-month follow-up post treatment.[122]

Summary

For most people with chronic pain conditions, pain is the only factor that truly affects their quality of life and disturbances in cognition and alterations in mood negatively affect our subjective experience of pain. Functional imaging is now able to capture not only real time activity in brain regions affected by pain but also changes in brain structure, where chronic pain shows temporal and spatial loss of gray and white matter relative to healthy controls. Fortunately imaging studies also show that these brain changes are reversible when pain is significantly relieved. Thus, people with chronic pain and those treating them can take hope from the ameliorating effects of comprehensive pain management involving education, exercise, mindfulness, lifestyle and social factors.

References

1. Apkarian AV, Bushnell MC, Treede RD, Zubieta JK. Human brain mechanisms of pain perception and regulation in health and disease. European Journal of Pain. 2005;9(4):463–84.

2. Melzack R. Pain and the neuromatrix in the brain. Journal of Dental Education. 2001;65(12):1378–82.

3. Ossipov MH, Dussor GO, Porreca F. Central modulation of pain. Journal of Clinical Investigation. 2010;120(11):3779–87.

4. Hadjipavlou G, Dunckley P, Behrens TE, Tracey I. Determining anatomical connectivities between cortical and brainstem pain processing regions in humans: a diffusion tensor imaging study in healthy controls. Pain. 2006;123(1–2):169–78.

5. Zambreanu L, Wise RG, Brooks JCW, Iannetti GD, Tracey I. A role for the brainstem in central sensitisation in humans. Evidence from functional magnetic resonance imaging. Pain. 2005;114(3):397–407.

6. Malisza KL, Gregorash L, Turner A, Foniok T, Stroman PW, Allman AA, et al. Functional MRI involving painful stimulation of the ankle and the effect of

physiotherapy joint mobilization. Magnetic Resonance Imaging. 2003;21(5):489–96.

7. Takamoto K, Sakai S, Hori E, Urakawa S, Umeno K, Ono T, et al. Compression on trigger points in the leg muscle increases parasympathetic nervous activity based on heart rate variability. Journal of Physiological Sciences. 2009;59(3):191–7.

8. Bender T, Nagy G, Barna I, Tefner I, Kadas E, Geher P. The effect of physical therapy on beta-endorphin levels. European Journal of Applied Physiology. 2007;100(4):371–82.

9. Willis WD, Westlund KN. Neuroanatomy of the pain system and of the pathways that modulate pain. Journal of Clinical Neurophysiology. 1997;14(1):2–31.

10. Patestas M, Gartner L. Ascending sensory pathways: a textbook of neuroanatomy. 2nd ed. New Jersey: Wiley-Blackwell; 2016.

11. Almeida TF, Roizenblatt S, Tufik S. Afferent pain pathways: a neuroanatomical review. Brain Research. 2004;1000(1–2):40–56.

12. Giesler GJ, Jr., Yezierski RP, Gerhart KD, Willis WD. Spinothalamic tract neurons that project to medial and/or lateral thalamic nuclei: evidence for a physiologically novel population of spinal cord neurons. Journal of Neurophysiology. 1981;46(6):1285–308.

13. Hodge CJ, Jr., Apkarian AV. The spinothalamic tract. Critical Reviews in Neurobiology. 1990;5(4):363–97.

14. Yezierski RP, Broton JG. Functional properties of spinomesencephalic tract (SMT) cells in the upper cervical spinal cord of the cat. Pain. 1991;45(2):187–96.

15. Mense S. Central nervous mechanisms of muscle pain: ascending pathways, central sensitization, and pain-modulating systems. In: Mense S, Gerwin RD, editors. Muscle pain: understanding the mechanisms. Berlin Heidelberg: Springer; 2010. p. 105–75.

16. Palecek J. The role of dorsal columns pathway in visceral pain. Physiological Research / Academia Scientiarum Bohemoslovaca. 2004;53(Suppl 1):S125–30.

17. Al-Chaer ED, Lawand NB, Westlund KN, Willis WD. Pelvic visceral input into the nucleus gracilis is largely mediated by the postsynaptic dorsal column pathway. Journal of Neurophysiology. 1996;76(4):2675–90.

18. Hwang SL, Lin CL, Lieu AS, Kuo TH, Yu KL, Ou-Yang F, et al. Punctate midline myelotomy for intractable visceral pain caused by hepatobiliary or pancreatic cancer. Journal of Pain and Symptom Management. 2004;27(1):79–84.

19. Nauta HJ, Soukup VM, Fabian RH, Lin JT, Grady JJ, Williams CG, et al. Punctate midline myelotomy for the relief of visceral cancer pain. Journal of Neurosurgery. 2000;92(2 Suppl):125–30.

20. Chung JM, Lee KH, Surmeier DJ, Sorkin LS, Kim J, Willis WD. Response characteristics of neurons in the ventral posterior lateral nucleus of the monkey thalamus. Journal of Neurophysiology. 1986;56(2):370–90.

21. Berkley KJ, Guilbaud G, Benoist JM, Gautron M. Responses of neurons in and near the thalamic ventrobasal complex of the rat to stimulation of uterus, cervix, vagina, colon, and skin. Journal of Neurophysiology. 1993;69(2):557–68.

22. Ab Aziz CB, Ahmad AH. The role of the thalamus in modulating pain. Malaysian Journal of Medical Sciences. 2006;13(2):11–8.

23. Ventral Posterior Inferior Nucleus. In: Gebhart GF, Schmidt RF, editors. Encyclopedia of Pain. Berlin, Heidelberg: Springer; 2013. p. 4159.

24. Monconduit L, Bourgeais L, Bernard JF, Le Bars D, Villanueva L. Ventromedial thalamic neurons convey nociceptive signals from the whole body surface to the dorsolateral neocortex. Journal of Neuroscience. 1999;19(20):9063–72.

25. Guilbaud G, Benoist JM, Jazat F, Gautron M. Neuronal responsiveness in the ventrobasal thalamic complex of rats with an experimental peripheral mononeuropathy. Journal of Neurophysiology. 1990;64(5):1537–54.

26. Kumar B, Kalita J, Kumar G, Misra UK. Central poststroke pain: a review of

pathophysiology and treatment. Anesthesia and Analgesia. 2009;108(5):1645–57.

27. Bowsher D, Leijon G, Thuomas KA. Central poststroke pain: correlation of MRI with clinical pain characteristics and sensory abnormalities. Neurology. 1998;51(5):1352–8.

28. Henry JL, Lalloo C, Yashpal K. Central poststroke pain: an abstruse outcome. Pain Research and Management: Journal of the Canadian Pain Society = Journal de la Société Canadienne pour le Traitement de la Douleur. 2008;13(1):41–9.

29. Andersen G, Vestergaard K, Ingeman-Nielsen M, Jensen TS. Incidence of central post-stroke pain. Pain. 1995;61(2):187–93.

30. Xie YF, Huo FQ, Tang JS. Cerebral cortex modulation of pain. Acta Pharmacologica Sinica. 2009;30(1):31–41.

31. Schnitzler A, Ploner M. Neurophysiology and functional neuroanatomy of pain perception. Journal of Clinical Neurophysiology. 2000;17(6):592–603.

32. Kenshalo DR, Jr., Chudler EH, Anton F, Dubner R. SI nociceptive neurons participate in the encoding process by which monkeys perceive the intensity of noxious thermal stimulation. Brain Research. 1988;454(1–2):378–82.

33. Kenshalo DR, Jr., Isensee O. Responses of primate SI cortical neurons to noxious stimuli. Journal of Neurophysiology. 1983;50(6):1479–96.

34. Kenshalo DR, Iwata K, Sholas M, Thomas DA. Response properties and organization of nociceptive neurons in area 1 of monkey primary somatosensory cortex. Journal of Neurophysiology. 2000;84(2):719–29.

35. Young GB, Blume WT. Painful epileptic seizures. Brain. 1983;106(3):537–54.

36. Tommerdahl M, Delemos KA, Favorov OV, Metz CB, Vierck CJ, Jr., Whitsel BL. Response of anterior parietal cortex to different modes of same-site skin stimulation. Journal of Neurophysiology. 1998;80(6):3272–83.

37. Rainville P, Duncan G, Price D, Carrier B, Bushnell M. Pain affect encoded in human

anterior cingulate but not somatosensory cortex. Science. 1997;277:968–77.

38. Bushnell MC, Duncan GH, Hofbauer RK, Ha B, Chen JI, Carrier B. Pain perception: Is there a role for primary somatosensory cortex? Proceedings of the National Academy of Sciences of the United States of America. 1999;96(14):7705–9.

39. Stevens RT, London SM, Apkarian AV. Spinothalamocortical projections to the secondary somatosensory cortex (SII) in squirrel monkey. Brain Research. 1993;631(2):241–6.

40. Del Gratta C, Della Penna S, Ferretti A, Franciotti R, Pizzella V, Tartaro A, et al. Topographic organization of the human primary and secondary somatosensory cortices: comparison of fMRI and MEG findings. NeuroImage. 2002;17(3):1373–83.

41. Chen TL, Babiloni C, Ferretti A, Perrucci MG, Romani GL, Rossini PM, et al. Human secondary somatosensory cortex is involved in the processing of somatosensory rare stimuli: an fMRI study. NeuroImage. 2008;40(4):1765–71.

42. Vogt BA. Pain and emotion interactions in subregions of the cingulate gyrus. Nature Reviews Neuroscience. 2005;6(7):533–44.

43. Treede R-D, Kenshalo DR, Gracely RH, Jones AKP. The cortical representation of pain. PAIN. 1999;79(2–3):105–11.

44. Toyoda H, Li X-Y, Wu L-J, Zhao M-G, Descalzi G, Chen T, et al. Interplay of amygdala and cingulate plasticity in emotional fear. Neural Plasticity. 2011;2011:9.

45. Bingel U, Lorenz J, Schoell E, Weiller C, Buchel C. Mechanisms of placebo analgesia: rACC recruitment of a subcortical antinociceptive network. Pain. 2006;120(1–2):8–15.

46. Zhang W, Liu X, Zhang Y, Song L, Hou J, Chen B, et al. Disrupted functional connectivity of the hippocampus in patients with hyperthyroidism: evidence from resting-state fMRI. European Journal of Radiology. 2014;83(10):1907–13.

47. Sikes RW, Vogt BA. Nociceptive neurons in area 24 of rabbit cingulate cortex. Journal of Neurophysiology. 1992;68(5):1720–32.

48. Zhang L, Zhang Y, Zhao ZQ. Anterior cingulate cortex contributes to the descending facilitatory modulation of pain via dorsal reticular nucleus. European Journal of Neuroscience. 2005;22(5):1141–8.

49. Cao Z, Wu X, Chen S, Fan J, Zhang R, Owyang C, et al. Anterior cingulate cortex modulates visceral pain as measured by visceromotor responses in viscerally hypersensitive rats. Gastroenterology. 2008;134(2):535–43.

50. Iwata K, Kamo H, Ogawa A, Tsuboi Y, Noma N, Mitsuhashi Y, et al. Anterior cingulate cortical neuronal activity during perception of noxious thermal stimuli in monkeys. Journal of Neurophysiology. 2005;94(3):1980–91.

51. Koyama T, Tanaka YZ, Mikami A. Nociceptive neurons in the macaque anterior cingulate activate during anticipation of pain. Neuroreport. 1998;9(11):2663–7.

52. Hutchison WD, Davis KD, Lozano AM, Tasker RR, Dostrovsky JO. Pain-related neurons in the human cingulate cortex. Nature Neuroscience. 1999;2(5):403–5.

53. Jones AK, Qi LY, Fujirawa T, Luthra SK, Ashburner J, Bloomfield P, et al. In vivo distribution of opioid receptors in man in relation to the cortical projections of the medial and lateral pain systems measured with positron emission tomography. Neuroscience Letters. 1991;126(1):25–8.

54. Starr CJ, Sawaki L, Wittenberg GF, Burdette JH, Oshiro Y, Quevedo AS, et al. Roles of the insular cortex in the modulation of pain: insights from brain lesions. Journal of Neuroscience. 2009;29(9):2684–94.

55. Berthier M, Starkstein S, Leiguarda R. Asymbolia for pain: a sensory-limbic disconnection syndrome. Annals of Neurology. 1988;24(1):41–9.

56. Ito SI. Possible representation of somatic pain in the rat insular visceral sensory cortex: a field potential study. Neuroscience Letters. 1998;241(2–3):171–4.

57. Zhang ZH, Dougherty PM, Oppenheimer SM. Monkey insular cortex neurons respond to baroreceptive and somatosensory convergent inputs. Neuroscience. 1999;94(2):351–60.

58. Lee MC, Tracey I. Imaging pain: a potent means for investigating pain mechanisms in patients. British Journal of Anaesthesia. 2013;111(1):64–72.

59. Coghill RC, Sang CN, Maisog JM, Iadarola MJ. Pain intensity processing within the human brain: a bilateral, distributed mechanism. Journal of Neurophysiology. 1999;82(4):1934–43.

60. Ohara PT, Granato A, Moallem TM, Wang BR, Tillet Y, Jasmin L. Dopaminergic input to GABAergic neurons in the rostral agranular insular cortex of the rat. Journal of Neurocytology. 2003;32(2):131–41.

61. Jasmin L, Burkey AR, Granato A, Ohara PT. Rostral agranular insular cortex and pain areas of the central nervous system: a tract-tracing study in the rat. Journal of Comparative Neurology. 2004;468(3):425–40.

62. Neugebauer V, Li W, Bird GC, Han JS. The amygdala and persistent pain. The Neuroscientist. 2004;10(3):221–34.

63. Rogan MT, Staubli UV, LeDoux JE. Fear conditioning induces associative long-term potentiation in the amygdala. Nature. 1997;390(6660):604–7.

64. Veinante P, Yalcin I, Barrot M. The amygdala between sensation and affect: a role in pain. Journal of Molecular Psychiatry. 2013;1(1):9.

65. Sarhan M, Freund-Mercier MJ, Veinante P. Branching patterns of parabrachial neurons projecting to the central extended amygydala: single axonal reconstructions. Journal of Comparative Neurology. 2005;491(4):418–42.

66. Neugebauer V, Li W. Processing of nociceptive mechanical and thermal information in central amygdala neurons with knee-joint input. Journal of Neurophysiology. 2002;87(1):103–12.

67. Han JS, Neugebauer V. Synaptic plasticity in the amygdala in a visceral pain model in rats. Neuroscience Letters. 2004;361(1–3):254–7.

68. Price JL. Comparative aspects of amygdala connectivity. Annals of the New York Academy of Sciences. 2003;985:50–8.

69. Shane R, Acosta J, Rossi GC, Bodnar RJ. Reciprocal interactions between the amygdala and ventrolateral periaqueductal gray in mediating of Q/N(1–17)-induced analgesia in the rat. Brain Research. 2003;980(1):57–70.

70. Pedersen LH, Scheel-Kruger J, Blackburn-Munro G. Amygdala GABA-A receptor involvement in mediating sensory-discriminative and affective-motivational pain responses in a rat model of peripheral nerve injury. Pain. 2007;127(1–2):17–26.

71. Ansah OB, Bourbia N, Goncalves L, Almeida A, Pertovaara A. Influence of amygdaloid glutamatergic receptors on sensory and emotional pain-related behavior in the neuropathic rat. Behavioural Brain Research. 2010;209(1):174–8.

72. Ohara PT, Vit JP, Jasmin L. Cortical modulation of pain. Cellular and Molecular Life Sciences. 2005;62(1):44–52.

73. Al Amin HA, Atweh SF, Baki SA, Jabbur SJ, Saade NE. Continuous perfusion with morphine of the orbitofrontal cortex reduces allodynia and hyperalgesia in a rat model for mononeuropathy. Neuroscience Letters. 2004;364(1):27–31.

74. Tang JS, Qu CL, Huo FQ. The thalamic nucleus submedius and ventrolateral orbital cortex are involved in nociceptive modulation: a novel pain modulation pathway. Progress in Neurobiology. 2009;89(4):383–9.

75. Zhang S, Tang JS, Yuan B, Jia H. Electrically-evoked inhibitory effects of the nucleus submedius on the jaw-opening reflex are mediated by ventrolateral orbital cortex and periaqueductal gray matter in the rat. Neuroscience. 1999;92(3):867–75.

76. Zhang YQ, Tang JS, Yuan B, Jia H. Inhibitory effects of electrical stimulation of thalamic nucleus submedius area on the rat tail flick reflex. Brain Research. 1995;696(1–2):205–12.

77. Grantham EG. Prefrontal lobotomy for relief of pain, with a report of a new operative technique. Journal of Neurosurgery. 1951;8(4):405–10.

78. Scarff JE. Unilateral prefrontal lobotomy for the relief of somatic pain. AMA Archives of Neurology and Psychiatry. 1950;64(5):740–1.

79. Quintero GC. Advances in cortical modulation of pain. Journal of Pain Research. 2013;6:713–25.

80. Lefaucheur JP, Drouot X, Cunin P, Bruckert R, Lepetit H, Creange A, et al. Motor cortex stimulation for the treatment of refractory peripheral neuropathic pain. Brain. 2009;132(6):1463–71.

81. Pagano RL, Fonoff ET, Dale CS, Ballester G, Teixeira MJ, Britto LR. Motor cortex stimulation inhibits thalamic sensory neurons and enhances activity of PAG neurons: possible pathways for antinociception. Pain. 2012;153(12):2359–69.

82. Pagano RL, Assis DV, Clara JA, Alves AS, Dale CS, Teixeira MJ, et al. Transdural motor cortex stimulation reverses neuropathic pain in rats: a profile of neuronal activation. European Journal of Pain. 2011;15(3):268.e1–14.

83. Passard A, Attal N, Benadhira R, Brasseur L, Saba G, Sichere P, et al. Effects of unilateral repetitive transcranial magnetic stimulation of the motor cortex on chronic widespread pain in fibromyalgia. Brain. 2007;130(10):2661–70.

84. Saitoh Y, Osaki Y, Nishimura H, Hirano S, Kato A, Hashikawa K, et al. Increased regional cerebral blood flow in the contralateral thalamus after successful motor cortex stimulation in a patient with poststroke pain. Journal of Neurosurgery. 2004;100(5):935–9.

85. Maarrawi J, Peyron R, Mertens P, Costes N, Magnin M, Sindou M, et al. Motor cortex stimulation for pain control induces changes in the endogenous opioid system. Neurology. 2007;69(9):827–34.

86. Kim S, Stephenson MC, Morris PG, Jackson SR. tDCS-induced alterations in GABA concentration within primary motor cortex predict motor learning and motor memory: a 7 T magnetic resonance spectroscopy study. NeuroImage. 2014;99:237–43.

87. Kuner R. Central mechanisms of pathological pain. Nature Medicine. 2010;16(11):1258–66.

88. Ossipov MH, Morimura K, Porreca F. Descending pain modulation and chronification of pain. Current Opinion in Supportive and Palliative Care. 2014;8(2):143–51.

89. Helmstetter FJ, Tershner SA, Poore LH, Bellgowan PS. Antinociception following opioid stimulation of the basolateral amygdala is expressed through the periaqueductal gray and rostral ventromedial medulla. Brain Research. 1998;779(1–2):104–18.

90. Eippert F, Bingel U, Schoell ED, Yacubian J, Klinger R, Lorenz J, et al. Activation of the opioidergic descending pain control system underlies placebo analgesia. Neuron. 2009;63(4):533–43.

91. Heinricher MM, Tavares I, Leith JL, Lumb BM. Descending control of nociception: specificity, recruitment and plasticity. Brain Research Reviews. 2009;60(1):214–25.

92. Fields HL, Anderson SD, Clanton CH, Basbaum AI. Nucleus raphe magnus: a common mediator of opiate- and stimulus-produced analgesia. Transactions of the American Neurological Association. 1976;101:208–10.

93. Fields HL, Anderson SD. Evidence that raphe-spinal neurons mediate opiate and midbrain stimulation-produced analgesias. Pain. 1978;5(4):333–49.

94. Ruda MA, Allen B, Gobel S. Ultrastructural analysis of medial brain stem afferents to the superficial dorsal horn. Brain Research. 1981;205(1):175–80.

95. Morgan MM, Whittier KL, Hegarty DM, Aicher SA. Periaqueductal gray neurons project to spinally projecting GABAergic neurons in the rostral ventromedial medulla. Pain. 2008;140(2):376–86.

96. Bruinstroop E, Cano G, Vanderhorst VGJM, Cavalcante JC, Wirth J, Sena-Esteves M,

et al. Spinal projections of the A5, A6 (locus coeruleus), and A7 noradrenergic cell groups in rats. Journal of Comparative Neurology. 2012;520(9):1985–2001.

97. Jones SL. Descending noradrenergic influences on pain. Progress in Brain Research. 1991;88:381–94.

98. Holden JE, Schwartz EJ, Proudfit HK. Microinjection of morphine in the A7 catecholamine cell group produces opposing effects on nociception that are mediated by alpha1- and alpha2-adrenoceptors. Neuroscience. 1999;91(3):979–90.

99. Lee Y-C, Chen P-P. A review of SSRIs and SNRIs in neuropathic pain. Expert Opinion on Pharmacotherapy. 2010;11(17):2813–25.

100. Hauser W, Urrutia G, Tort S, Uceyler N, Walitt B. Serotonin and noradrenaline reuptake inhibitors (SNRIs) for fibromyalgia syndrome. Cochrane Database of Systematic Reviews. 2013;1:Cd010292.

101. Le Bars D, Villanueva L, Bouhassira D, Willer JC. Diffuse noxious inhibitory controls (DNIC) in animals and in man. Patologicheskaia Fiziologiia i Eksperimental'naia Terapiia. 1992(4):55–65.

102. Villanueva L, Le Bars D. The activation of bulbo-spinal controls by peripheral nociceptive inputs: diffuse noxious inhibitory controls. Biological Research. 1995;28(1):113–25.

103. Bouhassira D, Bing Z, Le Bars D. Studies of the brain structures involved in diffuse noxious inhibitory controls: the mesencephalon. Journal of Neurophysiology. 1990;64(6):1712–23.

104. De Broucker TH, Cesaro P, Willer JC, Le Bars D. Diffuse noxious inhibitory controls in man: involvement of the spinoreticular tract. Brain. 1990;113(4):1223–34.

105. Piche M, Arsenault M, Rainville P. Cerebral and cerebrospinal processes underlying counterirritation analgesia. Journal of Neuroscience. 2009;29(45):14236–46.

106. Yarnitsky D, Arendt-Nielsen L, Bouhassira D, Edwards RR, Fillingim RB, Granot M, et al. Recommendations on terminology and practice of psychophysical DNIC testing. European Journal of Pain. 2010;14(4):339.

107. Lindstedt F, Berrebi J, Greayer E, Lonsdorf TB, Schalling M, Ingvar M, et al. Conditioned pain modulation is associated with common polymorphisms in the serotonin transporter gene. PloS one. 2011;6(3):e18252.

108. Lewis GN, Luke H, Rice DA, Rome K, McNair PJ. Reliability of the conditioned pain modulation paradigm to assess endogenous inhibitory pain pathways. Pain Research and Management. 2012;17(2):98–102.

109. Yarnitsky D, Bouhassira D, Drewes AM, Fillingim RB, Granot M, Hansson P, et al. Recommendations on practice of conditioned pain modulation (CPM) testing. European Journal of Pain. 2015;19(6):805–6.

110. Nijs J, Meeus M, Van Oosterwijck J, Roussel N, De Kooning M, Ickmans K, et al. Treatment of central sensitization in patients with 'unexplained' chronic pain: what options do we have? Expert Opinion on Pharmacotherapy. 2011;12(7):1087–98.

111. Williams ACdC, Eccleston C, Morley S. Psychological therapy for adults with longstanding distressing pain and disability. Cochrane Database of Systematic Reviews. 2012(11).

112. Nijs J, Malfliet A, Ickmans K, Baert I, Meeus M. Treatment of central sensitization in patients with 'unexplained' chronic pain: an update. Expert Opinion on Pharmacotherapy. 2014;15(12):1671–83.

113. Veehof MM, Oskam M-J, Schreurs KMG, Bohlmeijer ET. Acceptance-based interventions for the treatment of chronic pain: a systematic review and meta-analysis. PAIN®. 2011;152(3):533–42.

114. Shapiro SL, Carlson LE, Astin JA, Freedman B. Mechanisms of mindfulness. Journal of Clinical Psychology. 2006;62(3):373–86.

115. Reiner K, Tibi L, Lipsitz JD. Do mindfulness-based interventions reduce pain intensity? A critical review of the literature. Pain Medicine (Malden, Mass). 2013;14(2):230–42.

116. Bushnell MC, Case LK, Ceko M, Cotton VA, Gracely JL, Low LA, et al. Effect of environment on the long-term consequences of chronic pain. Pain. 2015;156(01):S42–S9.

117. McCracken LM, Vowles KE. Acceptance and commitment therapy and mindfulness for chronic pain: model, process, and progress. American Psychologist. 2014;69(2):178–87.

118. Wetherell JL, Afari N, Rutledge T, Sorrell JT, Stoddard JA, Petkus AJ, et al. A randomized, controlled trial of acceptance and commitment therapy and cognitive-behavioral therapy for chronic pain. PAIN. 2011;152(9):2098–107.

119. Kim Y-J, Byun J-H, Choi I-S. Effect of exercise on μ-opioid receptor expression in the rostral ventromedial medulla in neuropathic pain rat model. Annals of Rehabilitation Medicine. 2015;39(3):331–9.

120. Ellingson LD, Stegner AJ, Schwabacher IJ, Koltyn KF, Cook DB. Exercise strengthens central nervous system modulation of pain in fibromyalgia. Brain Sciences. 2016;6(1):8.

121. Nijs J, Paul van Wilgen C, Van Oosterwijck J, van Ittersum M, Meeus M. How to explain central sensitization to patients with 'unexplained' chronic musculoskeletal pain: practice guidelines. Manual Therapy. 2011;16(5):413–8.

122. Van Oosterwijck J, Meeus M, Paul L, De Schryver M, Pascal A, Lambrecht L, et al. Pain physiology education improves health status and endogenous pain inhibition in fibromyalgia: a double-blind randomized controlled trial. Clinical Journal of Pain. 2013;29(10):873–82.

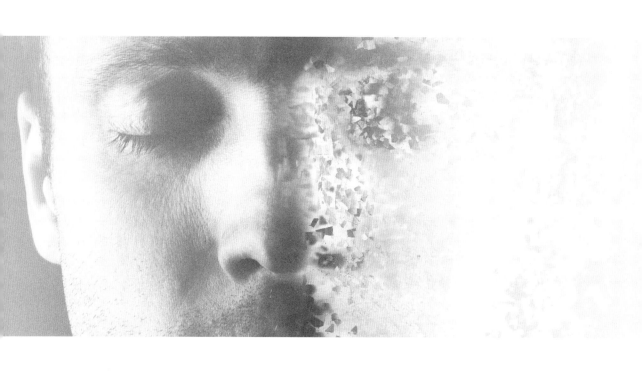

SECTION 2
Epidemiology, psychology, evaluation and treatment

Introduction

Although chronic pain (CP) is highly prevalent, with a significant impact on the health of individuals, only a small percentage of cases are associated with structural dysfunction. Epidemiological research is important as it provides key information on prevalence and factors associated with onset and persistence of pain. Understanding these factors helps to improve the clinical management of people living with CP. Studies show that all measured characteristics of health are worse in people with CP than in those with no pain, which for the most part is due to the physical, emotional and financial burden on patients, but also on society in general. The current cost of chronic pain in Europe is estimated to be more than €200 billion per annum[1] and in the USA $150 billion.[2] However, despite the enormous costs associated with both patient management and research, CP remains under-recognized and unacceptably managed.[3] Estimates of prevalence (actual number of cases alive with a condition) vary greatly in the general population, with figures ranging between 2% and 55%;[1, 4–7] however, the prevalence of CP among adults consulting primary care has been estimated at 22%[8] of the general population. Variation in prevalence is attributed to many factors; these include the types of population being studied, the survey methodology, and differing definitions of the term 'chronic pain'.[6] Few studies have examined the incidence (the rate of newly diagnosed cases in a given time period) of chronic pain conditions. However, a recent prospective study investigating occupational factors relating to chronic low back pain (CLBP) found that 22% of participants without any previous history of CLBP presented with the condition 5 years later.[9] Most studies use a pain duration lasting longer than 3–6 months, and the International Association for the Study of Pain suggests using the term 'chronic' if pain persists beyond normal tissue injury (normally 3 months); however, there is no generally accepted standard.

In order to understand CP in both general and specific populations, it is important to first understand the risk factors associated with both the presence and continuance of CP. Risk factors shown to be clinically relevant include sociodemographic, clinical, psychological, occupational and biological factors. Thus, this chapter will review and discuss current evidence and consider how these factors can be recognized and applied in the management of CP. CP is also associated with many sociodemographic factors across many different pain conditions. These include female gender, older age, social class and cultural background.[10] These risk factors are not directly responsive to medical intervention and thus not modifiable. However, while not modifiable, they should lead to further productive lines of inquiry in both research and patient management. Other modifiable risk factors, such as mental health, smoking, obesity, physical condition and employment status, can be managed through primary care, manual therapy and self-management settings. Table 4.1 shows modifiable and non-modifiable factors associated with CP.

Early life factors and adult-onset chronic pain

Overwhelming evidence shows that early life stress plays a key role in long-lasting alterations in pain processing.[11] However, although retrospective studies are subject to recall bias, long-term prospective studies show an increased risk of CP in adults with a history of childhood adversity,[12] with meta-analysis demonstrating that people who report childhood abuse or neglect are at increased risk of experiencing pain symptoms in adult life compared to those who have not been exposed to these adverse events.[13] Those reporting such early-life stressors show strong links with adult-onset low back pain,[14] fibromyalgia,[15] headache[16] and arthritis.[17] Risk factor experiences most commonly reported are those of emotional abuse, poverty, family separation, parental death and childhood neglect,[18] while premature birth weight and very low birth weights are also influences.

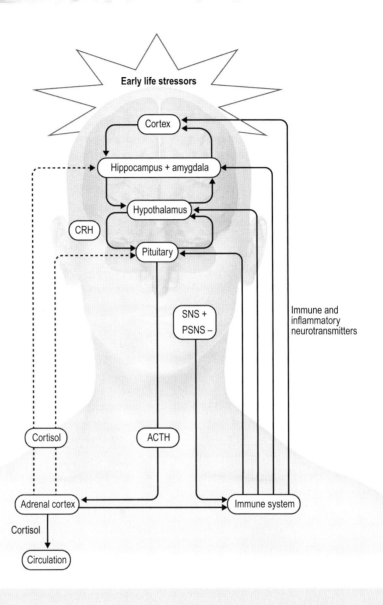

Figure 4.1
A schematic representation of the effect of early life stress on the HPA axis. Here, persistent activation of the HPA axis and the autonomic nervous system causes the increased release of glucocortiods from the adrenal cortex. Circulating glucocorticoids then downregulate central receptor sensitivity (negative feedback loop), thus increasing the release of CRH and ACTH. Circulating glucorticoids and increased SNS norepinepherine contribute to the release of inflammatory cytokines (e.g., TNF-α, IL-1, IL-6). Increases in the inflammatory response, combined with excessive sympathetic tone, further impact dorsal column processing of pain signals by contributing to activation of microglia and astroglia. Activated microglia exchange signals with astrocytes and nociceptive neurons, amplifying pain-related activity in the dorsal horn.

⟶ Positive feedback during normal function

---> Negative feedback during normal function

Table 4.1

Non-modifiable and modifiable factors associated with chronic pain (adapted from Van Hecke et al. 2013)[3]

Non-modifiable	• Age
	• Sex
	• Geographical and cultural background
	• Socioeconomic background
	• History of trauma
	• Heritable factors (genetics)
Modifiable	• Pain
	• Mental health
	• Obesity
	• Physical activity
	• Sleep
	• Employment status
	• Occupational factors

Experimental data

Although data are inconsistent, recent findings generally show that chronic low back pain patients presenting with a childhood history of physical and sexual abuse show lower pressure pain thresholds and increased temporal summation.[19] Similar findings have also been shown in adults presenting with functional gastrointestinal disorders (FGIDs). Here, FGID patients experiencing childhood trauma showed increased temporal summation compared to not only healthy controls but also people with FGIDs with no history of childhood trauma. Equally, FGID patients with childhood trauma also presented with greater gastrointestinal symptom severity, a greater number of CP sites, and greater symptom-related disability.[20] However, several studies show no differences in noxious stimuli testing between CP patients and controls.[18] For example, pain severity associated with rectal distension does not differ between women with a history of sexual abuse and controls[21]. It is suggested that experimentally induced pain sensitivity is not due to abuse history alone, but most likely due to additional psychological influences, with subjects reporting higher levels of psychological distress showing increased pain perception.[22]

Cross-sectional data

Many retrospective studies show childhood adversity to be associated with chronic conditions including pain. In a large sample of 18,303 people from the Americas, Europe, and Asia, Scott and colleagues examined whether childhood adversities and early-onset psychological disorders were independently associated with an increased risk of chronic physical conditions. Importantly, they found that the number of childhood adversities (three or more) was independently associated with conditions such as heart disease, diabetes mellitus, arthritis, chronic back pain and chronic headaches; neglect, family violence, and abuse were particularly associated[23]. Stickley and co-workers also found that an increased number of adversities correlated with a higher risk of CP in Japanese people suffering childhood adversities.[24]

It should be noted that the main limitation with these retrospective studies is recall bias. This bias does not specifically relate to people with chronic conditions over-reporting childhood adversity, rather to those free of pain likely under-reporting the occurrence of early-life adversity, thus exaggerating the perceived relationship between these two variables.[11] However, recent prospective studies show similar results. For example, in a Canadian study examining data from 3294 people between childhood in 1983 and follow-up in 2001, Gonzalez and colleagues also found that a greater number of childhood adversities significantly correlated with chronic physical and psychological conditions in adult life.[25]

Biological mechanisms

Although biological mechanisms facilitating the connection between early-life adversity and chronic conditions are not fully understood, animal and clinical studies suggest the role of several neuroimmune systems.[18] Current understanding suggests that alterations in function of the hypothalamic–pituitary–adrenal (HPA) axis, inflammatory mediators and endogenous pain modulation act as mediators between early-life adversity and the later onset of CP (Figure 4.2). A substantial review of these processes is beyond the scope of this chapter; a brief synopsis for each system is described below.

The hypothalamic–pituitary–adrenal axis and other brain responses

The HPA axis is activated by stress. Stress, of whatever kind, is an adverse environmental experience or a perceived threat that alters an organism's homeostasis, which stimulates a physiological response involving peripheral and central systems.[26] This occurs due to the release of glucocorticoids from the adrenal cortex, the end product of the HPA axis (Figure 4.1). Glucocorticoids bind to glucocorticoid receptors in many areas of the body, including the brain, and serve as a negative feedback of their own secretion, thus promoting recovery.[27] However, persistent activation of the HPA axis and autonomic nervous system decreases this negative feedback loop, thus increasing (1) the release of corticotropin-releasing hormone (CRH) from the hypothalamus and (2) increased plasma levels of adrenocorticotropic hormone[28].

Additionally, increased levels of glucocorticoids restrict energy utilization and alter metabolic hormones involved in energy metabolism such as insulin and glucose.[29] HPA axis dysfunction affects other parts of the brain, such as the hippocampus, amygdala, and prefrontal cortex, that undergo stress-induced structural remodeling, which further modifies behavioral and physiological responses. Evidence shows that early-life stress (from the prenatal period and into childhood) induces persistent changes in the capability of the HPA axis to respond to stress in adulthood.[30] Persistent HPA axis activity, especially the release of CRH, is also associated with pronociception. Animal studies find that rats persistently treated with CRH show both hyperalgesia and allodynia in response to noxious stimuli,[31] thus suggesting persistent HPA axis activation affects pain modulatory responses.

Inflammatory mediators

During the stress response, adrenergic stimulation triggers the release of inflammatory mediators that initially promote resistance to infection and repair to damaged tissue. The release of these proinflammatory mediators progressively stimulates the secretion of glucocorticoids that in turn reduce the inflammatory response.[32] This inhibitory influence of glucocorticoids is reduced during persistent HPA axis activity; thus, early-life stress is associated with increased levels of inflammatory markers not only during childhood but also

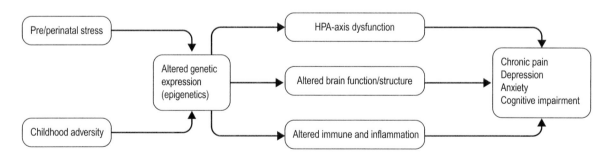

Figure 4.2
A Schematic representation of mechanisms connecting exposure to early life adversity to later life somatic and psychological outcomes

in adulthood.[32] Studies show that adults who report childhood adversity: (1) show reduced ability glucocorticoid signaling to control HPA axis function and (2) show an increased risk of disease with inflammatory origins.[33] Studies investigating these relationships in early-life stress assess levels of C-reactive protein, as it is shown to be both one of the most reliable indicators of inflammation[34, 35] and directly associated with somatic pain conditions.[18] Early-life stress also sensitizes the immune system by activating microglia in the central nervous system (Chapter 2). Animal studies show that exposure to stressful events during neonatal periods increases microglial activation and increased pain behaviors.[36] Additionally, evidence is now emerging on the effects of early-life stress on microglial function. Studies in this area suggest that, once activated, microglia have a long-lasting and significant impact on central processing and increased pain sensitivity in adults.[37]

Endogenous pain modulation

Because of immature descending pain pathways early in life, the neonatal cortex has little influence on pain control, and thus bio-behavioral responses to noxious stimuli are at this time due to spinal reflexes.[38] Studies show a relative delay in the development of endogenous pain modulatory pathways following neonatal injury that coincides with maturation of descending pathways from the brainstem.[39] Animal studies clearly demonstrate that opioid-mediated descending pathways via the rostral ventral medulla (RVM) (Chapter 3) primarily facilitate, rather than suppress, pain transmission during neonatal life.[40] Normally, the effects of activating this pain control system lead to it becoming more inhibitory, and thus pain facilitation and inhibition become more finely balanced. Studies also show that these pain modulatory pathways in the brainstem may be altered by early-life cutaneous pain experiences.[41] The periaqueductal gray (PAG) is also shown to undergo similar changes in early life; again, animal studies show that inflammatory pain leads to the increase of facilitatory beta-endorphins and long-lasting decreases in opioid receptor expression in the PAG in adult life.[42] These data suggest that early-life injury or stress can lead to permanent changes in RVM–PAG neurotransmitter-receptor signaling that ultimately bring about changes in descending control of spinal pain networks.

Sex differences underlying chronic pain

Epidemiological studies consistently find greater pain prevalence in women than in men[43]. Pain is reported more frequently by women and women show enhanced pain sensitivity.[44, 45] These observations are supported by a greater representation of females in many clinical pain disorders including tension-type headaches, fibromyalgia, migraine and irritable bowel syndrome (IBS).[46] Our understanding of sex, gender, and pain has significantly improved over recent years thanks to preclinical studies of mechanisms contributing to sex differences in both pain perception[45] and endogenous pain modulation.[47] Additionally, research also highlights contrasting effects of psychological variables on the experience of pain in men and women. In this area, studies show that pain-related catastrophizing, perceived disability, and lower self-efficacy are more

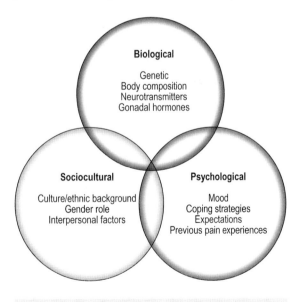

Figure 4.3

Interacting biopsychosocial factors relating to sex differences underlying chronic pain

prevalent in women,[48–50] while men experience higher levels of anxiety.[50] Although the exact mechanisms underlying sex differences are not fully understood, a series of interacting biopsychosocial variables have been suggested that are summarized in Figure 4.3 and described in detail in the following sections.

Psychosocial factors

Many studies suggest that differences in pain between genders also relate to psychological and social factors. However, although depression, anxiety, and pain catastrophizing are important factors in the development and maintenance of CP, associations between psychological factors and gender are less clear. Most studies fail to support any differential effects of depression, anxiety, and stress on experimentally provoked pain in male versus female subjects.[51] However, findings do suggest that cognitive and social factors may explain some sex-related differences.

Much attention has been given to the role of catastrophizing and various coping strategies, such as self-efficacy. As described in Chapter 5, pain catastrophizing is viewed as a mixture of rumination, magnification, and helplessness. The first two components relate to appraisal where people focus and exaggerate the threat of painful stimuli, while helplessness suggests a lack of ability to deal effectively with pain. While findings were inconsistent in earlier studies, more recent research shows sex difference in pain appraisal that is also associated with affective responsiveness to pain (pain unpleasantness rather than pain intensity).[52] Thus, catastrophizing may partly mediate sex differences in pain sensitivity but these are equally likely to be modulated by other psychological variables such as personality traits.[51]

Gender-specific beliefs and expectations about pain are in part gained through social learning. Here, the role of gender refers to stereotypical characteristics according to which women are more willing to report pain than men, while the masculine role is more associated with stoicism. However, although many studies have shown that women are more likely

to report pain or that their expectation of pain is greater, once gender was controlled during analysis, it was not a significant predictor of altered pain sensitivity.[51, 53] These studies show that gender plays only a small role in explaining differences in experimental pain experience. However, it is more likely that masculinity/femininity traits and their associations with emotional vulnerability may play a larger role in the contribution to sex differences in experimental pain perception.

Biological mechanisms

A number of mechanisms have been proposed for sex-related differences in pain perception, with the most obvious and most frequently researched being related to the possible influence of gonadal hormones. This is to be expected, given the distribution of sex hormones and their receptors in both the peripheral and central nervous systems pain pathways.[43] While precise neurobiological mechanisms are not fully established, animal and human studies show that estradiol and progesterone exert both pro- and anti-nociceptive effects on pain, while testosterone appears to be more anti-nociceptive.[46] Though experimental pain procedures in humans differ, meta-analysis shows that higher pain thresholds and tolerances are seen during the follicular compared to the periovulatory and luteal phases of the menstrual cycle.[54] However, much of this research suffers limitations in that studies do not include measurements of plasma levels of gonadal hormones which would have helped to determine associations between hormone activity and pain responses.

Sex hormones have also been implicated in differential brain activation during the processing of pain stimuli. While research is again limited, brain imaging studies show significant differences in central processing of pain between males and females. For example, more intense perception of noxious heat stimulation is found in female subjects, with greater activation in the prefrontal cortex, insula, and thalamus.[55] Moreover, functional magnetic resonance imaging (fMRI) studies also show sex-based differences in central processing in response to cutaneous pain, with greater activation in cingulate, insular, somatosensory, and cerebellar cortices shown in females.[56] Imaging studies also find male subjects to have greater activation of the contralateral prefrontal and secondary somatosensory cortices as well as bilateral parietal and insular cortices during noxious stimulation, while females show greater activation in ipsilateral perigenual and ventral cingulate cortex.[57]

Thus, while results are still inconsistent, activation patterns in males appear to occur predominantly in the somatosensory system, whereas females appear to show most activation in the cingulate cortex, which is more associated with affective processing. These findings may help to explain why women show a greater prevalence of (1) CP and (2) psychological comorbidities.[58]

Sex differences have also been found in descending pain modulation. Conditioned pain modulation studies generally show male subjects to have increased levels of endogenous analgesia[59]. However, meta-analyses of such studies suggest that gender differences in endogenous pain modulation may depend on both experimental methodology and modes of measurement (i.e., heat, mechanical pressure, etc.), as some types of pain stimuli are more gender-specific than others.[60]

Sex differences in pain are also shown with differences in the endogenous opioid system. Opioid neurotransmitters and mu-opioid receptors are centrally associated in the response to stress and the suppression of pain. For example, Zubieta and colleagues found that men show stronger activation of the mu-opioid system in the thalamus, basal ganglia, and amygdala than women.[61] All female subjects were scanned during the early follicular phase of their menstrual cycle, a time-period where levels of estradiol are low. Additionally, high estradiol states are associated with increases in mu-opioid receptor availability and increased activation of endogenous opioid transmission during painful stimuli.[62] Importantly, the same studies show significant reductions in endogenous opioid activation during low estradiol states that also correlate with hyperalgesic pain responses.

Sex differences in clinical pain

Population-based studies show consistent support for sex differences not only in the prevalence of pain generally but also for specific pain conditions.[45, 63] Conditions such as fibromyalgia, IBS, neuropathic pain, osteoarthritis, and a number of other musculoskeletal pain conditions are regularly shown to be more frequently reported by women.[63] However, given that many studies report on clinical samples from both primary care and pain treatment settings, bias may be associated with health care-seeking behavior.

Musculoskeletal pain

Many studies show that, irrespective of body region, both prevalence and severity of chronic musculoskeletal pain are greater in women.[63] For example, one large study that sampled 85,052 adults from seventeen countries across six continents showed not only higher prevalence rates of musculoskeletal pain among women (45%) than men (31%) but also higher prevalence rates of comorbid depression.[64] Most commonly, differences in the prevalence of low back pain between men and women are investigated. Studies in countries such as Sweden, Germany, China, Nigeria, and Turkey show that women report both higher current and higher lifetime prevalence of low back pain.[65-69]

Meta-analysis of sex differences in osteoarthritis also shows greater prevalence, incidence and degree of severity in women, especially in knees and after the age of menopause.[70] However, the same study found that no significant differences in the prevalence of hip osteoarthritis had been demonstrated, and that men were at higher risk for cervical spine degeneration, especially over the age of 55. Sex differences in fibromyalgia and widespread pain are also well studied. Several population studies over several cultures and ethnicity show approximately 90% of those presenting with fibromyalgia type symptoms are women,[71] especially those of low socioeconomic status.[72] However, although fatigue and widespread pain are significantly more prevalent in women, and the number of diagnostic trigger points is higher, perceived disability, global severity of symptoms, and psychological factors are similar in both sexes[73].

Abdominal pain

Epidemiological studies investigating the gender-related prevalence of abdominal pain are relatively scarce. Those studies examining abdominal pain have focused on pain associated with dysmenorrhea. However, even when dysmenorrheic pain is controlled, women still report more abdominal pain than men.[74] A number of population-based studies found that abdominal pain of unknown etiology shows increased prevalence rates among women. Although a meta-analysis shows higher abdominal pain prevalence rates for women in both the Netherlands and the United States,[51] some primary studies show no differences.[5] Recently, studies investigating the prevalence of IBS report that women are three times more likely to be diagnosed with the disorder. IBS is currently defined as a chronic disorder characterized by recurring or ongoing abdominal pain or pain, changes in bowel habit, and bloating in the absence of organic pathology.[75, 76] However, it should be noted that female predominance of IBS has mostly been studied in those who seek health care and not in the general population.[77] Most significant sex differences are related to sub-classifications of IBS where, interestingly, women are more likely to present with IBS with constipation, whereas IBS with diarrhea is more common in men.[78] IBS is discussed in more detail in Chapter 12.

Sex differences in response to non-pharmacological pain management

Gender differences in response to pain treatment are also an important consideration. Although many studies have investigated sex differences in responses to pharmacological treatments, only a few have looked at differences in responses to non-pharmacological treatments. Pieh and colleagues looked at gender differences in relation to outcomes after a multidisciplinary pain program consisting of individual physical therapy and psychotherapy, group relaxation techniques, cognitive behavioral therapy, and pain education. They found that women showed greater improvement in pain-related disability independent of pain duration, medication, and psychiatric comorbidities compared to men.[79] However, Keogh and co-workers found that although men and women show similar reductions in pain intensity immediately after a pain program, at three months following treatment only men maintained treatment gains, whereas for women, post treatment reduction in pain intensity disappeared[80]. In a study looking at sex differences in outcomes of physical therapy, Hansen and colleagues found that men responded best to general physiotherapy, while women responded best to intensive back exercises. Importantly, these findings may be reflective of occupational workload, as patients with hard physical occupations also responded best to physiotherapy, while subjects with sedentary or light jobs responded best to intensive back exercises.[81] However, further studies show that treatment gains are similar for men and women after active exercise rehabilitation for low back pain.[82, 83]

The impact of culture on chronic pain

Increased cultural diversity means health care professionals are often required to meet the needs of people from different ethnic backgrounds. It is therefore necessary to gain an understanding of the influence of race and ethnicity on the management of CP. Cultural factors influence beliefs, behavior, perception, and emotion, all of which affect the patient and impact health care. Several studies of experimental pain have found that patients' cultural and ethnic background is associated with significant variation in their pain intensity and attitudes to pain, as well as emotions and behaviors.[84] Historically, and in many contemporary cultural settings, pain has been, and is, inseparably bound up with its social and cultural significance: for example, pain may be seen as a test of faith or a means of redemption. However, in other settings, social and spiritual explanations have been discarded and the practice of medicine has been affirmed as the main authority for controlling and curing the symptoms of pain.[85] Some studies suggest that current biological explanations create more negative meanings for pain; for example, in conditions such as osteoarthritis, pain often generates anxiety as signifying ageing, or potential loss of career and/or family role.[85]

Cultural beliefs towards chronic pain

Beliefs around pain are strongly associated with psychological and physical functioning, coping abilities, and response to treatment.[86] Such beliefs are formed by the patient's cultural background, past experiences, and individual features, and are more related to pain and disability than disease processes.

The patient

Patients' culturally based responses often fall into two categories: the stoic and the emotive. Concerning pain perception, stoicism is associated with lower intensities of pain, resulting in under-reporting of not only mild pain but also moderate to severe pain.[87] Emotive patients are more likely to verbalize their expression of pain while also expecting people around them to react to their pain so as to validate their symptoms.[88] Patients from Northern Europe and Asian backgrounds have been found to show a more stoic response to pain while those from the Middle Eastern, African, Hispanic, and Mediterranean backgrounds tend to be more expressive.[89] Studies further suggest that stoical presentations of pain are associated with cultures that have been marginalized or exploited. Such patients are also more likely to come from deprived socioeconomic backgrounds.[90] Interestingly, these patients are also more likely to show lower expectations and more distrust of biomedical pain management.[84]

Concerning specific cultural variations in pain perception, clinical studies show higher levels of reported pain by African Americans compared to Caucasians for several pain conditions, including arthritis[91] and severe low back pain.[92] Similar findings also show those from Indian and Filipino backgrounds report higher pain tolerances than those living in the United States.[93] Some cultures promote positive acceptance of pain. For example, older Korean women describe positive acceptance of CP as an unavoidable quality of ageing and not a problem to be solved.[90] Hindu culture observes and accepts pain and suffering as a consequence of karma.

Differences in pain beliefs between a patient and their health care provider may also cause communication issues that are subsequently associated with reduced treatment outcomes. In a study comparing ethnic group differences in pain-related outcomes following a multidisciplinary program, both African Americans and Caucasian patients showed similar reductions in depressive symptoms.[94] However, Caucasian patients further reported reductions in pain severity while African Americans did not. This variation is shown to be due to cultural differences in self-care behaviors and differing preferences for pain management components. Additionally, cultural differences between patients and providers can burden patients further where they feel they are not being understood or believed. A Swedish study found that in addition to obvious language barriers, Muslim immigrant women perceived health care providers as doing their best, but also expressed feelings of not being believed, not examined properly, or not being offered optimal treatment for complaints of CP.[95]

The practitioner

In most health care settings, clinical formulations are heavily influenced by a provider dominant relationship. A provider is required to diagnose, counsel, treat, and often 'certify' a patient as 'sick' through discussion that in their mind is most appropriate for the patient's presentation.[96] Provider dominance may also introduce bias, leading to an ethnocentric view of what is wrong with the patient based on his or her background and social class. Indeed, studies show that clinicians may be culturally insensitive or have an inadequate cultural understanding from which to approach or effectively treat people with CP. For example, Chinese-Canadian patients respond more favorably to non-verbal communication of pain, and ethnic consideration of the patient was perceived to be beneficial by these patients.[97] Hispanic patients have been shown to be more likely to allow clinicians to take a predominant role in their diagnosis; however, for these patients faith and religion are also important forms of coping with CP.[98]

Cultural differences in musculoskeletal pain and disability

In Western countries, painful disorders of the musculoskeletal system are a major cause of disability and incapacity for work.[99] Although these disorders are attributed to occupational activities such as excessive computer use and repetitive manual work, such factors do not adequately explain the increasing incidence of disabling musculoskeletal pain experienced despite the decline in heavy physical labour. For example, in a recent worldwide study, Coggon and co-workers compared disabling low back pain and wrist/hand pain among diverse groups of workers from different cultural backgrounds. Overall, their findings showed large international variation in levels of pain-related disability among occupational groups that carry out similar tasks. However, although large differences in prevalence were observed, it could not be determined if they were due to the job, the person, or the culture.[100]

Relationships with patients from different cultural backgrounds

The experience of practicing in health care across cultural backgrounds was once far less common than it is today, when populations are more diverse in race, culture, language, religion, and ethnicity.[101] Individual patients may pursue health care that addresses their cultural and personal beliefs. Although health care is becoming more directed by evidence-based science, health care providers must develop knowledge and skills in order to both recognize and understand the beliefs and needs of patients coming from different cultural backgrounds. It is, however, often difficult for practitioners fully to understand and work effectively with a patient's explanatory model of health. Cultural differences can also unhelpfully affect interaction between the patient and practitioner when cultural misunderstandings lead to non-cooperation and/or mistrust. Such cultural issues include authority, communication style, gender, family, and, most importantly for manual therapy, physical contact.[102] To study every possible cultural factor that may influence a clinical

presentation is not possible, and Carrillo and colleagues therefore sensibly suggest a more practical approach of learning about the various types of problems that occur in cross-cultural clinical presentations so the practitioner is able to recognize and then deal with these as they arise.[102] Once they have been recognized, the practitioner can inquire further about the patient's beliefs and preferences regarding illness and disease.

In order to develop a simple explanatory model enabling clinicians to deal with patients from different backgrounds, Carrillo and colleagues summarize some useful questions developed by Kleinman,

---

Table 4.2

Methods for eliciting important patient information (adapted from Kleinman et al. 1978)

Eliciting patient information and negotiating
Explanatory model
What do you think has caused your problem? What do you call it?
Why do you think it started when it did?
How does it affect your life?
What worries you the most?
What kind of treatment do you think would work?
The patient's agenda
How can I be of most help to you?
What is most important for you?
Illness behavior
Have you seen anyone else about this problem besides a clinician/manual therapist?
Have you used any non-medical remedies or treatments for your problem?
Who normally advises you about your health?

Eisenberg and Good that not only help the practitioner to gain important information, but further, help the patient overcome their hesitancy in revealing their beliefs and fears (Table 4.2).[103]

Cross-culture cooperation

These questions can also be modified for use in the field of CP in that they help to determine what patients hope to achieve with treatment. The approach is also useful to elicit various folk beliefs and alternative medical practices that may influence the consultation. Here, the health care provider facilitates discussion with the patient regarding different cognitive and value orientations. Kleinman and colleagues describe the patient in these cases as a 'therapeutic ally' in the process of determining how differences in opinion may affect care.[103] For example, if the patient accepts the use of manual therapy but believes that a meeting with a fortune teller is also needed, the health care provider should understand this belief and not attempt to change it. However, a patient may be against more essential treatments such as antibiotics for acute infection; in such cases, the clinician must attempt to neutralize the meaning of the term 'antibiotic' and persuade the patient of the medication's value. Negotiations may require further mediation between the patient, the practitioner, and the patient's family: this is an important step in engaging a patient's trust.[103] In these cases, the clinician serves as the expert on disease, while the patient expresses their unique illness, based on their cultural background. Descriptions about 'what is wrong' are heavily tied to culture, which means that differing perceptions on presenting complaints and their causes may require compromise. Thus, if the patient does not 'buy in' to a biomedical explanation of their presenting complaint, negotiation of the problem in terms that reflect the patient's explanatory model often leads to compromise from both parties.[102] For example, a patient may not understand why they should take daily antihypertensive medicine when they believe their high blood pressure is episodic and related only to stress. Here, a compromise is reached by explaining that although their blood pressure fluctuates, their arteries are stressed the whole time which they do not notice. Thus, while the medication helps to relieve arterial stress it does not affect their life stress. As such, further treatment options including relaxation techniques or counseling may also be considered.

The influence of spirituality on chronic pain

Spirituality is becoming relevant to effective health care as it moves towards a more person-centered approach. Definitions of spirituality vary, but it is suggested that it should not be confined to religion but considered more broadly.[104] Spirituality is currently described as a dynamic and intrinsic aspect of humanity through which people seek meaning and purpose, as well as relationships, to self, family, others, community, society, nature, and the significant or sacred.[10] Spirituality is expressed through beliefs, values, traditions, and practices.[105] However, a person who becomes involved in therapeutic procedures often finds themselves in the realm of the unfamiliar. Here, they have time to think about their lives, its meaning, and the experience of a disease process. Factors associated with these circumstances may present as anxiety, pain, loneliness, and deprivation, resulting in challenges to values and beliefs.[106] Research shows, however, that a person's spiritual beliefs can positively impact health, longevity, and recovery from illness.[107]

People dealing with CP have often lost their jobs, and can experience both changes in family life and economic hardship, as well as struggling to obtain social and disability support.[108] People presenting with CP disorders have different religious and spiritual experiences compared to those facing terminal illness. Instead of struggling to stay alive, as, for example, in cases such as cancer, people with CP often wonder whether life is still worth living. Studies show that people with CP may report feelings of abandonment by others (including God)[108] while also demonstrating high levels of spiritual distress.[109] Additionally, CP patients also find it difficult to forgive or feel punished, especially if they have no community support. However, patients describe spirituality as an important aspect of how they cope with pain. Here, positive spirituality is associated with better psychological adjustment to CP, where strong levels of faith, meaning and purpose in life predict improved pain and disability-related outcomes.[109]

The impact of socioeconomic factors on chronic pain

Socioeconomic status (SES) and health are inseparably linked, and population studies consistently show that CP is prevalence is inversely related to SES. For research purposes, socioeconomic status is usually divided into four areas: occupation, income, educational achievement, and neighborhood. Gender differences, as described earlier in this chapter, are also recognized to interrelate with socioeconomic status and race. SES is therefore considered a latent model that cannot be measured with just a single parameter. When considering all the relevant factors, there is much debate about whether interrelations between the factors represent the sum of individual circumstances or whether these interrelations reflect factors functioning at a population or community level.[110]

Health-related conditions also have socioeconomic consequences that include both direct and indirect costs.[111] Direct costs arise due to the management of a condition and include diagnostic tests, medication, outpatient visits, and hospitalization. Indirect costs occur mainly due to the disability of patients and include lost wages due to sick leave, reduced work productivity, and additional costs of caregiving. Generally, studies show that low SES individuals experience and report more CP.[111-113] Specifically, low SES is also associated with increased levels of muscular pain and stiffness,[114] lumbar disc disorders,[111] and widespread musculoskeletal pain.[115] Moreover, psychological factors associated with SES are also strongly associated with widespread pain conditions such as fibromyalgia.[116] Thus, it is more likely that SES as a set of factors is more associated with the burden of altered physical and psychological function, especially regarding depression, anxiety, obesity, and diabetes.[117, 118]

Occupational status

Many studies have examined associations between CP and occupational factors.[119-121] In general, the prevalence of CP is highest among blue-collar workers of all ages whereas white-collar workers report less pain than other groups.[122] Additionally, low SES individuals are more likely to consult with a new occurrence of back pain within a year of their first consultation,[122] while those with jobs involving lifting and carrying heavy loads, or those working in extreme positions not only report higher incidences of musculoskeletal pain, but also file more claims using employers statutory insurance funds or workers compensation.[123]

Although research shows less reported pain among white-collar workers, they more frequently report neck, arm, and head pain. For example, keyboards users regularly report pain in the neck, shoulders, and upper limbs and headaches.[124] However, stronger neck pain and worse headaches are also significantly associated with fatigue and/or stress due to

Table 4.3

Common work and psychosocial variables associated with chronic pain

Work-related variables	Psychological variables
Blue-collar workers	
Heavy lifting/carrying	• Low job satisfaction
Extreme body position	• Monotonous
Body vibration	• Low social support
White-collar workers	
Excessive keyboard use	• High repetitive work-related demands
Ulnar deviation	• High psychological work-related demands
Head rotation	
Prolonged sitting postures	

high work-related demands.[125] Similarly, psychosocial factors strongly predict the onset of CP among people with jobs involving heavy lifting and repetitive movements.[116] Not surprisingly, psychosocial variables such as low job satisfaction, low social support and monotonous work are also significantly associated with the onset of widespread body pain.[113, 126] Thus, it is important that when investigating occupation for the onset and maintenance of musculoskeletal pain, attempts must be made to establish possible psychosocial factors. Table 4.3 gives a summary of work-related variables associated with CP in both blue- and white-collar workers.

Educational status

Educational attainment is considered a stable measurement of SES as it remains relatively constant during adulthood.[127] Data relating to education is also easy to collect and is unlikely to be affected by chronic disease that begins in adult life, as occupation and income may be.[128] Education also represents a marker for other traits such as awareness of health behavior, intelligence, and the ability to acquire adaptive skills.[129] Moreover, educational achievement is significantly related to health status and in observational studies is shown to be robustly correlated to morbidity and mortality across a range of musculoskeletal disorders[130] and other medical conditions.[127]

Concerning musculoskeletal pain, lower educational attainment (LEA) is strongly associated with higher prevalences of low back pain with more severe disability.[127, 130] Additionally, people diagnosed with fibromyalgia who report fewer years of education also report more severe pain and occupational disability.[131] Although the exact mechanisms mediating these associations are poorly understood, studies show that CP patients with LEA are at particular risk for developing maladaptive pain beliefs and coping strategies.[127] It is therefore important to ensure that patients are able to obtain and assimilate information relating to understanding and coping with pain before they finish their consultation. Roth and Geisser suggest that practitioners should consider assessing pain-relevant cognitive variables. They also suggest that in order to improve data collection in experimental settings, educational attainment should also be included as a robust independent variable in CP studies.[127]

Community status

The importance of communities for health has been observed over many years. They provide medical

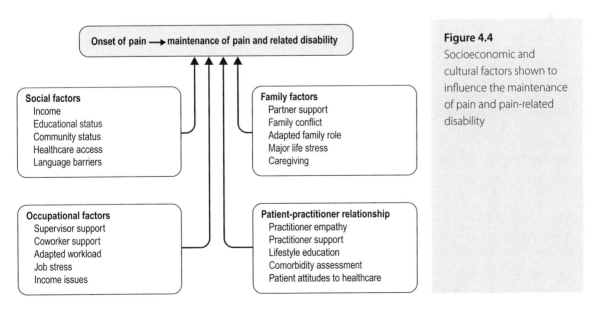

Figure 4.4

Socioeconomic and cultural factors shown to influence the maintenance of pain and pain-related disability

facilities, schools, housing and for many a place of work. These and other environmental factors such as air and water quality play an important role in our health and thus are important variables to consider epidemiologically. There have been only a few studies that have focused on these factors, even though consensus repeatedly suggests neighborhood status influences the health and quality of life of its residents.[132] For example, Winkleby and Cubbin examined the influence of neighborhood socioeconomic status on mortality among black, Mexican-American and white men and women in the USA. Not surprisingly, they found that mortality rates for gender, racial/ethnic groups were two to four times higher for those who lived in lowest SES neighborhoods.[132] Importantly, however, they also found that the effects of an individual's SES were significantly stronger than the effects of community SES.

Similar findings have been shown with people with musculoskeletal pain where those living in disadvantaged communities and who had been previously exposed to traumatic stress showed increased prevalence rates of pain, interference with life and daily function.[133] Interestingly, the same study showed the relationship between community disadvantage and musculoskeletal pain was also moderated by a common nucleotide polymorphism (where a phenotype of an individual is determined by environmental cues) for a gene (FKBP5) encoding a regulator of glucocorticoid receptor sensitivity and thus HPA axis function. These findings follow previous animal and human research showing polymorphisms of the gene FKBP5 to be associated with childhood trauma and stress-related psychiatric disorders.[134, 135]

Socioeconomic and cultural factors shown to influence the maintenance of pain and pain-related disability are summarized in Figure 4.4.

Musculoskeletal pain: epidemiological findings

Several studies show that people with lower socioeconomic backgrounds are more likely to report musculoskeletal pain and lower levels of health-related quality of life.[136, 137] For example, living in less affluent areas was found to be significantly associated with experiencing intense and widespread musculoskeletal pain with high levels of physical disability and mental illness, and also with low levels of life satisfaction.[136] Importantly, musculoskeletal disorders are not only significantly associated with SES, but additionally have strong independent associations with other chronic disease such as diabetes, cancer, and respiratory disorders.[138]

Possible explanations for these findings may relate to environmental factors such as sub-standard housing, the type of employment, and the influence of psychological stress on the musculoskeletal system. However, while psychological factors appear to be a major factor in the prevalence of musculoskeletal pain in lower SES, there are also biomechanical occupational factors that need to be considered. For example, persistent or recurrent low back pain conditions are also explained by biomechanical factors. It is suggested that reducing biomechanical occupational strains may help to reduce musculoskeletal pain among blue-collar workers and in so doing, reduce associated psychological factors.[139] Similarly, low back pain ranks as the primary cause of industrial pain in the USA. However, people reporting most severe disabling musculoskeletal pain are those working in areas such as sales, clerical roles, and precision production.[140]

Summary

Chronic pain is a very common clinical presentation, affecting individuals and their families, health services, and the wider society. Using the definition of CP as pain that has been suffered for the previous 3–6 months and several times in the previous week, a European study reports a prevalence of nearly 20% in the general population.[1] CP is more common in people living in socially deprived communities and in women. Pain management is shown to be unsatisfactory where therapeutic approaches are related mainly to providing immediate pain relief rather than to the more relevant concern of managing pain over a period of time. Thus, we need to first, recognize and second, understand the interaction of socioeconomic, gender, clinical, and genetic factors and their influences on people suffering persistent pain in order to identify and plan relevant therapeutic interventions. Blyth summarizes these issues nicely. She suggests that CP develops from interacting causal factors that may span different periods of time and act at different physical and psychological levels, and which may also be modified by individual protective factors.[110] Recognizing and assessing these factors is essential if we are to provide the best possible outcomes.

References

1. Breivik H, Collett B, Ventafridda V, Cohen R, Gallacher D. Survey of chronic pain in Europe: prevalence, impact on daily life, and treatment. European Journal of Pain. 2006;10(4):287–333.

2. Bureau of the Census. Statistical abstracts of the United States. Washington DC; 1996.

3. van Hecke O, Torrance N, Smith BH. Chronic pain epidemiology – where do lifestyle factors fit in? British Journal of Pain. 2013;7(4):209–17.

4. Blyth FM, March LM, Brnabic AJ, Jorm LR, Williamson M, Cousins MJ. Chronic pain in Australia: a prevalence study. Pain. 2001;89(2–3):127–34.

5. Catala E, Reig E, Artes M, Aliaga L, Lopez JS, Segu JL. Prevalence of pain in the Spanish population: telephone survey in 5000 homes. European Journal of Pain. 2002;6(2):133–40.

6. Johannes CB, Le TK, Zhou X, Johnston JA, Dworkin RH. The prevalence of chronic pain in United States adults: results of an Internet-based survey. Journal of Pain. 2010;11(11):1230–9.

7. Dureja GP, Jain PN, Shetty N, Mandal SP, Prabhoo R, Joshi M, et al. Prevalence of chronic pain, impact on daily life, and treatment practices in India. Pain Practice. 2014;14(2):E51–62.

8. Gureje O, Von Korff M, Simon GE, Gater R. Persistent pain and well-being: a world health organization study in primary care. JAMA. 1998;280(2):147–51.

9. Esquirol Y, Niezborala M, Visentin M, Leguevel A, Gonzalez I, Marquie JC. Contribution of occupational factors to the incidence and persistence of chronic low back pain among workers: results from the longitudinal VISAT study. Occupational and Environmental Medicine. 2017;74(4):243–51.

10. Roudsari RL, Allan HT, Smith PA. Looking at infertility through the lens of religion and spirituality: a review of the literature. Human Fertility. 2007;10(3):141–9.

11. Burke NN, Finn DP, McGuire BE, Roche M. Psychological stress in early life as a predisposing factor for the development of chronic pain: clinical and preclinical evidence and neurobiological mechanisms. Journal of Neuroscience Research. 2017;95(6):1257–70.

12. Macfarlane GJ. The epidemiology of chronic pain. Pain. 2016;157(10):2158–9.

13. Davis DA, Luecken LJ, Zautra AJ. Are reports of childhood abuse related to the experience of chronic pain in adulthood? A meta-analytic review of the literature. Clinical Journal of Pain. 2005;21(5):398–405.

14. Nickel R, Egle UT, Hardt J. Are childhood adversities relevant in patients with chronic low back pain? European Journal of Pain. 2002;6(3):221–8.

15. Imbierowicz K, Egle UT. Childhood adversities in patients with fibromyalgia and somatoform pain disorder. European Journal of Pain. 2003;7(2):113–9.

16. Lee S, Tsang A, Von Korff M, de Graaf R, Benjet C, Haro JM, et al. Association of headache with childhood adversity and mental disorder: cross-national study. British Journal of Psychiatry. 2009;194(2):111–6.

17. Scott KM, Von Korff M, Angermeyer MC, Benjet C, Bruffaerts R, de Girolamo G, et al. The association of childhood adversities and early onset mental disorders with adult onset chronic physical conditions. Archives of General Psychiatry. 2011;68(8):838–44.

18. Burke NN, Finn DP, McGuire BE, Roche M. Psychological stress in early life as a predisposing factor for the development of chronic pain: clinical and preclinical evidence and neurobiological mechanisms. Journal of Neuroscience Research. 2017;95(6):1257–70.

19. Tesarz J, Eich W, Treede RD, Gerhardt A. Altered pressure pain thresholds and increased wind-up in adult patients with chronic back pain with a history of childhood maltreatment: a quantitative sensory testing study. Pain. 2016;157(8):1799–809.

20. Sherman AL, Morris MC, Bruehl S, Westbrook TD, Walker LS. Heightened temporal summation of pain in patients with functional gastrointestinal disorders and history of trauma. Annals of Behavioral Medicine. 2015;49(6):785–92.

21. Whitehead WE, Crowell MD, Davidoff AL, Palsson OS, Schuster MM. Pain from rectal distension in women with irritable bowel syndrome: relationship to sexual abuse. Digestive Diseases and Sciences. 1997;42(4):796–804.

22. Fillingim RB, Edwards RR. Is self-reported childhood abuse history associated with pain perception among healthy young women and men? Clinical Journal of Pain. 2005;21(5):387–97.

23. Scott KM, Von Korff M, Angermeyer MC, Benjet C, Bruffaerts R, de Girolamo G, et al. Association of childhood adversities and early-onset mental disorders with adult-onset chronic physical conditions. Archives of General Psychiatry. 2011;68(8):838–44.

24. Stickley A, Koyanagi A, Kawakami N. Childhood adversities and adult-onset chronic pain: Results from the World Mental Health Survey, Japan. European Journal of Pain. 2015;19(10):1418–27.

25. Gonzalez A, Boyle MH, Kyu HH, Georgiades K, Duncan L, MacMillan HL. Childhood and family influences on depression, chronic physical conditions, and their comorbidity: findings from the Ontario Child Health Study. Journal of Psychiatric Research. 2012;46(11):1475–82.

26. Maniam J, Antoniadis C, Morris MJ. Early-Life Stress, HPA Axis Adaptation, and mechanisms contributing to later health outcomes. Frontiers in Endocrinology. 2014;5:73.

27. Herman JP, McKlveen JM, Solomon MB, Carvalho-Netto E, Myers B. Neural regulation of the stress response: glucocorticoid feedback mechanisms. Brazilian Journal of Medical and Biological Research. 2012;45(4):292–8.

28. McEwen BS. Physiology and neurobiology of stress and adaptation: central role of the brain. Physiological Reviews. 2007;87(3):873–904.

29. Dallman MF, Akana SF, Pecoraro NC, Warne JP, la Fleur SE, Foster MT. Glucocorticoids, the etiology of obesity and the metabolic syndrome. Current Alzheimer Research. 2007;4(2):199–204.

30. Juruena MF. Early-life stress and HPA axis trigger recurrent adulthood depression. Epilepsy and Behavior. 2014;38:148–59.

31. Goncharova ND. Stress responsiveness of the hypothalamic–pituitary–adrenal axis: age-related features of the vasopressinergic regulation. Frontiers in Endocrinology. 2013;4:26.

32. Danese A, Pariante CM, Caspi A, Taylor A, Poulton R. Childhood maltreatment predicts adult inflammation in a life-course study. Proceedings of the National Academy of Sciences of the United States of America. 2007;104(4):1319–24.

33. Dong M, Giles WH, Felitti VJ, Dube SR, Williams JE, Chapman DP, et al. Insights into causal pathways for ischemic heart disease: adverse childhood experiences study. Circulation. 2004;110(13):1761–6.

34. Pearson TA, Mensah GA, Alexander RW, Anderson JL, Cannon RO, 3rd, Criqui M, et al. Markers of inflammation and cardiovascular disease: application to clinical and public health practice: A statement for healthcare professionals from the Centers for Disease Control and Prevention and the American Heart Association. Circulation. 2003;107(3):499–511.

35. Raposa EB, Bower JE, Hammen CL, Najman JM, Brennan PA. A developmental pathway from early life stress to inflammation: the role of negative health behaviors. Psychological Science. 2014;25(6):1268–74.

36. Wang KC, Wang SJ, Fan LW, Cai Z, Rhodes PG, Tien LT. Interleukin-1 receptor antagonist ameliorates neonatal lipopolysaccharide-induced long-lasting hyperalgesia in the adult rats. Toxicology. 2011;279(1–3):123–9.

37. Burke NN, Fan CY, Trang T. Microglia in health and pain: impact of noxious early life events. Experimental Physiology. 2016;101(8):1003–21.

38. Hatfield LA. Neonatal pain: what's age got to do with it? Surgical Neurology International. 2014;5(Suppl 13):S479-S89.

39. Schwaller F, Fitzgerald M. The consequences of pain in early life: injury-induced plasticity in developing pain pathways. European Journal of Neuroscience. 2014;39(3):344–52.

40. Hathway GJ, Vega-Avelaira D, Fitzgerald M. A critical period in the supraspinal control of pain: opioid-dependent changes in brainstem rostroventral medulla function in preadolescence. Pain. 2012;153(4):775–83.

41. Zhang Y-H, Wang X-M, Ennis M. Effects of neonatal inflammation on descending modulation from the rostroventromedial medulla. Brain Research Bulletin. 2010;83(1–2):16–22.

42. LaPrairie JL, Murphy AZ. Neonatal injury alters adult pain sensitivity by increasing opioid tone in the periaqueductal gray. Frontiers in Behavioral Neuroscience. 2009;3:31.

43. Bartley EJ, Fillingim RB. Sex differences in pain: a brief review of clinical and experimental findings. BJA: British Journal of Anaesthesia. 2013;111(1):52–8.

44. Gerdle B, Bjork J, Coster L, Henriksson K, Henriksson C, Bengtsson A. Prevalence of widespread pain and associations with work status: a population study. BMC Musculoskeletal Disorders. 2008;9:102.

45. Kindler LL, Valencia C, Fillingim RB, George SZ. Sex differences in experimental and clinical pain sensitivity for patients with shoulder pain. European Journal of Pain. 2011;15(2):118–23.

46. Fillingim RB, Ness TJ. Sex-related hormonal influences on pain and analgesic responses. Neuroscience and Biobehavioral Reviews. 2000;24(4):485–501.

47. Quiton RL, Greenspan JD. Sex differences in endogenous pain modulation by distracting and painful conditioning stimulation. Pain. 2007;132(Suppl 1):S134-S49.

48. Keefe FJ, Brown GK, Wallston KA, Caldwell DS. Coping with rheumatoid arthritis pain: catastrophizing as a maladaptive strategy. Pain. 1989;37(1):51–6.

49. Edwards RR, Haythornthwaite JA, Sullivan MJ, Fillingim RB. Catastrophizing as a mediator of sex differences in pain: differential effects for daily pain versus laboratory-induced pain. Pain. 2004;111(3):335–41.

50. Jackson T, Iezzi T, Gunderson J, Nagasaka T, Fritch A. Gender differences in pain perception: the mediating role of self-efficacy beliefs. Sex Roles. 2004;47(11):561–8.

51. Racine M, Tousignant-Laflamme Y, Kloda LA, Dion D, Dupuis G, Choiniere M. A systematic literature review of 10 years of research on sex/gender and pain perception - part 2: do biopsychosocial factors alter pain sensitivity differently in women and men? Pain. 2012;153(3):619–35.

52. Forsythe LP, Thorn B, Day M, Shelby G. Race and sex differences in primary appraisals, catastrophizing, and experimental pain outcomes. Journal of Pain. 2011;12(5):563–72.

53. Robinson ME, Gagnon CM, Riley JL, 3rd, Price DD. Altering gender role expectations: effects on pain tolerance, pain threshold, and pain ratings. Journal of Pain. 2003;4(5):284–8.

54. Riley JL, 3rd, Robinson ME, Wise EA, Price DD. A meta-analytic review of pain perception across the menstrual cycle. Pain. 1999;81(3):225–35.

55. Paulson PE, Minoshima S, Morrow TJ, Casey KL. Gender differences in pain perception and patterns of cerebral activation during noxious heat stimulation in humans. Pain. 1998;76(1–2):223–9.

56. Henderson LA, Gandevia SC, Macefield VG. Gender differences in brain activity evoked by muscle and cutaneous pain: a retrospective study of single-trial fMRI data. NeuroImage. 2008;39(4):1867–76.

57. Derbyshire SWG, Nichols TE, Firestone L, Townsend DW, Jones AKP. Gender differences in patterns of cerebral activation during equal experience of painful laser stimulation. Journal of Pain. 2002;3(5):401–11.

58. Unruh AM. Gender variations in clinical pain experience. Pain. 1996;65(2–3):123–67.

59. Granot M, Weissman-Fogel I, Crispel Y, Pud D, Granovsky Y, Sprecher E, et al. Determinants of endogenous analgesia magnitude in a diffuse noxious inhibitory control (DNIC) paradigm: do conditioning stimulus painfulness, gender and personality variables matter? Pain. 2008;136(1–2):142–9.

60. Popescu A, LeResche L, Truelove EL, Drangsholt MT. Gender differences in pain modulation by diffuse noxious inhibitory controls: a systematic review. Pain. 2010;150(2):309–18.

61. Zubieta JK, Smith YR, Bueller JA, Xu Y, Kilbourn MR, Jewett DM, et al. Mu-opioid receptor-mediated antinociceptive responses differ in men and women. Journal of Neuroscience. 2002;22(12):5100–7.

62. Smith YR, Stohler CS, Nichols TE, Bueller JA, Koeppe RA, Zubieta JK. Pronociceptive and antinociceptive effects of estradiol through endogenous opioid neurotransmission in women. Journal of Neuroscience. 2006;26(21):5777–85.

63. Fillingim RB, King CD, Ribeiro-Dasilva MC, Rahim-Williams B, Riley JL. Sex, gender, and pain: a review of recent clinical and experimental findings. Journal of Pain. 2009;10(5):447–85.

64. Tsang A, Von Korff M, Lee S, Alonso J, Karam E, Angermeyer MC, et al. Common chronic pain conditions in developed and developing countries: gender and age differences and comorbidity with depression-anxiety disorders. Journal of Pain. 2008;9(10):883–91.

65. Bingefors K, Isacson D. Epidemiology, co-morbidity, and impact on health-related quality of life of self-reported headache and musculoskeletal pain – a gender perspective. European Journal of Pain. 2004;8(5):435–50.

66. Schneider S, Randoll D, Buchner M. Why do women have back pain more than men? A representative prevalence study in the federal republic of Germany. Clinical Journal of Pain. 2006;22(8):738–47.

67. Barrero LH, Hsu YH, Terwedow H, Perry MJ, Dennerlein JT, Brain JD, et al. Prevalence and physical determinants of low back pain in a rural Chinese population. Spine. 2006;31(23):2728–34.

68. Oksuz E. Prevalence, risk factors, and preference-based health states of low back pain in a Turkish population. Spine. 2006;31(25):E968–72.

69. Gureje O, Akinpelu AO, Uwakwe R, Udofia O, Wakil A. Comorbidity and impact of chronic spinal pain in Nigeria. Spine. 2007;32(17):E495–500.

70. Srikanth VK, Fryer JL, Zhai G, Winzenberg TM, Hosmer D, Jones G. A meta-analysis of sex differences prevalence, incidence and severity of osteoarthritis. Osteoarthritis and Cartilage. 2005;13(9):769–81.

71. Wolfe F, Ross K, Anderson J, Russell IJ, Hebert L. The prevalence and characteristics of fibromyalgia in the general population. Arthritis and Rheumatism. 1995;38(1):19–28.

72. Assumpcao A, Cavalcante AB, Capela CE, Sauer JF, Chalot SD, Pereira CA, et al. Prevalence of fibromyalgia in a low socioeconomic status population. BMC Musculoskeletal Disorders. 2009;10:64.

73. Yunus MB. Gender differences in fibromyalgia and other related syndromes. Journal of Gender Specific Medicine. 2002;5(2):42–7.

74. Unruh AM. Gender variations in clinical pain experience. Pain. 1996;65(2–3):123–67.

75. Manning AP, Thompson WG, Heaton KW, Morris AF. Towards positive diagnosis of the irritable bowel. British Medical Journal. 1978;2(6138):653–4.

76. Quigley EM. Overlapping irritable bowel syndrome and inflammatory bowel disease: less to this than meets the eye? Therapeutic Advances Gastroenterology. 2016;9(2):199–212.

77. Drossman DA, Camilleri M, Mayer EA, Whitehead WE. AGA technical review on irritable bowel syndrome. Gastroenterology. 2002;123(6):2108–31.

78. Talley NJ, Zinsmeister AR, Melton LJ, 3rd. Irritable bowel syndrome in a community: symptom subgroups, risk factors, and health care utilization. American Journal of Epidemiology. 1995;142(1):76–83.

79. Pieh C, Altmeppen J, Neumeier S, Loew T, Angerer M, Lahmann C. Gender differences in outcomes of a multimodal pain management program. Pain. 2012;153(1):197–202.

80. Keogh E, McCracken LM, Eccleston C. Do men and women differ in their response to interdisciplinary chronic pain management? Pain. 2005;114(1–2):37–46.

81. Hansen FR, Bendix T, Skov P, Jensen CV, Kristensen JH, Krohn L, et al. Intensive, dynamic back-muscle exercises, conventional physiotherapy, or placebo-control treatment of low-back pain. A randomized, observer-blind trial. Spine. 1993;18(1):98–108.

82. Mannion AF, Junge A, Taimela S, Muntener M, Lorenzo K, Dvorak J. Active therapy for chronic low back pain: part 3. Factors influencing self-rated disability and its change following therapy. Spine. 2001;26(8):920–9.

83. George SZ, Fritz JM, Childs JD, Brennan GP. Sex differences in predictors of outcome in selected physical therapy interventions for acute low back pain. Journal of Orthopaedic and Sports Physical Therapy. 2006;36(6):354–63.

84. Bates MS, Edwards WT, Anderson KO. Ethnocultural influences on variation in chronic pain perception. Pain. 1993;52(1):101–12.

85. Monsivais D, McNeill J. Multicultural influences on pain medication attitudes and beliefs in patients with nonmalignant chronic pain syndromes. Pain Management Nursing. 2007;8(2):64–71.

86. Turk DC, Okifuji A. Psychological factors in chronic pain: evolution and revolution. Journal of Consulting and Clinical Psychology. 2002;70(3):678–90.

87. Helme R, Gibson S. Pain in older people. In: Crombie I, editor. Epidemiology of pain. Seattle: IASP Press; 1999.

88. Moore A, Grime J, Campbell P, Richardson J. Troubling stoicism: sociocultural influences and applications to health and illness behaviour. Health (London). 2013;17(2):159–73.

89. Fortier MA, Anderson CT, Kain ZN. Ethnicity matters in the assessment and treatment of children's pain. Pediatrics. 2009;124(1):378–80.

90. Pillay T, Zyl HAv, Blackbeard D. Chronic pain perception and cultural experience. Procedia - Social and Behavioral Sciences. 2014;113:151–60.

91. Creamer P, Lethbridge-Cejku M, Hochberg MC. Determinants of pain severity in knee osteoarthritis: effect of demographic and psychosocial variables using 3 pain measures. Journal of Rheumatology. 1999;26(8):1785–92.

92. Selim AJ, Fincke G, Ren XS, Deyo RA, Lee A, Skinner K, et al. Racial differences in the use of lumbar spine radiographs: results from the Veterans Health Study. Spine. 2001;26(12):1364–9.

93. Callister LC. Cultural influences on pain perceptions and behaviors. Home Health Care Management and Practice. 2003;15(3):207–11.

94. Merry B, Campbell CM, Buenaver LF, McGuire L, Haythornthwaite JA, Doleys DM, et al. Ethnic group differences in the outcomes of multidisciplinary pain treatment. Journal of Musculoskeletal Pain. 2011;19(1):24–30.

95. Mullersdorf M, Zander V, Eriksson H. The magnitude of reciprocity in chronic pain management: experiences of dispersed ethnic populations of Muslim women. Scandinavian Journal of Caring Sciences. 2011;25(4):637–45.

96. Putsch RW. Dealing with patients from other cultures. In: Walker H, editor. The history, physical, and laboratory examinations. 3rd ed. Boston: Butterworths; 1990.

97. Hsieh AY, Tripp DA, Ji LJ. The influence of ethnic concordance and discordance on verbal reports and nonverbal behaviours of pain. Pain. 2011;152(9):2016–22.

98. Katz JN, Lyons N, Wolff LS, Silverman J, Emrani P, Holt HL, et al. Medical decision-making among Hispanics and non-Hispanic whites with chronic back and knee pain: a qualitative study. BMC Musculoskeletal Disorders. 2011;12:78.

99. Madan I, Reading I, Palmer KT, Coggon D. Cultural differences in musculoskeletal symptoms and disability. International Journal of Epidemiology. 2008;37(5):1181–9.

100. Coggon D, Ntani G, Palmer KT, Felli VE, Harari R, Barrero LH, et al. Disabling musculoskeletal pain in working populations: is it the job, the person, or the culture? Pain. 2013;154(6):856–63.

101. Rothschild SK. Cross-cultural issues in primary care medicine. Disease-a-Month. 1998;44(7):293–319.

102. Carrillo JE, Green AR, Betancourt JR. Cross-cultural primary care: a patient-based approach. Annals of Internal Medicine. 1999;130(10):829–34.

103. Kleinman A, Eisenberg L, Good B. Culture, illness, and care: clinical lessons from anthropologic and cross-cultural research. Annals of Internal Medicine. 1978;88(2):251–8.

104. Speck. P. Spiritual care in health care. Scottish Journal of Healthcare Chaplaincy. 2004;7(1):21–5.

105. Puchalski CM, Vitillo R, Hull SK, Reller N. Improving the spiritual dimension of whole person care: reaching national and international consensus. Journal of Palliative Medicine. 2014;17(6):642–56.

106. Austin P, Macleod R, Siddall P, McSherry W, Egan R. The ability of hospital staff to recognise and meet patients' spiritual needs: a pilot study (In press). Journal for the Study of Spirituality 2016;6:20–37; 10.1080/20440243.2016.1158453.

107. Moreira-Almeida A, Koenig HG. Religiousness and spirituality in fibromyalgia and chronic pain patients. Current Pain and Headache Reports. 2008;12(5):327–32.

108. Rippentrop EA, Altmaier EM, Chen JJ, Found EM, Keffala VJ. The relationship between religion/spirituality and physical health, mental health, and pain in a chronic pain population. Pain. 2005;116(3):311–21.

109. Siddall P, McIndoe L, Austin P, Wrigely P. The impact of pain on spiritual well-being in people with a spinal cord injury. Spinal Cord. 2017;55(1):105–11.

110. Blyth FM. The demography of chronic pain: an overview. In: Croft P, Blyth FM, Van der Windt D, editors. Chronic pain epidemiology: from aetiology to public health. Oxford: Oxford University Press; 2010.

111. Katz JN. Lumbar disc disorders and low-back pain: socioeconomic factors and consequences. Journal of Bone and Joint Surgery American volume. 2006;88(Suppl 2):21–4.

112. Aggarwal VR, Macfarlane TV, Macfarlane GJ. Why is pain more common

amongst people living in areas of low socio-economic status? A population-based cross-sectional study. British Dental Journal. 2003;194(7):383–7; discussion 380.

113. Davies KA, Silman AJ, Macfarlane GJ, Nicholl BI, Dickens C, Morriss R, et al. The association between neighbourhood socio-economic status and the onset of chronic widespread pain: results from the EPIFUND study. European Journal of Pain. 2009;13(6):635–40.

114. Brekke M, Hjortdahl P, Kvien TK. Severity of musculoskeletal pain: relations to socioeconomic inequality. Social Science and Medicine. 2002;54(2):221–8.

115. Brekke M, Hjortdahl P. Musculo-skeletal pain among 40- and 45-year olds in Oslo: differences between two socioeconomically contrasting areas, and their possible explanations. International Journal for Equity in Health. 2004;3:10.

116. McBeth J, Harkness EF, Silman AJ, Macfarlane GJ. The role of workplace low-level mechanical trauma, posture and environment in the onset of chronic widespread pain. Rheumatology (Oxford). 2003;42(12):1486–94.

117. Everson SA, Maty SC, Lynch JW, Kaplan GA. Epidemiologic evidence for the relation between socioeconomic status and depression, obesity, and diabetes. Journal of Psychosomatic Research. 2002;53(4):891–5.

118. Dany L, Roussel P, Laguette V, Lagouanelle-Simeoni MC, Apostolidis T. Time perspective, socioeconomic status, and psychological distress in chronic pain patients. Psychology, Health and Medicine. 2016;21(3):295–308.

119. Latza U, Kohlmann T, Deck R, Raspe H. Influence of occupational factors on the relation between socioeconomic status and self-reported back pain in a population-based sample of German adults with back pain. Spine. 2000;25(11):1390–7.

120. Latza U, Kohlmann T, Deck R, Raspe H. Can health care utilization explain the association between socioeconomic status and back pain? Spine. 2004;29(14):1561–6.

121. Feyer A, Herbison P, Williamson A, de Silva I, Mandryk J, Hendrie L, et al. The role of physical and psychological factors in occupational low back pain: a prospective cohort study. Occupational and Environmental Medicine. 2000;57(2):116–20.

122. Papageorgiou AC, Macfarlane GJ, Thomas E, Croft PR, Jayson MI, Silman AJ. Psychosocial factors in the workplace – do they predict new episodes of low back pain? Evidence from the South Manchester Back Pain Study. Spine. 1997;22(10):1137–42.

123. Baur X, Weber K, Zaghow M. Regulations on occupational diseases and the current situation in Germany. Scandinavian Journal of Work, Environment and Health. 1996;22(4):306–10.

124. Palmer KT, Cooper C, Walker-Bone K, Syddall H, Coggon D. Use of keyboards and symptoms in the neck and arm: evidence from a national survey. Occupational Medicine. 2001;51(6):392–5.

125. Leroux I, Brisson C, Montreuil S. Job strain and neck–shoulder symptoms: a prevalence study of women and men white-collar workers. Occupational Medicine. 2006;56(2):102–9.

126. Harkness EF, Macfarlane GJ, Nahit E, Silman AJ, McBeth J. Mechanical injury and psychosocial factors in the work place predict the onset of widespread body pain: a two-year prospective study among cohorts of newly employed workers. Arthritis and Rheumatism. 2004;50(5):1655–64.

127. Roth RS, Geisser ME. Educational achievement and chronic pain disability: mediating role of pain-related cognitions. Clinical Journal of Pain. 2002;18(5):286–96.

128. Heistaro S, Vartiainen E, Heliovaara M, Puska P. Trends of back pain in eastern Finland, 1972–1992, in relation to socioeconomic status and behavioral risk factors. American Journal of Epidemiology. 1998;148(7):671–82.

129. Dionne CE, Von Korff M, Koepsell TD, Deyo RA, Barlow WE, Checkoway H. Formal education and back pain: a review. Journal of Epidemiology and Community Health. 2001;55(7):455–68.

130. Cunningham LS, Kelsey JL. Epidemiology of musculoskeletal impairments and associated disability. American Journal of Public Health. 1984;74(6):574–9.

131. Turk DC, Okifuji A, Sinclair JD, Starz TW. Differential responses by psychosocial subgroups of fibromyalgia syndrome patients to an interdisciplinary treatment. Arthritis and Rheumatism. 1998;11(5):397–404.

132. Winkleby MA, Cubbin C. Influence of individual and neighbourhood socioeconomic status on mortality among black, Mexican-American, and white women and men in the United States. Journal of Epidemiology and Community Health. 2003;57(6):444–52.

133. Ulirsch JC, Weaver MA, Bortsov AV, Soward AC, Swor RA, Peak DA, et al. No man is an island: living in a disadvantaged neighborhood influences chronic pain development after motor vehicle collision, and this effect is moderated by common genetic variation influencing HPA axis function. Pain. 2014;155(10):2116–23.

134. Klengel T, Mehta D, Anacker C, Rex-Haffner M, Pruessner JC, Pariante CM, et al. Allele-specific FKBP5 DNA demethylation mediates gene-childhood trauma interactions. Nature Neuroscience. 2013;16(1):33–41.

135. Lee RS, Tamashiro KL, Yang X, Purcell RH, Harvey A, Willour VL, et al. Chronic corticosterone exposure increases expression and decreases deoxyribonucleic acid methylation of Fkbp5 in mice. Endocrinology. 2010;151(9):4332–43.

136. Brekke M, Hjortdahl P, Kvien TK. Severity of musculoskeletal pain: relations to socioeconomic inequality. Social Science and Medicine. 2002;54(2):221–8.

137. Thomas E, Silman AJ, Croft PR, Papageorgiou AC, Jayson MIV, Macfarlane GJ. Predicting who develops chronic low back pain in primary care: a prospective study. BMJ: British Medical Journal. 1999;318(7199):1662–7.

138. Putrik P, Ramiro S, Chorus AM, Keszei AP, Boonen A. Socioeconomic inequities in perceived health among patients with musculoskeletal disorders compared with other chronic disorders: results from a cross-sectional Dutch study. RMD Open. 2015;1(1):e000045.

139. Plouvier S, Leclerc A, Chastang J-F, Bonenfant S, Goldberg M. Socioeconomic position and low-back pain – the role of biomechanical strains and psychosocial work factors in the GAZEL cohort. Scandinavian Journal of Work, Environment and Health. 2009;35(6):429–36.

140. Katz WA. Musculoskeletal pain and its socioeconomic implications. Clincal Rheumatology. 2002;21(Suppl 1):S2–4.

Introduction

All too often, chronic pain (CP) is difficult to manage. It is now established that pain is a complex experience influenced by a multitude of psychological and social factors that are shaped by emotions, social and environmental circumstances, attitudes, beliefs, expectations, and, of course, biological factors. Pain is further influenced by previous experience. Learning from such experiences helps a person to cope with pain while also maintaining good health and is thus essential for survival.[1] However, pain that persists for long periods of time will influence both physical and psychological features, and understanding this is crucial to understanding a person in pain. Thus, as practitioners, our awareness of these features is essential for the management of people with CP.

Patients often appear to report irrational or inexplicable beliefs to describe their pain and its existence. However, if investigated, these beliefs often have backgrounds that are simple to explain, given the patient's history and experience, culturally, socially and, equally important, medically. This is especially true concerning musculoskeletal pain where patients given a diagnosis from imaging findings base their understanding of their pain and disability on these results. These beliefs form part of a psychosocial perspective that helps to predict the extent of pain-associated disability.[3] However, in many cases the extent, or lack, of damage does not correlate well with the experience or level of pain. Very often, in cases such as headache, neck and low back pain, people report pain symptoms where no identifiable lesion is found. Even in laboratory conditions where the intensity of pain stimuli are controlled, there is a large amount of variability in patient response.[3]

As manual therapy moves towards biopsychosocial (BPS) models of pain, the influence of psychological factors must be considered. Those involved in physical therapy need to conduct and understand biomedical evaluation within a BPS setting. Here, reported anxiety and fear or indeed behavioral indicators need to be evaluated.[4]

In other words, manual therapists must additionally manage the patient's pain behavior and distress as well as peripheral nociceptive factors and thus must consider adjunct/complementary psychological treatment approaches. This chapter discusses beliefs and emotions associated with CP and evidence-based interventions shown to be effective for the psychological features apparent in those suffering with CP.

The biopsychosocial model of pain

Early models of nociception followed the Cartesian view of a linear relationship between pain and tissue injury. These models relate to specific receptor mechanisms or pathways from peripheral tissue to the spinal cord and up to the brain, or a more 'patterned' response in which nociception is due to a pattern of responses in many afferent systems.[5] However, these sensory and affective models do not explain most of what is observed clinically and experimentally, or the frequent failure of treatment to resolve pain symptoms.

The BPS model of illness developed by George Engel describes the interaction between psychological, social, and pathophysiological variables. This model hypothesizes that functioning of the mind affecting the body has a reciprocal affect on the mind. Such a model has long since been recognized in explaining many CP conditions.[6] The BPS model was further developed by Turk and Flor, whose model presumes some form of physical pathology or changes in musculoskeletal tissues and nerves that initiate nociceptive input to the brain. Appraisal of this input involves personal significance that is attributed to the pain and thus influences consequent behaviors. These appraisals are further influenced by the beliefs each person has acquired over their lifetime.[7] Based on these beliefs, a person may ignore the pain and continue to work and remain both physically and socially active, or they may withdraw from all these activities and assume a sick role. Additionally, beliefs about pain are also formed by the responses of close family and/or friends that may promote either a healthy, active response or a sick role.[7]

Illness versus disease

The BPS model also considers disease and illness. Disease is defined as an objective identifiable biological phenomenon that affects specific body structures or systems caused by anatomical, pathological, or physiological changes.[5] Illness, on the other hand, refers to the subjective experience or belief that disease is present. Gatchel and colleagues suggest that illness also refers to how a sick person and their close family and friends live with and respond to symptoms of disability. Interestingly, they further suggest that the distinction between illness and disease is comparable to distinctions between nociception and pain. Nociception, as described in Chapter 1, involves stimulation of nerves that relay information about real or potential tissue damage to the brain. Alternatively, pain is the subjective 'processed' awareness that results from transduction, transmission, and modulation of sensory information,[5] which is formed by prior learning and sociocultural and psychological influences (Figure 5.1). Additionally, the term 'sickness' in chronic pain refers to social and cultural beliefs and reactions not only of patients but also of their friends and family (Figure 5.2).

Psychosocial risk factors

Previous physical and psychological trauma

As described in Chapter 4, previous trauma and adverse events, either in childhood or in adult life, have a strong association with the onset of CP.[8] Many studies show that a history of physical, sexual, and/or verbal abuse is significantly more likely to be present in adults with CP; for example, previous childhood adversity is reported to be over 50% in people with chronic pain, compared to 20% in control subjects.[9] Childhood abuse and stressful life events are

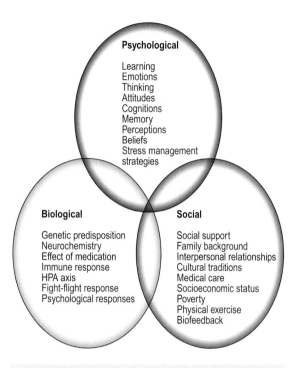

Figure 5.1

A biopsychosocial framework showing the interactions between biological, psychological and social factors, which in combination influence the onset, maintenance and management of people with chronic pain

especially associated with functional gastrointestinal disorders,[10] chronic pelvic pain in women,[11] and fibromyalgia.[12] Additionally, current literature relating to post-traumatic stress disorder (PTSD) suggests that CP and PTSD are mutual maintaining conditions. For example, affective and avoidance mechanisms of PTSD exacerbate and maintain CP, while cognitive, affective, and behavioral components of CP exacerbate and maintain PTSD.[13]

Social dysfunction

Social disconnection or exclusion has also been shown to be associated with the development and maintenance of physical pain. In fact, evidence from a wide range of psychological studies suggests that physical and social pain operate via common neurobiological mechanisms; both are necessary to help in the survival of social animals in directing them away from threats and towards supportive others.[14] Brain regions shown to be most associated with physical-social pain are the anterior cingulate and insular cortices. For example, people who are more sensitive to social disconnection or rejection are more likely to show activation in the anterior cingulate and insular cortices in addition to increases in sympathetic and inflammatory-related conditions.[15] Importantly, these processes have the potential to reinforce pain-related behaviors, especially in childhood, when the early social interactions of children with family and school are so important.[16]

Gender

A number of psychosocial mechanisms are reported to play a fundamental role in gender differences in pain. For example, sociocultural beliefs about femininity and masculinity appear to define pain responses between the sexes, with pain expression being more socially accepted in women than in men.[17] Coping strategies also appear to be different between sexes: men are most likely to use behavioral distraction to manage pain; women most often use social support, emotion-focused techniques, and attentional focus.[18] Thus, it is not surprising that research shows women more often engage in catastrophizing,[19] a form of attention that is associated with pain severity and pain-related disability. Socioculturally, owing to beliefs about masculine and stoic roles, men are also noted by both sexes as more unwilling to report pain.[20] Bartley and Fillingim suggest that these factors may contribute to sex differences in experimental pain.[17] Psychological comorbidities are also thought to play a part; for example, female gonadal hormones have been implicated in depression.[21]

Alterations in psychological processes

Psychological mechanisms involved in the perception of pain are highly interconnected and function together as a system. As described in Chapter 3, the limbic system modulates the amount of pain experienced for any given noxious stimulus. Imaging studies show pain-provoked limbic neural responses throughout the prefrontal, orbitofrontal, and cingulate cortices.[22,23]

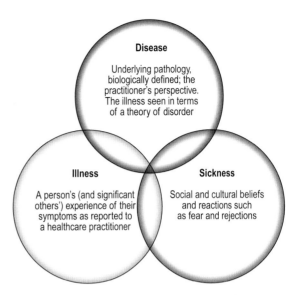

Figure 5.2
A conceptual model of associations between disease, illness, and sickness

It has also been shown that the affective mechanisms of pain can be completely blocked. Cancer patients undergoing frontal lobectomy still acknowledge severe pain, but display no emotion or attention, showing that pain without perception is merely a signal that something is wrong somewhere in the body.[24]

Cognition and attention to pain

Cognition is defined as a process of acquiring knowledge and understanding through thought, experiences, and the senses;[25] it includes awareness, perception, reasoning, decision-making and judgment.[16] Cumulative work shows these processes to be altered in people with CP in brain regions such as the anterior cingulate cortex and prefrontal cortex.[26] Synaptic plasticity in the dorsal horn and other cortical regions contribute to long-term potentiation in these brain regions due to increased and prolonged glutamate release potentiating increased responses in both AMPA and NMDA receptors.[26] It is therefore suggested that persistent pain is responsible for alterations in cortical function resulting in reduced cognitive abilities.[16] Focusing attention on pain makes pain feel worse. Conversely, people who are distracted from their pain report significantly lower ratings in pain. One function of pain is to demand attention, especially when it is viewed as a warning signal, when pain is considered a threat.[2] Additionally, attention to pain is often associated with fear and anxiety when taking action to either escape or avoid further insult. However, due to emotion and cognitive processes involved in pain perception, abnormal focus on pain, or 'hypervigilance,' explains why apparently small injuries may cause abnormally high levels of pain.[27]

Hypervigilance

Hypervigilance is an important feature of anxiety and is associated with protective and/or preventative behaviors that include avoidance of activity.[3] Avoiding activity after an injury is an adaptive response but, in CP states, is most often maladaptive. The belief that activity may cause further damage reduces anxiety in the short term, but is often counterproductive in the long term. Such hypervigilance often predisposes CP patients to pay close attention to trivial musculoskeletal symptoms that may otherwise be ignored, with avoidance of further activity contributing to further problems, chiefly due to deconditioning.[7] Many studies show that undue attention to pain is dependent on the level of pain-related fear and pain severity.[28] For example, using quantitative sensory testing in people with knee osteoarthritis, Herbert and colleagues showed that levels of pain vigilance were not only significantly associated with pain severity, but were also a predictor of temporal summation (Chapter 2).[29] Additionally, using a series of self-reporting measures, Crombez and co-workers showed that increased vigilance was best predicted by the interaction of pain severity and pain-related fear.[30] Pain hypervigilance is measured using the Pain Vigilance and Awareness Questionnaire (PVAQ) developed by McCracken and colleagues.[31] Items assess awareness, consciousness, vigilance, and observations of pain. Key points of hypervigilance are summarized in Box 5.1.

Catastrophizing

To catastrophize is to view or present a situation as considerably worse than it actually is.[25] Repeated and

---

> **Box 5.1**
>
> Key points: hypervigilance
>
> - Hypervigilance is associated with increased:
>   - attention to symptoms
>   - health care-seeking behavior
>   - anxiety
> - Assessed with the Pain Vigilance and Awareness Questionnaire (PVAQ)
> - Attention management using cognitive behavioral therapy (CBT) treatments aiming to increase patient skills in managing pain and reduce pain-related anxiety.[1]

habitual evaluation of pain-related situations as wholly catastrophic has shown to be a strong predictor of pain severity.[3] Here, initial catastrophizing about the relevance of pain is key to the onset and maintenance of not only pain but also associated fear avoidance behaviors, described below. Importantly, pain catastrophizing (PC) is characterized by the tendency to magnify the threat of pain and to feel helpless in pain situations, and by an inability to prevent pain-related thoughts either in anticipation of, during, or after a painful encounter.[32] Given that PC is associated with negative affective and behavioral responses to pain, it is not surprising that investigators have focused specifically on limbic brain regions associated with the processing of the unpleasantness of pain. Functional imaging techniques show increased pain catastrophizing thoughts correlate with increased activity within the prefrontal cortex and ACC.[33] These findings suggest alterations in supraspinal endogenous pain modulatory pathways in response to severe pain. Indeed, both conditioned pain modulation and temporal summation have subsequently been shown to be negatively correlated with levels of PC.[34] Additionally, PC has tentatively been shown to be associated with hypothalamic-pituitary-adrenal axis dysfunction.[35] However, the significance of this finding and the robustness of these data require further study.

PC is typically viewed as a trait-like disposition in which those with such feelings report more negative thoughts, more distress, and higher pain intensity compared to non-catastrophizers.[36] Sullivan and colleagues have developed a measurement tool, the Pain Catastrophizing Scale (PCS), which incorporates items that assess dimensions of helplessness, pessimism, rumination, and magnification-all shown to be key predictors of PC.[37] Thus, given that PC has associations with pain and suffering, it is not surprising that reductions in PC during multidisciplinary pain programs are related to decreases in pain severity and disability. Jenson and colleagues found that reductions in PC over cognitive-based multidisciplinary pain programs correlate with 6–12 month improvements in disability, pain intensity, and depression.[38] The same authors, in a later study, found that these improvements were most strongly associated with long-term changes in pain beliefs.[39] These data suggest that multidisciplinary pain programs in which CBT is a principal component can lead to reductions in aberrant pain beliefs, including PC, and to reductions in pain, disability, and depression. Interestingly, catastrophizing is shown to be specifically related to chronic low back pain. Quartana and colleagues found PC to be positively correlated with lower paraspinal muscle tension but not trapezius muscle responses.[40] These associations are given further support by the work of Wolff and co-workers, who showed not only high resting lumbar paraspinal muscle tension but also high blood pressure and heart rate in subjects with high PC scores.[41] These results suggest that both self-reporting and standard physiological measures can help identify pain catastrophizers and thus improve therapeutic intervention for those suffering chronic and, very often, disabling pain. Key points of pain catastrophizing are summarized in Box 5.2.

Self-efficacy

Self-efficacy is a widely investigated psychological factor affecting people with CP and is related to functional outcomes pain management (Figure 5.3). The term self-efficacy (SE) describes the confidence a person has in his or her own ability to achieve a desired outcome in a given situation,[42] with CP often being

---

Box 5.2

Key points: pain catastrophizing

- Described as a tendency to magnify the threat value of pain

- PC is associated with increased:
  - pain severity
  - health care-seeking behavior
  - disability
  - activity interference
  - muscle tone

- Pain catastrophizing represents a robust cognitive process variable in multidisciplinary treatment or in stand-alone manual therapy for chronic musculoskeletal pain disorders

- Assessed with the Pain Catastrophizing Scale (PCS)

---

associated with level of confidence in performing daily physical activities. Bandura further proposes that SE determines the level of effort and persistence people show when faced with obstacles or aversive situations.[43] Thus, low pain SE is defined by a feeling that pain is uncontrollable and, given the physical demands of daily life, unthinkable.[2] Studies show that lower levels of SE are associated with higher levels of pain and disability.[44–46] Encouragingly, however, SE ratings are shown to improve following cognitive behavioral management for low back pain and also associated with improvement in other outcomes such as pain-related disability.[47]

SE is also strongly associated with fear avoidance beliefs, especially concerning movement. Interestingly, in a study investigating whether SE or fear of movement mediate the relationship between pain intensity and disability in chronic LBP patients, Costa and co-workers found that only improvements in SE beliefs determined changes in pain and disability and not fear avoidance beliefs.[44] Thus, SE does play a major role in fear avoidance. Graded exposure to feared activities without negative consequences may reduce fear while also increasing perceived SE. However, in order to predict methods of improving SE beliefs, Warner and colleagues evaluated sources of SE for physical activity. In a large study of 1,406 subjects they found that mastery experience of performing a physical task successfully, self-persuasion, and reduction in negative affective states are the most important predictors for levels of SE.[48]

SE can be accurately measured using the Pain Self-Efficacy Questionnaire (PSEQ). The PSEQ is a reliable and valid self-reporting measure that correlates strongly with pain-related disability and beliefs described above. Importantly, the PSEQ relates to several behaviors including work status, medication use, and interference with daily activities.[49] Key points of self-efficacy are summarized in Box 5.3.

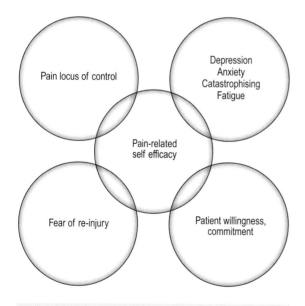

Figure 5.3

A representation of self-efficacy factors common in people with chronic pain

Box 5.3

Key points: pain self-efficacy

- Self-efficacy reflects a resilient self-belief system in the face of obstacles
- Low self-efficacy is associated with:
  - fear avoidance beliefs
  - pain behavior
  - high levels of disability
  - drop-out from pain management programs
  - interference with daily activity
  - strong predictor of functional outcomes
- Assessed with the Pain Self-Efficacy Questionnaire

Pain-related learning

Pain is a significant emotional stressor that can trigger learning behaviors that can be both implicit and explicit.[16] Implicit learning processes are mostly unconscious and thus are difficult to manage. The most commonly observed include operant conditioning (negative reinforcement of pain behaviors such as inactivity and medication intake), social learning and classical conditioning (reactive muscular tension).[50,51] For example, pain behaviors such as limping are sustained in an attempt to escape from anticipated noxious stimulation, while the 'sick-role' allows increased attention and thus the potential for help and sympathy. However, often the most disabling type of pain-related learning is fear. Experimentally, fear is learnt quickly as repetitions of noxious stimuli increase heart rate and anticipation.[52] However, in people with CP, fear learning leads to avoidance of many normal everyday activities and exaggerated pain perception.[53]

Fear avoidance

The influence of fear avoidance on pain-related psychological function is a recurring theme throughout this chapter. Avoidance refers to behavior aimed at preventing a potentially painful situation from occurring or recurring. Avoidance is a natural consequence in the presence of acute pain stimuli but serves to hinder recovery under CP conditions.[7] While it is not possible to avoid pain in CP conditions, it is possible to avoid perceived threats or activities presumed to reinjure or increase pain severity.[24] Thus, in 'fear avoidance' situations, when presented with a physical task such as gentle exercise or climbing stairs, there is a determined effort to escape and avoid recurrence or aggravation of injury, perceived or otherwise.[54] Not surprisingly, avoidance of physical activities and work tasks is strongly associated with loss of work and disability.[55]

Importantly, using the Fear Avoidance Beliefs Questionnaire (FABQ), Grotte and colleagues showed that patients with chronic low back pain have significantly more fear avoidance beliefs than patients with acute low back pain. FABQ scores further predicted levels of pain and disability at 12 month follow-up.[56] George and co-workers also found that fear avoidance beliefs are similar across different anatomical regions. Encouragingly, they also found that those with higher pain and lower function showed largest improvement in both pain and function following physical therapy.[57] Importantly, fear avoidance behavior has been observed in patients with osteoarthritis[58], neuropathic pain,[59] and fibromyalgia.[60] In a recent systematic review, Wertli and colleagues showed evidence that fear avoidance beliefs are prognostic for poor outcomes in people with subacute low back pain. Not surprisingly, they suggest early treatment and therapies to reduce such beliefs to avoid delayed recovery.[61] Figure 5.4 shows the cognitive processes through which fear avoidance develops.

Emotions and pain

Emotional distress is probably the most disruptive feature of pain perception and is a key consideration when assessing people with CP, with anxiety, fear, anger, and depression the most common emotions.[2] Importantly, how these emotions are controlled by those in pain has significant consequences on their impact on pain. It has been widely shown, in both

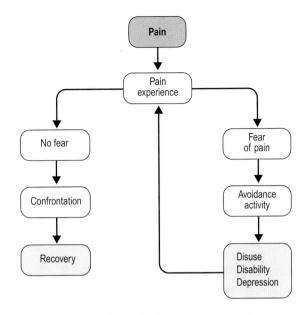

Figure 5.4

The fear avoidance model of chronic pain (W. Vlaeyen and S. J. Linton, 2000, *Pain*, 85, p. 329); with permission from IASP

people with pain conditions and healthy volunteers, that positive emotions are associated with reduced pain and negative mood is associated with amplification of pain.[62–64] Such negative effects are the key reason why pain is associated with suffering. Indeed, visually induced analgesia is associated with the affective content of pleasurable, neutral or unpleasant images. Pain responses are shown to depend on primal and appraisal processes.[65] However, all too often, practitioners elect to focus more on sensory-discriminatory features of pain (intensity and character) rather than the emotional effects. Indeed, as with the increase in pain intensity, negative mood is also associated with poor treatment outcomes.[66,67]

Pain and anxiety

People with persistent pain typically have higher levels of anxiety and this is a common reason for health care-seeking behavior.[2] In a study aiming to explore descriptions of worry in CP patients, Eccleston and colleagues found that worry about pain is an emotion that is more difficult to dismiss, more distracting, more attention grabbing, more intrusive, and more distressing than non-pain-related worry.[68] These findings support previous work in which Borkovec found significant correlations between levels of somatic awareness as measured with the Modified Somatic Perceptions Questionnaire (MSPQ) and current state of general anxiety using the State-Trait Anxiety Inventory (STAI-state).[69] This pattern of results suggest that worrying in CP patients does not arise from a general disposition to anxiety, but anxiety is a natural process initiated by increases in pain severity and suffering.[68] However, anxiety about the threat of pain also increases vigilance that further serves to increase fear and distress. Moreover, continued pain-related fear and catastrophic thoughts during the CP experience, as described earlier in this chapter, serve to initiate and maintain pain-related disability.

Pain-related anxiety is also shown to significantly impact on how patients respond to physical therapy.[70,71] Anxious patients are more likely to report worry about health, injury and greater experience of pain. Moreover, pain-anxious people may show attention to sensations and catastrophic misinterpretation to pain sensations during therapy. Thus, physical therapists need to evaluate anxiety levels in patients both before and during physical therapy. Several studies have developed methods to quantify anxiety in people with CP. In particular, McCracken and co-workers developed a questionnaire measuring fear of pain across cognitive, behavioral, and physiological areas. Here, they showed that the Pain Anxiety Symptoms Scale (PASS) as a reliable and valid tool in predicting anxiety-related disability and interference due to pain that contribute to health behaviors.[72] Furthermore, in a later study, the same authors found that PASS scores significantly predict pain severity and complaint pain behaviors.[73] Box 5.4 summarizes key points in pain-related anxiety.

Pain and depression

Depression is also a common and powerful emotional state that affects how we experience pain.[2] Depression

Box 5.4

Key points: pain-related anxiety

- Pain-related anxiety and worry play a significant role in the experience of chronic pain
- Anxiety is associated with the following symptoms:
  - restlessness
  - easily fatigued
  - poor concentration
  - muscle tension
  - sleep disturbance
- High levels of anxiety are associated with the following behaviors:
  - pain severity
  - fear avoidance
  - increased vigilance
  - catastrophic thoughts
- High levels of anxiety respond poorly to physical therapy
- Most reliably assessed using the Pain Anxiety Symptoms Scale (PASS)

is characterized by negative mood, hopelessness, and despair, and about 50% of people with chronic pain meet the criteria for mild to moderate levels of depression.[74] It has been widely shown that pain and depression coexist where both conditions respond to similar treatments, exacerbate one another, and share similar physiological pathways and neurotransmitters.[74,75] More than any other comorbidity, patients present with a complex set of overlapping psychological and physical symptoms that are typically unexplained.[76] Additionally, people with depression complain of significantly more physical symptoms such as pain and fatigue and seek health care resources more than non-depressed patients. In a review, Blair and colleagues found that on average, 65% of patients with depression also present with pain.[74] Importantly, they also found that depression is infrequently diagnosed where clinicians focus exclusively on physical symptoms.

Depression complicates the management of patients with pain and is strongly associated with poor outcomes. As such, an important role of manual therapists is to exclude conditions that may contraindicate or reduced the effectiveness of physical treatment. As for other areas of psychological function described above, initial screening tools for depression should be used. For example, depression is common in low back pain and is associated with increased pain severity, physical disability, increased medication use, and likelihood of unemployment.[77] Thus, if left unmanaged, it is expensive in terms of medical costs as well as losses of productivity in the workplace.[78] However, while the comorbidity of depression with CP conditions is well recognized, many health care providers do not routinely screen for psychological function, including depression. Manual therapists therefore need to be able to identify those patients with depression in primary or secondary care settings or where patients are referred post-surgically. These observations are highlighted by Haggman and colleagues, who showed that manual therapists are relatively poor at screening for symptoms of depression in patients with low back pain.[79]

There are several depression self-reporting measures available. Those seen as most reliable in manual therapy practice are the Depression Anxiety Stress Scale (DASS)[80] and the Beck Depression Inventory (BDI).[81] However, in contrast to the BDI, DASS is able to discriminate between depression and other affective states, those of anxiety and the related state of tension/stress.[82] The ability of DASS to separately measure these three related states is shown to be of significant use for manual therapists in dealing with complicated links between environmental demands and emotional and physical disorder.[82] Box 5.5 summarizes key points in pain-related depression.

Box 5.5

Key points: pain-related depression

- The negative mood of depression significantly affects how we experience pain
- Characterized by:
  - hopelessness
  - despair
  - constant fatigue
  - worthlessness
  - significant impairment in social, occupational, and family functioning
- Depression complicates the treatment of patients with chronic pain
- Depression is infrequently screened by manual therapists
- Most reliably assessed using the BDI and DASS (includes discriminating against other psychological variables)

Pain and stress

Stress is often seen in people suffering with CP. Stress is a normal human emotion that may be both productive in situations where stress is necessary for performance, or unproductive, as in situations where too much stress worsens performance.[83] However, 'stress' is an ambiguous word that can be used to define either environmental disruption ('stressor') or the range of physiological responses ('stress'). Nevertheless, people react to 'stressors' by showing emotions such as anger, anxiety, depression, or features of all three. Clinically, increased stress, or more appropriately, psychological distress, is defined as an alteration of emotion and mood in which psychological and physical symptoms occur.[84]

Concerning low back pain, Main and Waddell describe three categories of stress history that significantly contribute to presenting physical symptoms. First, and most commonly, patients become distressed about seeing health professionals if, as happens in many cases, no observable pathology can be found as a cause of pain. Opinions may then differ between practitioners, or patients are told that their pain is imaginary. Second, if patients have been involved in serious injury or ongoing conflict, they should be evaluated for post-traumatic stress symptoms such as repeated experiencing of a traumatic event(s), avoiding activities associated with particular traumas, and experiencing psychological distress and physiological arousal. Third, a small but important group have a history of physical, psychological, and/or sexual abuse, either in childhood or as an ongoing problem.[84] Importantly, Lampe and colleagues show that patients with idiopathic chronic low back pain present with significantly more episodes of previous stressful events compared to patients with low back pain with an organic etiology. The authors also found people with idiopathic low back pain show more difficulties in coping with pain and exhaustion, leading to feelings of helplessness.[11] Patients in distress also show increased bodily awareness and sensations indicative of heightened sympathetic activity, such as increased sweating in specific body areas, shallow breathing, increased heart rate, and the sensation of 'butterflies'.

Emotions due to stress, such as anxiety and depression, are evaluated using self-reporting measures, as described in previous sections. However, the construct of stress can also be measured using both physiological measurements as well as self-reporting questionnaires. Briefly, physiological measurements include cortisol screening of people suffering CP. Cortisol is an end product of hypothalamic-pituitary-adrenal (HPA) axis stimulation due to an acute pain episode. Often, when acute pain turns chronic, stimulation of the HPA axis continues, resulting in elevated serum cortisol levels.[85] Stress can also be measured subjectively using various self-reporting measures such as the DASS, as previously mentioned the Stressful Life Event Screening Questionnaire[86] and the Davidson trauma scale.[87] Box 5.6 summarizes key points in pain-related stress.

Box 5.6

Key points: pain-related stress

- Life stress is a significant contributor to the onset and maintenance of chronic pain disorders

- Significant features of stress are:
  - chronic fatigue
  - poor concentration
  - irritability and impatience
  - generalized body aches
  - increased sweating
  - trembling
  - difficulty sleeping

- Generally assessed with the DASS, which is able to discriminate between specific emotional symptoms and more general emotional states

Pain and perceived disability

Disability is a term that refers to difficulties in performing daily life tasks and activities at home and at work. People with CP hold various beliefs about pain based mostly on prior learning and social influences, including health care delivery. Studies show that in many cases beliefs about pain are associated with physical dysfunction, in which pain signifies harm, with people believing they have little personal control over pain, and where pain is considered an enduring part of future life.[88] Disability appears to be a consequence of prolonged avoidance of physical activity that in time impacts daily life functioning. For example, people are required to perform work-related physical activities such as prolonged standing, lifting, carrying, pushing, and pulling. Several studies show that fear of pain is a better predictor of disability than pain itself.[89] Concerning chronic low back pain, Pensri and colleagues found that people who show high levels of fear avoidance and past history of low back pain also show high levels of perceived disability.[90]

As pain becomes more chronic, increasing fear about pain leads people to persistently avoid activities, which in turn leads to further disability. Furthermore, pain catastrophizing has been shown to influence disability both occupationally and socially.[32] However, whether pain-related fear and disability is mediated by avoidance or hypervigilance has not yet been determined. Patients often have beliefs about the cause of their pain, the anticipated effects of treatment, and likely outcomes[91]. The belief that pain will never improve or is constant over time is associated with poor compliance from the patient in both physical and psychological treatments. These beliefs further lead patients to think that pain is controlled by powerful others, such as family doctors, therapists, and/or family members. However, BPS approaches have been shown to reduce levels of disability and distress. As part of multidisciplinary pain programs, cognitive behavioral therapy and education help the patients both to reconceptualize and to better understand their problem.[88]

Several questionnaires have been developed to evaluate disability. The Roland Morris Disability Questionnaire (RMDQ) and the Oswestry Disability Index (ODI) are widely used measures of disability in people with low back pain;[92,93] and the Physical Functioning Scale of the Short Form-36 (SF-36) also provides a valid measure of general functional disability.[94,95] These questionnaires address the effect of pain on typical daily activities including personal care, walking, climbing stairs, sleeping, sex, and social life. Importantly, such questionnaires show the ability to predict treatment outcomes when taken at baseline in patients with a variety of occupational musculoskeletal complaints. Box 5.7 summarizes the key points in pain-related disability. Figure 5.5 is a schematic diagram showing how dysfunctional beliefs about pain affect mood, behavior, and vigilance in people suffering chronic pain

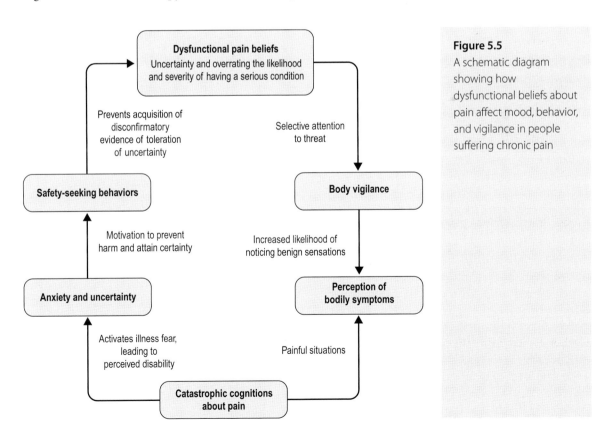

Figure 5.5

A schematic diagram showing how dysfunctional beliefs about pain affect mood, behavior, and vigilance in people suffering chronic pain

Box 5.7

Key points: pain-related disability

- Disability affects approximately 40% of people with chronic pain

- Pain disability beliefs characterized by:

  - prolonged avoidance of physical activity

  - increased use of passive coping strategies

  - psychological distress as a poor predictor for pain relief with active therapy

- Changes in fear avoidance and psychological distress account for changes in disability following therapy

- Most reliably assessed using the Roland Morris Disability Questionnaire (RMDQ), the Oswestry Disability Index (ODI), and the Short Form-36 (SF-36)

Psychological intervention in the management of chronic pain

Psychological approaches to the management of CP became popular in the 1960s, after the development of Melzack and Wall's gate-control theory of pain[96] and the ensuing 'neuromatrix' pain theory.[97] These theories were the first to suggest that the interaction of physiological and psychosocial processes affects the transmission, perception, and appraisal of pain. Thus, the BPS model of pain is now probably the most widely accepted approach to understanding pain. In this approach, CP is viewed as an illness and thus recognized as a subjective experience, with treatment aimed at managing rather than curing CP. Recent studies show that as a part of multidisciplinary pain programs, psychologically based interventions show promising results.[98,99] Current psychological treatments for the management of CP are chiefly aimed at achieving behavioral and cognitive changes as well as increases in self-management.

As described previously in this chapter, pain-related fear has significant implications for both increased pain intensity and disability. Pain-related fear thus contributes to passive pain coping behaviors that in turn contribute to physical deconditioning. Recently, the notion of psychological flexibility as an ability to engage in the present moment that allows patients to adjust their behavior has been shown to improve CP treatment outcomes.[100] Here, pain acceptance helps to acknowledge pain, curb maladaptive attempts to control pain and helps people to learn to live a richer life by engaging in valued activities despite the presence of pain.[101]

Behavioral approaches

Operant behavior therapy

Operant behavior therapy for CP is aimed at recognizing and avoiding maladaptive behaviors used to avoid painful situations.[102] Behavioral drive to avoid pain leads to people evading situations that may be painful, but that may, paradoxically, sustain physical and psychological health. Such avoidance thus contributes not only to the maintenance of pain, but also to physical deconditioning and depression.[100] For example, many CP sufferers learn through repeated associations that taking medication helps to remove or reduce the sensation of pain. Generally, behavioral treatments are aimed at graded activation, with patients being instructed to break the cycle of inactivity and deconditioning and engage in activities in a stepwise manner that allows gradual increases in the length of time and intensity of activity. Progress is overseen by the clinician and appropriate reinforcement of compliance with activities or correction of misunderstandings about pain are applied. Operant behavioral therapy has been shown to be effective in low back pain[103] and fibromyalgia[104] populations.

Cognitive behavioral therapy

Cognitive behavioral therapy (CBT) is a BPS treatment approach to CP that not only targets maladaptive behaviors but also cognitive responses and evaluation (understanding) of pain. Intervention includes education about pain and the patient's pain condition, coping skills training, problem solving, and behavioral skills such as relaxation and activity-based instruction.[105] Unlike operant behavioral approaches, CBT further addresses maladaptive beliefs about pain, especially catastrophizing thoughts, through the use of identifying, reorganizing, and replacement of unhelpful and unrealistic thoughts about pain and its effects. CBT is now widely considered as a 'gold-standard' psychological treatment for CP. CBT-related changes in catastrophizing and helplessness are predictive of future changes in pain severity and interference in daily function.[106] Concerning the effects of CBT on fear avoidance, counter conditioning by means of graded exposure to feared stimuli (e.g., movement of a specific limb) has recently been shown to be an effective CBT treatment for reducing disabling fear and has been applied in different CP settings.[59,107] These studies strongly suggest that graded exposure helps to modify the meaning that people attach to their pain and painful experiences. De Jong and colleagues suggest that such therapies activate cortical neuronal networks that resolve motor output and sensory feedback. CBT has been shown to be effective in the treatment of low back pain[108] and whiplash-associated disorders,[109] but is not as effective with patients with fibromyalgia.[100] A recent Cochrane review showed that CBT provides a small incremental benefit in reducing pain and pain-related disability and improving mood at the end of treatment.[110]

Mindfulness

Mindfulness is a form of meditation developed in Eastern philosophy and adapted to Western therapies. Mindfulness promotes awareness and acceptance of physical, cognitive, and emotional states and aims to separate psychological reactions from uncontrollable experiences associated with persistent pain. Recently, mindfulness-based interventions have been developed and introduced to encourage detached awareness of both somatic and psychological sensations within the body.[111] Through mindful awareness and meditation, thoughts about pain may be observed as a distinct event as opposed to a sign of underlying tissue damage that warrants a maladaptive response. Thus, a person can then recognize sensations as something familiar, which in turn can serve to relieve emotional and behavioral responses to episodes of pain. Recently, mindfulness therapies have shown efficacy in reducing both pain severity and psychological symptoms in conditions ranging from irritable bowel syndrome,[112] migraine,[113] fibromyalgia,[114] and chronic low back pain.[115] However, McCracken and Vowles point out that mindfulness studies have mostly focused on mental health outcomes such as symptoms of anxiety, and have rarely addressed pain severity, physical activity, and social role performance.[116] Thus, investigations into how mindfulness practice can affect behavioral patterns that are easily translated to reduced pain severity and improved physical and social function are currently required.

Acceptance and commitment therapy

Acceptance and commitment therapy (ACT) includes a combination of acceptance and mindfulness methods in association with behavioral change approaches. ACT promotes the importance of assisting a patient's progress toward achieving more valued and enjoyable life by increasing psychological flexibility as opposed to only focusing on reorganizing understandings of CP. Here, ACT targets unproductive coping and avoidance strategies by developing and practicing techniques that establish psychological flexibility.[100] Such techniques encourage CP patients to actively embrace pain and its effects rather than promoting a futile attempt at eradicating their pain. ACT uses six core principles:[117]

- acceptance
- defusing maladaptive cognitions
- being present
- self as context
- values
- committed action.

ACT-based interventions for the severity of pain and coping with stress and pain have shown promise, especially in achieving improvements in pain catastrophizing, pain-related disability, fear avoidance, and life satisfaction.[118] For example, in a recent pilot study using CP patients in a primary care setting, McCracken and colleagues found that ACT helped to lower levels of depression and pain-related disability and helped to significantly increase pain acceptance immediately after treatment and at three month follow-up.[119] Additionally, in a study of people with chronic whiplash-associated disorders, Wicksell and colleagues found that ACT approaches show improvements in the above problems immediately after treatment and at seven month follow-up.[120]

Factors affecting outcomes of psychological interventions

The most challenging aspect in managing CP is the high prevalence of comorbid emotional distress described throughout this chapter. Evidence shows upward of three times more prevalence of anxiety and depression in CP patients than among the general population.[74] Baseline levels of pain, depression, and anxiety are shown to predict both rates of progression and drop-out rates in some samples.[110] Furthermore, patients also describe different levels of interpersonal stress, such as a lack of support from co-workers and/ or loved ones. Indeed pain-related disability is significantly higher in those who lack social support.

Additionally, to prevent avoidable flare-ups, 'pacing' of treatment and self-management are also recommended. Interestingly, Turk suggests that the lack of satisfactory treatment outcomes is accounted for by the myth that all patients with the same medical conditions are similar in all clinically important variables.[121] He proposes identification of patient subgroups using (1) self-reporting measures and (2) detailed assessments of pain conditions, socioeconomic status, cultural and ethnic background. Additionally, patients' readiness to adopt self-management approaches towards their pain has also been shown to have a significant bearing on treatment response. Here, Kerns and co-workers show four factors: (1) precontemplation, (2) contemplation, (3) action, and (4) maintenance, to be internally stable.[122] They suggest that patients who are 'precontemplative' may benefit more from insight-focused therapy as opposed to patients in an 'action' stage, who would get greater benefit from relaxation and active coping-based strategies. The presence of other medical comorbidities should also be considered. For example, comorbid symptoms of obesity and fatigue are also common in people with CP.

Summary

Manual therapists commonly treat CP patients with significant comorbid psychological features and

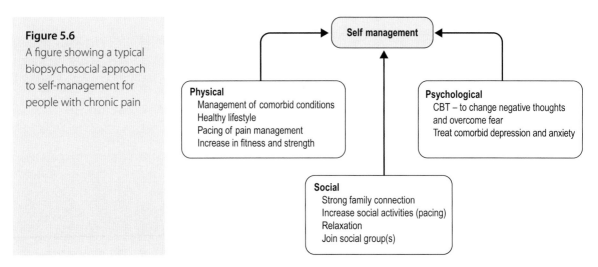

Figure 5.6
A figure showing a typical biopsychosocial approach to self-management for people with chronic pain

Self management

Physical
Management of comorbid conditions
Healthy lifestyle
Pacing of pain management
Increase in fitness and strength

Psychological
CBT – to change negative thoughts and overcome fear
Treat comorbid depression and anxiety

Social
Strong family connection
Increase social activities (pacing)
Relaxation
Join social group(s)

thus must have an understanding of BPS models of pain. Previously, manual therapy placed considerable reliance on the patient's report of pain, concerning both diagnosis and subsequent management. Reported pain is assumed to show strong associations with peripheral nociceptive input. However, CP is influenced by a number of 'non-peripheral' factors that are driven from limbic system brain regions. Additionally, manual therapists make their clinical diagnoses through replication of the patient's pain using active and/or passive mechanical stress tests. As described in this chapter, pain provocation can be affected by fear and apprehension of re-injury or an increase in pain intensity. Thus a patient's global rating of pain is broadly influenced by extra-nociceptive factors. Cumulative evidence now suggests that in addition to biomedical assessments, manual therapists must incorporate specific assessments of subjectively reported anxiety, stress, and fear in addition to behavioral signs such as protected movement. Therefore, a combination of physical and psychological treatment is recommended for patients presenting with significant levels of pain-related disability and/or psychological distress.

References

1. Elomaa MM, de CWAC, Kalso EA. Attention management as a treatment for chronic pain. European Journal of Pain. 2009;13(10):1062–7.

2. Linton SJ, Shaw WS. Impact of psychological factors in the experience of pain. Physical Therapy. 2011;91(5):700–11.

3. Eccleston C. Role of psychology in pain management. British Journal of Anaesthesia. 2001;87(1):144–52.

4. Main CJ, Watson PJ. Psychological aspects of pain. Manual Therapy. 1999;4(4):203–15.

5. Gatchel RJ, Peng YB, Peters ML, Fuchs PN, Turk DC. The biopsychosocial approach to chronic pain: scientific advances and future directions. Psychological Bulletin. 2007;133(4):581–624.

6. Engel GL. The need for a new medical model: a challenge for biomedicine. Science. 1977;196(4286):129–36.

7. Turk DC, Okifuji A. Psychological factors in chronic pain: evolution and revolution. Journal of Consulting and Clinical Psychology. 2002;70(3):678–90.

8. Goldberg RT, Pachas WN, Keith D. Relationship between traumatic events in childhood and chronic pain. Disability and Rehabilitation. 1999;21(1):23–30.

9. Goldberg RT, Goldstein R. A comparison of chronic pain patients and controls on traumatic events in childhood. Disability and Rehabilitation. 2000;22(17):756–63.

10. Leserman J, Drossman DA, Li Z, Toomey TC, Nachman G, Glogau L. Sexual and physical abuse history in gastroenterology practice: how types of abuse impact health status. Psychosomatic Medicine. 1996;58(1):4–15.

11. Lampe A, Sollner W, Krismer M, Rumpold G, Kantner-Rumplmair W, Ogon M, et al. The impact of stressful life events on exacerbation of chronic low-back pain. Journal of Psychosomatic Research. 1998;44(5):555–63.

12. Walker EA, Keegan D, Gardner G, Sullivan M, Bernstein D, Katon WJ. Psychosocial factors in fibromyalgia compared with rheumatoid arthritis: II. Sexual, physical, and emotional abuse and neglect. Psychosomatic Medicine. 1997;59(6):572–7.

13. Sharp TJ, Harvey AG. Chronic pain and posttraumatic stress disorder: mutual maintenance? Clinical Psychology Review. 2001;21(6):857–77.

14. MacDonald G, Leary MR. Why does social exclusion hurt? The relationship between social and physical pain. Psychological Bulletin. 2005;131(2):202–23.

15. Slavich GM, O'Donovan A, Epel ES, Kemeny ME. Black sheep get the blues: a psychobiological model of social rejection and depression. Neuroscience and Biobehavioral Reviews. 2010;35(1):39–45.

16. Simons L, Elman I, Borsook D. Psychological processing in chronic pain: a neural systems approach. Neuroscience and Biobehavioral Reviews. 2014;39:61–78.

17. Bartley EJ, Fillingim RB. Sex differences in pain: a brief review of clinical and experimental findings. BJA: British Journal of Anaesthesia. 2013;111(1):52–8.

18. Unruh AM, Ritchie J, Merskey H. Does gender affect appraisal of pain and pain coping strategies? Clinical Journal of Pain. 1999;15(1):31–40.

19. Forsythe LP, Thorn B, Day M, Shelby G. Race and sex differences in primary appraisals, catastrophizing, and experimental pain outcomes. Journal of Pain. 2011;12(5):563–72.

20. Robinson ME, Riley JL, 3rd, Myers CD, Papas RK, Wise EA, Waxenberg LB, et al. Gender role expectations of pain: relationship to sex differences in pain. Journal of Pain. 2001;2(5):251–7.

21. Fernandez-Guasti A, Fiedler JL, Herrera L, Handa RJ. Sex, stress, and mood disorders: at the intersection of adrenal and gonadal hormones. Hormone and Metabolic Research = Hormon- und Stoffwechselforschung = Hormones et metabolisme. 2012;44(8):607–18.

22. Seifert F, Bschorer K, De Col R, Filitz J, Peltz E, Koppert W, et al. Medial

prefrontal cortex activity is predictive for hyperalgesia and pharmacological antihyperalgesia. Journal of Neuroscience. 2009;29(19):6167–75.

23. Lorenz J, Minoshima S, Casey KL. Keeping pain out of mind: the role of the dorsolateral prefrontal cortex in pain modulation. Brain. 2003;126(5):1079–91.

24. Hansen GR, Streltzer J. The psychology of pain. Emergency Medicine Clinics of North America. 2005;23(2):339–48.

25. 2017 [cited Mar 2017]. Available from: https://en.oxforddictionaries.com/definition/catastrophize.

26. Zhuo M. Long-term potentiation in the anterior cingulate cortex and chronic pain. Philosophical Transactions of the Royal Society B: Biological Sciences. 2014;369(1633):20130146.

27. Leeuw M, Goossens ME, Linton SJ, Crombez G, Boersma K, Vlaeyen JW. The fear-avoidance model of musculoskeletal pain: current state of scientific evidence. Journal of Behavioral Medicine. 2007;30(1):77–94.

28. Crombez G, Eccleston C, Vlaeyen JW, Vansteenwegen D, Lysens R, Eelen P. Exposure to physical movements in low back pain patients: restricted effects of generalization. Health Psychology. 2002;21(6):573–8.

29. Herbert MS, Goodin BR, Pero ST, Schmidt JK, Sotolongo A, Bulls HW, et al. Pain hypervigilance is associated with greater clinical pain severity and enhanced experimental pain sensitivity among adults with symptomatic knee osteoarthritis. Annals of Behavioral Medicine. 2014;48(1):50–60.

30. Crombez G, Eccleston C, Baeyens F, Van Houdenhove B, Van Den Broeck A. Attention to chronic pain is dependent upon pain-related fear. Journal of Psychosomatic Research. 1999;47(5):403–10.

31. McCracken LM. 'Attention' to pain in persons with chronic pain: a behavioral approach. Behavior Therapy. 1997;28(2):271–84.

32. Quartana PJ, Campbell CM, Edwards RR. Pain catastrophizing: a critical review. Expert Review of Neurotherapeutics. 2009;9(5):745–58.

33. Seminowicz DA, Davis KD. Cortical responses to pain in healthy individuals depends on pain catastrophizing. Pain. 2006;120(3):297–306.

34. Weissman-Fogel I, Sprecher E, Pud D. Effects of catastrophizing on pain perception and pain modulation. Experimental Brain Research. 2008;186(1):79–85.

35. Pruessner M, Hellhammer DH, Pruessner JC, Lupien SJ. Self-reported depressive symptoms and stress levels in healthy young men: associations with the cortisol response to awakening. Psychosomatic Medicine. 2003;65(1):92–9.

36. Sullivan MJL, Bishop SR, Pivik J. The Pain Catastrophizing Scale: development and validation. Psychological Assessment. 1995;7(4):524–32.

37. Sinclair VG. Predictors of pain catastrophizing in women with rheumatoid arthritis. Archives of Psychiatric Nursing. 2001;15(6):279–88.

38. Jensen MP, Turner JA, Romano JM. Changes in beliefs, catastrophizing, and coping are associated with improvement in multidisciplinary pain treatment. Journal of Consulting and Clinical Psychology. 2001;69(4):655–62.

39. Jensen MP, Turner JA, Romano JM. Changes after multidisciplinary pain treatment in patient pain beliefs and coping are associated with concurrent changes in patient functioning. Pain. 2007;131(1–2):38–47.

40. Quartana PJ, Burns JW, Lofland KR. Attentional strategy moderates effects of pain catastrophizing on symptom-specific physiological responses in chronic low back pain patients. Journal of Behavioral Medicine. 2007;30(3):221–31.

41. Wolff B, Burns JW, Quartana PJ, Lofland K, Bruehl S, Chung OY. Pain catastrophizing, physiological indexes, and chronic pain severity: tests of mediation and moderation

models. Journal of Behavioral Medicine. 2008;31(2):105–14.

42. Bandura A. Self-efficacy: toward a unifying theory of behavioral change. Psychological Review. 1977;84(2):191–215.

43. Bandura A. Self-efficacy mechanism in human agency. American Psychologist. 1982;37(2):122–47.

44. Costa Lda C, Maher CG, McAuley JH, Hancock MJ, Smeets RJ. Self-efficacy is more important than fear of movement in mediating the relationship between pain and disability in chronic low back pain. European Journal of Pain. 2011;15(2):213–9.

45. Woby SR, Urmston M, Watson PJ. Self-efficacy mediates the relation between pain-related fear and outcome in chronic low back pain patients. European Journal of Pain. 2007;11(7):711–8.

46. Dixon G, Thornton EW, Young CA. Perceptions of self-efficacy and rehabilitation among neurologically disabled adults. Clinical Rehabilitation. 2007;21(3):230–40.

47. Altmaier EM, Russell DW, Kao CF, Lehmann TR, Weinstein JN. Role of self-efficacy in rehabilitation outcome among chronic low back pain patients. Journal of Counseling Psychology. 1993;40(3):335–9.

48. Warner LM, Schuz B, Wolff JK, Parschau L, Wurm S, Schwarzer R. Sources of self-efficacy for physical activity. Health Psychology. 2014;33(11):1298–308.

49. Nicholas MK. The pain self-efficacy questionnaire: taking pain into account. European Journal of Pain. 2007;11(2):153–63.

50. Schneider C, Palomba D, Flor H. Pavlovian conditioning of muscular responses in chronic pain patients: central and peripheral correlates. Pain. 2004;112(3):239–47.

51. Flor H, Knost B, Birbaumer N. The role of operant conditioning in chronic pain: an experimental investigation. Pain. 2002;95(1–2):111–18.

52. Jenewein J, Moergeli H, Sprott H, Honegger D, Brunner L, Ettlin D, et al.

Fear-learning deficits in subjects with fibromyalgia syndrome? European Journal of Pain. 2013;17(9):1374–84.

53. Fuchs X, Becker S, Kleinböhl D, Diers M, Flor H. Respondent learning in chronic pain: how precise is imprecision? Pain. 2015;156(10):2108–9.

54. Kamper SJ, Apeldoorn AT, Chiarotto A, Smeets RJ, Ostelo RW, Guzman J, et al. Multidisciplinary biopsychosocial rehabilitation for chronic low back pain. Cochrane Database of Systematic Reviews. 2014;9:Cd000963.

55. Waddell G, Newton M, Henderson I, Somerville D, Main CJ. A Fear-Avoidance Beliefs Questionnaire (FABQ) and the role of fear-avoidance beliefs in chronic low back pain and disability. Pain. 1993;52(2):157–68.

56. Grotle M, Vollestad NK, Veierod MB, Brox JI. Fear-avoidance beliefs and distress in relation to disability in acute and chronic low back pain. Pain. 2004;112(3):343–52.

57. George SZ, Stryker SE. Fear-avoidance beliefs and clinical outcomes for patients seeking outpatient physical therapy for musculoskeletal pain conditions. Journal of Orthopaedic and Sports Physical Therapy. 2011;41(4):249–59.

58. Scopaz KA, Piva SR, Wisniewski S, Fitzgerald GK. Relationships of fear, anxiety, and depression with physical function in patients with knee osteoarthritis. Archives of Physical Medicine and Rehabilitation. 2009;90(11):1866–73.

59. de Jong JR, Vlaeyen JWS, Onghena P, Cuypers C, Hollander Md, Ruijgrok J. Reduction of pain-related fear in complex regional pain syndrome type I: the application of graded exposure in vivo. Pain. 2005;116(3):264–75.

60. Martinez MP, Sanchez AI, Miro E, Medina A, Lami MJ. The relationship between the fear-avoidance model of pain and personality traits in fibromyalgia patients. Journal of Clinical Psychology in Medical Settings. 2011;18(4):380–91.

61. Wertli MM, Rasmussen-Barr E, Weiser S, Bachmann LM, Brunner F. The role of fear avoidance beliefs as a prognostic factor for outcome in patients with nonspecific low back pain: a systematic review. Spine Journal. 2014;14(5):816–36.e4.

62. Kamping S, Bomba IC, Kanske P, Diesch E, Flor H. Deficient modulation of pain by a positive emotional context in fibromyalgia patients. Pain. 2013;154(9):1846–55.

63. Jensen KB, Petzke F, Carville S, Fransson P, Marcus H, Williams SC, et al. Anxiety and depressive symptoms in fibromyalgia are related to poor perception of health but not to pain sensitivity or cerebral processing of pain. Arthritis and Rheumatism. 2010;62(11):3488–95.

64. de Tommaso M, Calabrese R, Vecchio E, De Vito Francesco V, Lancioni G, Livrea P. Effects of affective pictures on pain sensitivity and cortical responses induced by laser stimuli in healthy subjects and migraine patients. International Journal of Psychophysiology. 2009;74(2):139–48.

65. De Wied M, Verbaten MN. Affective pictures processing, attention, and pain tolerance. Pain. 2001;90(1–2):163–72.

66. Lumley MA, Cohen JL, Borszcz GS, Cano A, Radcliffe AM, Porter LS, et al. Pain and emotion: a biopsychosocial review of recent research. Journal of Clinical Psychology. 2011;67(9):942–68.

67. Hooten WM, Townsend CO, Sletten CD, Bruce BK, Rome JD. Treatment outcomes after multidisciplinary pain rehabilitation with analgesic medication withdrawal for patients with fibromyalgia. Pain Medicine. 2007;8(1):8–16.

68. Eccleston C, Crombez G, Aldrich S, Stannard C. Worry and chronic pain patients: a description and analysis of individual differences. European Journal of Pain. 2001;5(3):309–18.

69. Borkovec TD. The nature, functions, and origins of worry. In: Tallis GCLDF, editor. Worrying: perspectives on theory, assessment and treatment. Wiley Series in Clinical Psychology. Oxford, England: John Wiley & Sons; 1994. p. 5–33.

70. Hadjistavropoulos HD, Hadjistavropoulos T, Quine A. Health anxiety moderates the effects of distraction versus attention to pain. Behaviour Research and Therapy. 2000;38(5):425–38.

71. Main CJ, Waddell G. Psychometric construction and validity of the Pilowsky Illness Behaviour Questionnaire in British patients with chronic low back pain. Pain. 1987;28(1):13–25.

72. McCracken LM, Zayfert C, Gross RT. The pain anxiety symptoms scale: development and validation of a scale to measure fear of pain. Pain. 1992;50(1):67–73.

73. McCracken LM, Gross RT, Aikens J, Carnrike Jr CLM. The assessment of anxiety and fear in persons with chronic pain: a comparison of instruments. Behaviour Research and Therapy. 1996;34(11–12):927–33.

74. Bair MJ, Robinson RL, Katon W, Kroenke K. Depression and pain comorbidity: a literature review. Archives of Internal Medicine. 2003;163(20):2433–45.

75. Gallagher RM, Verma S. Managing pain and comorbid depression: a public health challenge. Seminars in Clinical Neuropsychiatry. 1999;4(3):203–20.

76. Wessely S, White PD. There is only one functional somatic syndrome. British Journal of Psychiatry. 2004;185(2):95–6.

77. Sullivan MJ, Reesor K, Mikail S, Fisher R. The treatment of depression in chronic low back pain: review and recommendations. Pain. 1992;50(1):5–13.

78. Panzarino PJ, Jr. The costs of depression: direct and indirect; treatment versus nontreatment. Journal of Clinical Psychiatry. 1998;59(Suppl 20):11–4.

79. Haggman S, Maher CG, Refshauge KM. Screening for symptoms of depression by physical therapists managing low back pain. Physical Therapy. 2004;84(12):1157–66.

80. Brown TA, Chorpita BF, Korotitsch W, Barlow DH. Psychometric properties of the Depression Anxiety Stress Scales (DASS) in clinical samples. Behaviour Research and Therapy. 1997;35(1):79–89.

81.   Beck AT, Steer RA, Carbin MG. Psychometric properties of the Beck Depression Inventory: twenty-five years of evaluation. Clinical Psychology Review. 1988;8(1):77–100.

82.   Lovibond PF, Lovibond SH. The structure of negative emotional states: comparison of the Depression Anxiety Stress Scales (DASS) with the Beck Depression and Anxiety Inventories. Behaviour Research and Therapy. 1995;33(3):335–43.

83.   Manchikanti L, Fellows B, Singh V. Understanding psychological aspects of chronic pain in interventional pain management. Pain Physician. 2002;5(1):57–82.

84.   Main C, Waddell G. Psychololigcal distress. In: Waddell G, editor. The back pain revolution. Philadelphia: Churchill Livingstone; 1998. p. 173–86.

85.   Vachon-Presseau E, Roy M, Martel MO, Caron E, Marin MF, Chen J, et al. The stress model of chronic pain: evidence from basal cortisol and hippocampal structure and function in humans. Brain. 2013;136(3):815–27.

86.   Goodman LA, Corcoran C, Turner K, Yuan N, Green BL. Assessing traumatic event exposure: general issues and preliminary findings for the Stressful Life Events Screening Questionnaire. Journal of Traumatic Stress. 1998;11(3):521–42.

87.   McDonald SD, Beckham JC, Morey RA, Calhoun PS. The validity and diagnostic efficiency of the Davidson Trauma Scale in military veterans who have served since September 11th, 2001. Journal of Anxiety Disorders. 2009;23(2):247–55.

88.   Walsh DA, Radcliffe JC. Pain beliefs and perceived physical disability of patients with chronic low back pain. Pain. 2002;97(1–2):23–31.

89.   Crombez G, Vlaeyen JW, Heuts PH, Lysens R. Pain-related fear is more disabling than pain itself: evidence on the role of pain-related fear in chronic back pain disability. Pain. 1999;80(1–2):329–39.

90.   Pensri P, Janwantanakul P, Worakul P, Sinsongsook T. Biopsychosocial factors and perceived disability in saleswomen with concurrent low back pain. Safety and Health at Work. 2010;1(2):149–57.

91.   Schwartz DP, DeGood DE, Shutty MS. Direct assessment of beliefs and attitudes of chronic pain patients. Archives of Physical Medicine and Rehabilitation. 1985;66(12):806–9.

92.   Roland M, Morris R. A study of the natural history of back pain. Part I: development of a reliable and sensitive measure of disability in low-back pain. Spine. 1983;8(2):141–4.

93.   Fairbank JC, Couper J, Davies JB, O'Brien JP. The Oswestry Low Back Pain Disability Questionnaire. Physiotherapy. 1980;66(8):271–3.

94.   Gandek B, Sinclair SJ, Kosinski M, Ware JE. Psychometric evaluation of the SF-36(*) Health Survey in Medicare Managed Care. Health Care Financing Review. 2004;25(4):5–25.

95.   Ware JE. Health Survey: manual and interpretation guide. Boston, MA: Health Institute; 1993.

96.   Melzack R, Wall PD. Pain mechanisms: a new theory. Survey of Anesthesiology. 1967;11(2):89–90.

97.   Melzack R. Pain and stress: a new perspective. In: Gatchel DC, Turk RJ, editors. Psychosocial factors in pain: critical perspectives. New York, NY: Guilford Press; 1999. p. 89–106.

98.   Hildebrandt J, Pfingsten M, Saur P, Jansen J. Prediction of success from a multidisciplinary treatment program for chronic low back pain. Spine. 1997;22(9):990–1001.

99.   Gatchel RJ, Okifuji A. Evidence-based scientific data documenting the treatment and cost-effectiveness of comprehensive pain programs for chronic nonmalignant pain. Journal of Pain. 2006;7(11):779–93.

100. Sturgeon JA. Psychological therapies for the management of chronic pain. Psychology Research and Behavior Management. 2014;7:115–24.

101. Kranz D, Bollinger A, Nilges P. Chronic pain acceptance and affective well-being: a coping perspective. European Journal of Pain. 2010;14(10):1021–5.

102. Fordyce W. Behavioral methods for chronic pain and illness. In: Main C, Keefe F, Jensen M, Vlaeyen J, Vowles K, editors. Fordyce's behavioral methods for chronic pain and illness. St Louis: Mosby; 1976.

103. Nicholas MK, Wilson PH, Goyen J. Operant-behavioural and cognitive-behavioural treatment for chronic low back pain. Behaviour Research and Therapy. 1991;29(3):225–38.

104. Thieme K, Flor H, Turk DC. Psychological pain treatment in fibromyalgia syndrome: efficacy of operant behavioural and cognitive behavioural treatments. Arthritis Research and Therapy. 2006;8(4):R121.

105. Roditi D, Robinson ME. The role of psychological interventions in the management of patients with chronic pain. Psychology Research and Behavior Management. 2011;4:41–9.

106. Sullivan MJL, Adams H, Ellis T. Targeting catastrophic thinking to promote return to work in individuals with fibromyalgia. Journal of Cognitive Psychotherapy. 2012;26(2):130–42.

107. Meulders A, Karsdorp PA, Claes N, Vlaeyen JWS. Comparing counterconditioning and extinction as methods to reduce fear of movement-related pain. Journal of Pain. 16(12):1353–65.

108. Gatchel RJ, Rollings KH. Evidence informed management of chronic low back pain with cognitive behavioral therapy. Spine Journal. 2008;8(1):40–4.

109. Dunne RL, Kenardy J, Sterling M. A randomized controlled trial of cognitive-behavioral therapy for the treatment of PTSD in the context of chronic whiplash. Clinical Journal of Pain. 2012;28(9):755–65.

110. Williams AC, Eccleston C, Morley S. Psychological therapies for the management of chronic pain (excluding headache) in adults. Cochrane Database of Systematic Reviews. 2012;11:Cd007407.

111. Kabat-Zinn J. An outpatient program in behavioral medicine for chronic pain patients based on the practice of mindfulness meditation: theoretical considerations and preliminary results. General Hospital Psychiatry. 1982;4(1):33–47.

112. Zernicke KA, Campbell TS, Blustein PK, Fung TS, Johnson JA, Bacon SL, et al. Mindfulness-based stress reduction for the treatment of irritable bowel syndrome symptoms: a randomized wait-list controlled trial. International Journal of Behavioral Medicine. 2013;20(3):385–96.

113. Oberg EB, Rempe M, Bradley R. Self-directed mindfulness training and improvement in blood pressure, migraine frequency, and quality of life. Global Advances in Health and Medicine. 2013;2(2):20–5.

114. Schmidt S, Grossman P, Schwarzer B, Jena S, Naumann J, Walach H. Treating fibromyalgia with mindfulness-based stress reduction: results from a 3-armed randomized controlled trial. Pain. 2011;152(2):361–9.

115. Cramer H, Haller H, Lauche R, Dobos G. Mindfulness-based stress reduction for low back pain. A systematic review. BMC Complementary and Alternative Medicine. 2012;12:162.

116. McCracken LM, Vowles KE. Acceptance and commitment therapy and mindfulness for chronic pain: model, process, and progress. The American Psychologist. 2014;69(2):178–87.

117. Hayes SC, Luoma JB, Bond FW, Masuda A, Lillis J. Acceptance and commitment therapy: model, processes and outcomes. Behaviour Research and Therapy. 2006;44(1):1–25.

118. Veehof MM, Oskam MJ, Schreurs KM, Bohlmeijer ET. Acceptance-based interventions for the treatment of chronic pain: a systematic review and meta-analysis. Pain. 2011;152(3):533–42.

119. McCracken LM, Sato A, Taylor GJ. A Trial of a brief group-based form of acceptance and commitment therapy (ACT) for chronic pain in general practice: pilot outcome and process results. Journal of Pain. 2013;14(11):1398–406.

120. Wicksell RK, Ahlqvist J, Bring A, Melin L, Olsson GL. Can exposure and acceptance strategies improve functioning and life satisfaction in people with chronic pain and whiplash-associated disorders (WAD)? A randomized controlled trial. Cognitive Behaviour Therapy. 2008;37(3):169–82.

121. Turk DC. The potential of treatment matching for subgroups of patients with chronic pain: lumping versus splitting. Clinical Journal of Pain. 2005;21(1):44–55; discussion 69–72.

122. Kerns RD, Rosenberg R, Jamison RN, Caudill MA, Haythornthwaite J. Readiness to adopt a self-management approach to chronic pain: the Pain Stages of Change Questionnaire (PSOCQ). Pain. 1997;72(1–2):227–34.

Introduction

Despite the high prevalence and costs associated with chronic pain (CP), significant relief for the vast majority remains elusive. For most people suffering CP, the resolution of pain symptoms is uncommon, while the experience of pain may impair quality of life and cause significant physical disability and emotional distress.[1] Importantly, how practitioners think about pain significantly influences the way they evaluate and treat patients. For example, clinicians may assume that underlying pathology is required to cause symptoms. A pathology-directed case history and physical examination are undertaken, and, when considered appropriate, diagnostic imaging and laboratory tests are performed. Alternatively, in the absence of organic pathology, manual therapists may assume that biomechanical dysfunction is necessary to cause musculoskeletal pain. Assessment may therefore be primarily focused on orthopedic testing and diagnostic imaging if deemed appropriate. Only in the absence of physical findings are psychological mechanisms considered, and thus a patient's symptoms are dichotomously characterized as being either somatic or psychogenic.

It is rare that the severity of pain correlates with the significance of observable pathology. For example, mechanisms of pain and disability in people suffering severe pain with conditions such as fibromyalgia or irritable bowel syndrome are unobservable and relatively unknown. On the other hand, patients presenting with structural abnormalities such as life-threatening space occupying lesions or herniated discs are often asymptomatic. Effective treatment can only occur if there is patient-centered evaluation of biological factors in combination with the patient's psychosocial and behavioral presentation.[1] A comprehensive assessment of interacting factors that can influence pain severity and related disability using both verbal and non-verbal cues is therefore essential. One of the first steps in a manual therapist's assessment of people with CP is to identify the basis for symptoms and their occurrence. Importantly, the effects of manual therapy have been shown to extend beyond physical factors related to symptom control and has moved towards behavioral and quality of life domains of therapeutic care.[2] This chapter will review and discuss current evidence relating to CP evaluation, in particular evaluation of musculoskeletal pain, beginning with the case history and clinical examination. The following sections will review current standardized pain assessment methods as well as tools available to evaluate the effect of pain on quality of life and levels of disability.

The clinical approach to the pain experience

The patient's own pain description is invaluable as it gives the practitioner information about location, intensity, and character of the pain. However, the subjective reporting of pain is affected by numerous psychological and behavioral factors, and so the evaluation of CP patients requires more time and effort compared to those presenting with acute pain. In addition to gathering information regarding the description of pain, practitioners must also collect data concerning the patient's (and significant others') thoughts, feelings, such as depression, and other psychosocial factors.[3] Thus, pain is a multidimensional experience in which the simplest categorization is that of sensory intensity, emotional and cognitive factors, and interference with everyday life.[4] Dansie and Turk[1] neatly summarize these issues with the acronym ACT-UP (Activity, Coping, Think, Upset, Peoples responses), which can be used to guide practitioners through the initial interview process (Table 6.1).

Table 6.1: A brief psychosocial screen (ACT-UP)[1]

1 Activities	How is pain affecting your life (i.e., sleep, physical activities, and relationships)?
2 Coping	How do you cope with your pain (what relieves or aggravates your pain)?
3 Think	Do you think your pain will ever get better?
4 Upset	Are you worried (anxious) and/or depressed (down, blue)?
5 People	How do other people respond when you have pain?

Critical first steps

The primary objectives of pain assessment in a clinical setting are to make a differential diagnosis and determine the impact of pain on the patient's quality of life (Table 6.2). CP has a major impact on physical, emotional, and cognitive function, on family and social life, and on the person's ability to work.[5] Thus, a pain history must not only make clear location, intensity, pain characteristics and time course of pain, but also any concerns about potential pathophysiological causes and psychological effects it may have on the patient. Thus, the practitioner must have the skills necessary to recognize symptoms and behaviors of both 'bottom-up' and 'top-down' pain mechanisms.

Simply listening to the patient will help, for example in identifying clues as to how a problem developed from a local pain issue to a more generalized pain experience. Initial documentation must include information of pain location, intensity, quality, onset/duration/variations/rhythms, pain relief, aggravating triggers, effects of pain (sleep, appetite, physical activity, emotions, concentration, etc.), personal expression of pain, and response to previous treatment.[5,6] Several initial pain assessment tools have been developed, and a good example is one developed by Breivik and colleagues,[7] shown in Table 6.3. Pain is often described as a private experience. However, it is also a public one, particularly with regard to facial expression,[8] which is often missed and more difficult to accurately assess.

Additionally, as reviewed in previous chapters, psychological and cultural beliefs must also be considered and evaluated. Here, the ability to listen and respond to the expressed concerns of patients is helpful in identifying more latent factors related to the maintenance of pain.

Problems surrounding the assessment of pain

Unfortunately, there is no objective tool able to measure how much pain a person experiences. Thus, pain intensity is measured using verbal and non-verbal communication to describe the person's subjective experience.[9] Generally, issues arise because patients are asked to quantify their pain on a unidimensional numerical scale where they must average out their experience both temporally and situationally. Additionally, most pain ratings are retrospective, a circumstance in which patients have been shown to over- or underestimate levels of pain, as it varies over time.[9] Given these factors, there is considerable variation in how patients discriminate between points on a scale. For example, one person's 4/10 may have a significantly different meaning to another person with the same score. Thus, the choice of dimension in the pain experience depends on

Table 6.2: Aims and steps taken during a clinical pain assessment (adapted from Turk and Melzack, Handbook of Pain Assessment)[9]

Aims of clinical pain assessment	
1	Make a differential diagnosis
2	Predict a treatment response
3	Evaluate the characteristics of pain
4	Evaluate the impact of pain on the patient Determine levels of disability Determine limitations in physical capacity
5	Monitor progress following initial treatment
6	Assess effectiveness of treatment program
7	Evaluate the need to continue/modify treatment

Table 6.3: Taking a specific case history for patients presenting with musculoskeletal pain (adapted from Breivik et al.)[7]

Chronic pain case history	
1	Where is your pain?
2	How intense is your pain?
3	How would you describe your pain? (e.g., aching, throbbing, burning, shooting, stabbing)
4	How did your pain start?
5	How has your pain progressed since it started?
6	What relieves your pain (e.g., movement, body position, rest, medication, specific activities)
7	What aggravates your pain (e.g., movement, body position, rest, specific activities, medication)
8	How does your pain affect: • sleep • physical function • your ability to work • your ability to be physically active • your economy • your mood • your family life • your social life • your sex life
9	What (if any) treatments are/have you received? • positive effects • adverse effects
10	Are you depressed or anxious?
11	Do you worry about the consequences of your pain condition on your general health?
12	Are you involved in any litigation and/or compensation processes?

the purpose of the assessment.[8] Concerning ongoing evaluation, it is recommended that CP patients should be encouraged to rate their pain at the same time of day, in the same place, and in the presence of the same people at each assessment period, using the same measures.[10] Reporting of pain intensity is also related to other variables such as cultural background, the meaning of the situation, personality variables and emotions, and past experiences.[11] Thus, the dimension of pain itself does not reflect either psychological or physical dysfunction caused by a specific disorder.

Location of pain is also oversimplified in that only the main site(s) of pain are usually recorded. However, the number of sites has been shown to have significant implications for pain-related disability. Using only the main site of pain thus conceals other factors related to pain disability, such as psychological distress and self-reported health.[12] Additionally, other symptoms such as fatigue, sleep disturbance, and changes in weight are further associated with CP. Each of these symptoms may be due to pain itself, to emotional distress, or to any treatment prescribed to control pain.[1] Thus, instruments have been developed specifically for CP patients to assess the impact of pain on the themselves and on their life. Self-reporting measures help to further validate relevant contributing and maintaining factors. These measures evaluate attitudes, beliefs, emotions, cognitions, quality of life, and expectations relating to their own unique pain experience. Moreover, these inexpensive and easy-to-administer measures may gain data about behaviors that patients may feel uncomfortable about revealing during an interview.[1] However, little research interest has been shown in how patients decide on a particular description of pain. It appears that people quantify CP using references to both function and mood (e.g., awful, unpleasant).[13] Thus, it is important to understand that these measures do not replace, but rather complement the interview process, by obtaining invaluable information that may help to determine a more significant diagnosis and/or further assessments if required.

Measuring the pain experience

Levels of measurement

Pain is measured in terms of intensity, quality, and affect, with quantitative estimates of the pain experience being gathered as perceived by the patient. Before discussing methods of measuring pain intensity, it is first important to understand the properties of different types of scale. Generally, measurement scales are used to quantify and/or categorize variables. The type/level of measurement always refers to the relationship among the values that are allocated to the characteristics for a variable. Thus, the level of measurement helps decide how to interpret the data from that variable. Measurement scales must satisfy one or more of the following:

- *Identity*: each value on a scale has a unique meaning.

- *Magnitude*: values on a scale have an ordered relationship to each other. Thus some values are larger and some smaller, but the distance between them is not necessarily equal.

- *Equal intervals*: scale units along a scale (continuum) so they have equal distance from each other – the difference between 1 and 2 is the same as between 19 and 20. However, no true zero point exists.

- *A minimum value of zero*: the scale has a true zero point below which no values exist.

Concerning analysis of data, knowing the level of measurement helps to decide what statistical analysis is appropriate for the values on a given scale. There are four types of measurement defined by the above properties and each is relevant to the measurement of pain intensity (Figure 6.1). For further reading concerning clinical data analysis, *Statistics in Medicine* is recommended.[14]

Nominal scales

A nominal scale only satisfies the 'identity' property and is the crudest form of measurement that classifies variables (e.g., gender, blood group), with no order along a continuum being required. It simply needs a count of frequency for each case.[15]

Ordinal scales

Ordinal scales satisfy both identity and magnitude properties and involve the ranking of values, attitudes or items (first to last or high to low) along a continuum of a characteristic being measured. However, there

Figure 6.1

A diagram showing the four different levels of measurement used in the evaluation of clinical and experimental data

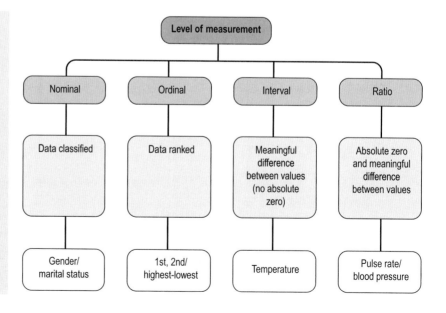

is no information determining the interval between points on ordinal scales. For example, if using a Likert scale of attitude, the distance between 'very strong agreement' and 'strong agreement' may be different to that between 'undecided' and 'disagree'.

Interval scales

Interval scales have properties of identity, magnitude, and equal intervals. For example, a Celsius scale measuring temperature is made up of equal intervals: the distance between 20 and 30 degrees is the same as between 80 and 90 degrees. However, the zero point on interval scales is arbitrary concerning temperature, since values exist below the zero point.

Ratio scales

The highest level of measurement is the ratio scale. In addition to the interval scale, the ratio scale has an absolute zero. Examples of ratio variables include weight, length, and time. Ratio scale data allow comparisons such as time: 20 minutes is twice as long as 10 minutes.

Evaluating pain intensity

Four types of scale commonly used to assess pain intensity are briefly described below. They are the visual analog scale (VAS), the numerical rating scale (NRS), the verbal rating scale (VRS), and the faces pain scale (FPS), previously used with children but now commonly used in adults, particularly the elderly.

The visual analog scale (VAS)

The VAS is shown as a 10 cm line anchored by verbal descriptors, from 'no pain' to 'worst possible pain' (Figure 6.2). A VAS may have specific points labeled along the line, usually in millimeters. The VAS is therefore considered to have 101 response levels, making it very sensitive to changes in pain intensity compared to other measures with a limited number of response points.[16] However, because the VAS can only be administered on paper or electronically, photocopying and differences in computer screen size can lead to changes in its length.[17] Additionally, orientation of the VAS also affects results, since horizontal orientation shows normally distributed ratings which are not shown when it is used vertically.[18] However, this discrepancy may be connected to language, as a Chinese study showed the opposite to happen, with less error noted when employing the VAS vertically.[19] Surprisingly, some studies investigating experimental and clinical pain show VAS to have ratio scale properties.[20] However, opinions differ, with some arguing that VAS shows no true unit of measurement and therefore shows non-linear properties, thus functioning like an ordinal scale.[21] However, Price and colleagues show the VAS to have an accurate stimulus–response curve, reflecting accurate ratios of pain intensity with a true zero point.[22,23]

The numerical rating scale (NRS)

The NRS involves asking patients to rate their pain on a 0 to 10 (11-point scale), 0 to 20 (21-point scale) or 0 to 100 (101-point scale), where one end is anchored with a verbal descriptor of 'no pain' and the other 'worst pain possible' (see Figure 6.2). One advantage of the NRS over the VAS is that it can be administered verbally, with a patient simply stating their pain intensity on the type of NRS administered. Otherwise, using a paper version, patients are asked to circle the number that best describes their pain intensity. Unlike the VAS, the NRS surprisingly does not show ratio scale properties. Price and colleagues argue that the NRS lacks a true zero point as it inaccurately predicts discriminations of pain intensity ratios while also repeatedly showing artificially high ratings at the lower end of the scale.[20,24] However, Jensen and Karoly argue that while the NRS does not have ratio data type qualities, this issue does not impact its reliability, validity or sensitivity especially with treatment outcomes.[10]

The verbal rating scale (VRS)

The VRS contains a list of adjectives used to represent increasing pain intensities, the most commonly used being: no pain, mild pain, moderate pain, and severe pain (see Figure 6.2). These descriptors may also be assigned numbers denoting the place on a scale; however, it should be noted that unlike the VAS and NRS, intervals between descriptors on the VRS are not necessarily equal, thus data taken from VRS scales are

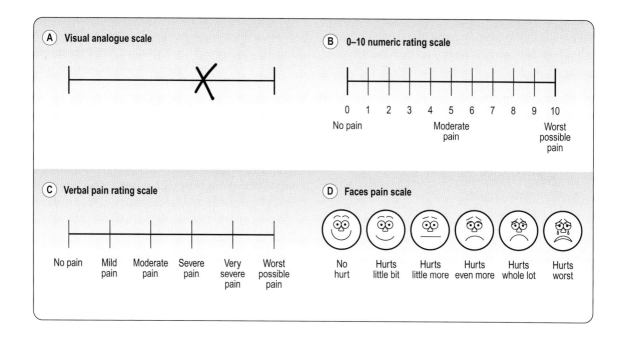

Figure 6.2

Pain rating scales: (A) the visual analog scale, (B) the 0–10 numerical rating scale, (C) the verbal pain rating scale and (D) the faces scale

considered ordinal and may only be ranked (i.e., highest to lowest or best to worst). For example, the interval between 'no pain' and 'mild pain' may be significantly smaller than between 'moderate pain' and 'severe pain'.[10] Thus, interpretation of the degree of difference is difficult. Because of this issue, the use of the VRS in experimental settings is not recommended. Additionally, the VRS requires patients to read and select from a finite number of adjectives and in many cases patients are unable to find a descriptor that accurately describes their pain intensity.[26] Given that the VRS uses adjectives to describe levels of pain, these categories cannot be presented in an equidistant manner, either on VAS or NRS, and are thus ranked in levels of severity that offer measurement as ordinal data.[27,28]

The faces pain scale (FPS)

The FPS uses drawings to illustrate facial expressions representing a person's experience of different levels of pain severity (see Figure 6.2).[29] Although the faces

scale was developed for assessing pain in children or for those with difficulty with written language, it has been shown to be equally reliable when evaluating pain in older adults.[30] Thus the FPS is a reliable measure of pain with cognitively impaired and end-of-life non-verbal patients because it does not require reading, writing, or energy. While there are several well-tested versions of the FPS, with the number of faces ranging between six and nine faces, Kim and Buschmann found that an 11 face scale using both NRS and VAS was also appropriate to assess pain in older adults.[30] The FPS alone provides ordinal data where each faces category is ordered (ranked) in a specific order.

Pain intensity scale reliability and validity

The VAS is shown to be reliable in acute and CP settings when repeated within a short space of time.[31] However, people with cognitive impairment do not score on VAS so consistently.[17] Experimental studies show that the experience of pain varies over time, although the strength of physical stimulus remains the same.[32] Overall, however, the VAS has been shown to make significant predictions in pain reduction in people with CP.[33] Interestingly, the VAS has also been investigated as a tool measuring levels of disability in people with CP. These findings are particularly relevant given strong associations between CP and perceived disability. Here, Boonstra and colleagues showed significant correlations between the VAS and the Roland Morris Disability Questionnaire.[34]

The NRS is also reliable for measuring pain intensity. In particular, a two-point change in NRS scoring before and after rehabilitation exceeds statistical measurement error and thus is reliable for use in evaluating the effectiveness of interventions for people with low back pain.[35] Although the VRS has also been shown to be a reliable assessment of postoperative pain,[36] when compared to the NRS it shows lower reproducibility when measuring pain exacerbations in CP in people with chronic cancer pain.[37] Interestingly, although the FPS is less sensitive in responsiveness than the VAS and NRS, it is nevertheless shown to be reliable and valid not only for use in adults and children but also in people with cognitive and communication disabilities in cases such as dementia.[38]

Evaluating pain affect

While the assessment of pain intensity is important, experimental and clinical evidence shows pain to be both sensory-discriminative and motivational-affective. Put simply, pain intensity is defined as how severe pain is perceived, whereas the effect of pain is defined as the emotional arousal and discomfort felt and described by the patient. Thus, scales measuring only pain intensity are considered inaccurate given there is no way of knowing which dimension of pain a patient is rating.[39] Several measures have been developed to measure pain affect that are shown to be reliable and valid in many languages.

The McGill Pain Questionnaire

The McGill Pain Questionnaire (MPQ) evaluates (1) sensory, (2) affective-emotional and (3) evaluative aspects of pain and is one of the most widely used multidimensional

measures for evaluating pain.[40] In its original form, the MPQ contains 78 pain descriptors within 20 groups of words that are divided into three main categories, as above. The affective subscale provides information in terms of tension, fear, and autonomic features that are part of the pain experience; it includes descriptors such as 'fearful,' 'miserable,' 'annoying,' and 'nauseating.'[41] The MPQ and its short-form (SF-MPQ) have become gold standards in the assessment of various qualities of CP. The patient is required to indicate the intensity of each descriptor on a scale from 0 to 3 (severe). The three pain subscales are calculated individually together with the total pain score.[42]

The verbal rating scale

The VRS has also been developed to assess suffering associated with pain. These scales consist of descriptors that define increasing levels of discomfort and distress using terms such as 'bearable', 'unpleasant', 'miserable,' and 'intolerable' and respondents choose a single word that represents the degree of unpleasantness related to their pain.[10] Like VRS intensity scales, in these scales levels of affect are ranked and can be examined in relation to pain intensity and other constructs such as mood. However, like the VRS and pain intensity, Jensen and Karoly recommend that a simpler ranking method be used to evaluate the relationship between pain intensity and other pain dimensions.[43]

Affective features of pain are complex and more difficult to evaluate than pain intensity; thus, there are fewer valid and reliable measures available to evaluate these influences. While it is yet to be seen if multidimensional or unidimensional measures are more reliable in assessing pain affect, it could be suggested that in using a multidimensional pain measure, one may be able to capture which domain of pain is most influential for the patient. However, it is presently unknown whether single measures are more or less reliable than multidimensional measures in this regard.

Evaluating pain quality

Evaluating pain quality is useful in distinguishing various pain mechanisms and/or conditions. In the absence of diagnostic gold standards for pain diagnoses, pain quality measures are particularly useful in differentiating between non-neuropathic and neuropathic pain conditions and between peripheral nociceptive and central sensitization-based mechanisms.[44,45] In a Delphi study among pain experts, consensus revealed nociceptive pain to have:[46]

- a clear stimulus response relationship with aggravating and relieving factors in clinical testing

- relief with the action of anti-inflammatory medications

- pain local to injury/dysfunction

- localized pain on palpation

- absence of allodynia and hyperalgesia.

Conversely, peripheral neuropathic pain presents with:

- symptoms associated with allodynia and hyperalgesia

- dermatomal/cutaneous nerve distribution

- pain provocation associated with subjective aggravating and relieving factors

- pain provocation associated with disturbance of neural tissue.

Additionally, central pain was suggested to be typified by:

- diffuse locations of pain

- exaggerations in stimulus–response relationships

- spontaneous pain ('life of its own') and paroxysmal pain (intermittent pain with no association with any precursor)

- strong associations with emotional disorders and altered cognition.

There are a number self-reporting questionnaires and classifications, some of which are described below, and most of which identify neuropathic pain.

The Leeds Assessment of Neuropathic Symptoms and Signs

The Leeds Assessment of Neuropathic Symptoms and Signs (LANSS) is a simple, reliable, and valid seven-item measure for identifying patients with neuropathic pain.[47] Although the LANSS consists of only five symptoms and two examination items (allodynia and pin-prick testing), the need for clinical examination has limited its use in research.[48] However, more recently, the self-completed LANSS (7-item) has been shown to be equally reliable and valid in the general population and against previously validated neuropathic pain tools.

The pain quality assessment scale (PQAS)

Originally the neuropathic pain scale (NPS) was also considered to be sensitive to treatments known to affect neuropathic pain.[49] However, several pain qualities common in people with neuropathic and non-neuropathic pain are not assessed by the NPS. These include 'electric', 'tingling', 'pins and needles', 'radiating', and 'numbness'.[50] As these symptoms have been shown to be important qualities associated with neuropathic pain,[51] Jensen and colleagues added 10 further neuropathic and non-neuropathic descriptors ('achy', 'throbbing', 'cramping') to the NPS. With these additional items the NPS was shown to be a valid measure useful for additionally assessing non-neuropathic pain.[45] Because of this, the measure was renamed the pain quality assessment scale (PQAS). Further studies have also demonstrated that the PQAS identifies the effects of pain treatment on different types of pain quality.[10]

Identifying pain modifiers

Aggravating and relieving factors

Although the above assessment scales are shown to be both reliable and valid, one of the major issues is that of dimensionality.[13] It is widely recognized that pain is multidimensional; however, there is no agreement on the dimensions.[1] Generally, for people with CP, pain severity varies depending on a number of obvious and latent (hidden) physical and psychosocial variables. Thus, asking the patient about what makes their pain worse helps to identify factors that may have initiated, maintained, or amplified painful episodes. For example, do specific activities contribute to the initiation or exacerbation of pain, such as repetitive lifting or static work postures? Similarly, do certain situations initiate or aggravate episodes of pain, such as work and/or interpersonal conflicts? Pain may also vary depending on the time of day; for example, continuous joint loading and/or muscle activation may increase the chances of pain later in the day. Equally, it is also important to identify factors that alleviate pain. Is pain relieved with certain types of medication? For instance, does movement or rest help to ease symptoms, or does warmth or cold help to reduce the severity of pain? Although case history taking is able to elicit more obvious aggravating variables, self-reporting measures are more valuable in identifying more latent (hidden) variables or those which may be private to the patient, who may not wish to report them verbally. There are several useful measures that have been shown to elicit information about functional capacity and activity interferences such as the Short-Form Health Survey (SF-36)[52] and the back pain function scale (BPFS).[53]

Emotional distress

As described in Chapter 5, emotional distress, particularly anxiety, stress, anger, and depression, are strongly associated with CP. Emotional distress-related symptoms such as fatigue, sleep disturbance, poor concentration, memory deficit, and decreased libido further present challenges when evaluating people with CP. Self-reporting questionnaires that measure psychological distress have also been developed specifically for people with pain. For example, mood and personality variables can be elicited with a number of scale measures. The most commonly used scales include the System Checklist-90 (SCL-90), which measures emotional stress,[54] and the depression, anxiety, and stress scale (DASS), also shown to be a reliable measure of depression, anxiety, and stress in people with CP across all age groups.[55] More specifically, the Beck Depression Inventory-II (BDI-II) is a reliable and valid measure of depressive symptoms[56] across several different languages.[57]

Pain beliefs

As reviewed in Chapter 5, pain-related beliefs and coping methods are shown to significantly influence physical and psychological dysfunction in people with CP.[58] For example, as previously described, catastrophizing about pain leads to negative concerns about painful situations that paradoxically may result in increased pain intensity and psychological distress. Likewise, fear behaviors lead to avoidance of both physical and social activities for fear of recurrence or exacerbation of symptoms. Furthermore, self-efficacy beliefs (confidence, or lack of confidence, in ability to perform tasks when in pain) has not only been shown to be associated with higher levels of pain disability, but also found to be a more important factor of disability than fear avoidance and pain catastrophizing in chronic musculoskeletal pain.[59,60] These pain beliefs can be assessed using well-validated measures such as the pain catastrophizing scale (PCS),[61] the Fear Avoidance Beliefs Questionnaire (FABQ)[62] and the Pain Self-Efficacy Questionnaire (PSEQ).[63]

Mechanism-based evaluation of musculoskeletal pain

Although investigation into the etiology of a person's pain presentation is important in the clinical management of people living with CP, understanding pain mechanisms is also important to clinical reasoning and decision-making processes. Indeed, in the absence of gold standard assessment, the accurate identification of mechanisms is probably best achieved by the identification of information clusters based on a combination of findings from the history, examination, and other investigations.[64] However, while clinical areas such as pain medicine and palliative care use pain mechanisms in the clinical reasoning and decision-making processes, Smart and colleagues found that physical therapists are less likely to do so.[65] These studies also show that manual therapists are less likely to consider cognitive-affective mechanisms in their clinical reasoning process for the evaluation of pain in their patients.[66] Thus, researchers within physical therapy[44,66,67] now propose the teaching and application of mechanism-based decision-making for pain.

Classifying underlying pathophysiological mechanisms is a common sense method that is well-suited to pain. The studies of various authors[46,65,67,68] propose mechanism-based clinical reasoning for pain, where it is now evident that there are five general mechanisms of pain:[2]

- peripheral nociceptive mechanisms

- peripheral neuropathic mechanisms

- central sensitization/central neuropathic mechanisms

- sympathetically maintained pain mechanisms

- cognitive-affective maintained pain mechanisms.

Whilst many patients present with pain that may be attributable to a combination of nociceptive, peripheral neuropathic and central mechanisms, evidence suggests that pain arises from the relative dominance of specific mechanisms.[69]

Classification of peripheral nociceptive pain mechanisms

This type of pain commonly presents to manual therapists when pain arises from small diameter afferent fibers (C and Aδ fibers) in musculoskeletal tissue in response to noxious chemical (inflammatory), mechanical, or thermal stimuli (Chapter 1). Peripheral nociceptors are activated by proinflammatory mediators resulting from injury or by lowered pH cased by ischemia, or normally because of prolonged mechanical loading,[70] especially seen in people presenting with mechanical low back and neck pain. The clinical features of nociceptive pain follow a typical anatomical pattern that corresponds to the area of dysfunction/injury. Pain is also likely to be associated with additional signs of inflammation such as warmth, redness, swelling, and reduced function and responsive to nonsteroidal anti-inflammatory and opioid medication.[71] Aggravating and relieving factors are often related to movements or postures that can be reproduced on passive, active, and resisted isometric movement testing of the painful area. Thus, diagnosis and differentiation of injury may be made between contractile (muscle, tendon) tissue from inert

Table 6.4: Clinical indictors of nociceptive pain (adapted from Smart et al.)

Subjective
• Pain that is localized to the area of dysfunction/injury (with or without somatic referral)
• Pain that is clearly proportional to the anatomical/movement nature of aggravating and relieving factors
• Pain that is usually intermittent and sharp with movement/mechanical provocation
• Pain that may be a more constant dull ache or throb at rest

• Pain in the absence of:
  • dysesthesias (e.g., electrical, coldness, burning)
  • night pain/disturbed sleep

Objective
• Observed antalgic postures/movements

(osseo-capsular-ligamentous) tissues.[2] Furthermore, if aggravating inputs continue (e.g., ongoing inflammatory mechanisms), sensitization of pain receptors may lead to lowering of pain thresholds (hyperalgesia/allodynia) (discussed in Chapter 1).

While clinical features of nociceptive pain have not been widely studied, pain consultants and musculoskeletal physiotherapists in a Delphi study identified a list of eight symptoms and four signs that are indicative nociceptive pain. These criteria were further assessed in 464 low back pain patients and regression analysis showed six symptoms and one sign to have significantly high levels of classification accuracy[70] (Table 6.4).

Classification of peripheral neuropathic/peripheral sensitization pain mechanisms

Peripheral neuropathic pain is caused by pathology/dysfunction affecting the somatosensory system[72] due to trauma, sports injuries, compression, inflammation, and ischemia[73]. Symptoms in such cases include spontaneous pain, paresthesia and dysthesia, in addition to pain provoked by normally innocuous stimuli (allodynia) and exaggerated or prolonged pain to noxious stimuli (hyperalgesia). Studies suggest that many patients with musculoskeletal pain present with symptoms suggestive of neuropathic pain, especially in those presenting with neck, shoulder, and low back pain.[74,75] People with presenting neuropathic pain components also show higher ratings of pain intensity in addition to comorbid affective disorders and poorer health-related quality of life.[70]

Mechanical irritation of peripheral nerves can lead to musculoskeletal tissue dysfunction. Repetitive compressive, tensile, shear and vibration forces acting on or adjacent to neural tissue passing through anatomically narrow tissue spaces can lead to mechanical (e.g., strain, contraction) irritation of neural tissue (Figure 6.3). Equally, injured somatic tissue releasing inflammatory mediators in or adjacent to peripheral nerves may also lead to chemically irritated neural tissue[76]. However, peripheral neuropathic pain is not a single mechanism, but a result of pathophysiological processes that alter the structure and function of peripheral nerves and their central terminals.[70] As with nociceptive pain, there

Table 6.5: Clinical indictors of peripheral neuropathic pain (adapted from Smart and Colleagues)

Subjective
• Pain that is referred in a dermatomal or cutaneous distribution
• History of nerve injury, pathology, or mechanical compromise
Objective
• Pain that is provoked by mechanical movement tests that compress neural tissue

are no gold standard tests which diagnose peripheral neuropathic pain. Thus, classification is gained by gaining subjective information on pain-related symptoms and signs reflective of neuropathic pain mechanisms.

Several assessment tools have been developed to help discriminate neuropathic pain from non-neuropathic pain, the most widely used being the painDETECT[75] and the Standardized Evaluation of Pain (StEP).[68] However, like their work concerning the clinical features of nociceptive pain, Smart and

Table 6.6: Clinical indictors of central sensitization pain (adapted from Smart and colleagues)

Subjective
• Pain that is:
• disproportionate
• non-mechanical
• unpredictable
in response to nonspecific/multiple aggravating factors
• Pain that is disproportionate to the nature and extent of injury/dysfunction/pathology
• Pain that is strongly associated with maladaptive psychosocial factors
Objective
• Pain that is diffuse/non-anatomical on palpation

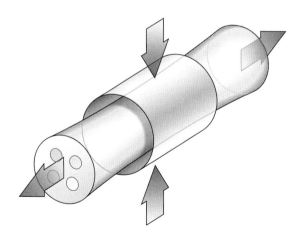

Figure 6.3
A schematic representation of physical stresses placed on a peripheral nerve

colleagues also developed a set of symptoms and signs that predicted peripheral neuropathic pain in people presenting with low back pain[77] (Table 6.5).

Classification of central sensitization pain mechanisms

Central sensitization refers to enhanced neurophysiological processes occurring throughout the central nervous system including the spinal cord and supraspinal areas of the brain that contribute to up-regulation of the nociceptive system[78] (discussed in Chapters 2 and 3). However, central sensitization also refers to the increased responsiveness of central spinal neurons to input from peripheral large and small diameter fibers.[79] Thus, it is important to understand that both 'top-down' and 'bottom-up' pathophysiological mechanisms exist. For example, the presence of non-segmental diffuse areas of pain on palpation (allodynia) is considered clinically to reflect central nervous system dysfunction. Here, increased synaptic excitability and expanded receptive fields within the dorsal horn allow non-nociceptive afferent input to activate second order neurons.[80] CP disorders such as chronic whiplash disorders, temporomandibular joint disorder, chronic low back pain, and fibromyalgia frequently present with symptoms that reflect central sensitization.[79]

In such disorders, pain is more widespread, persists beyond expected healing times, pain severity is disproportionate to objective clinical testing, and there is hypersensitivity to other sensory stimuli (light, sound, temperature). These symptoms are further associated with cognitive-affective dysfunction.[81] Therefore, the ability to recognize patients with symptoms suggestive of central sensitization would help in deciding on suitable management strategies. However, it is

Table 6.7: Additional signs and symptoms often seen in patients with central sensitization[82]

Sign or symptom	Description (questioning/examination)
Inconsistent clinical findings	Inconsistent findings across clinical tests
Muscle weakness	Subjective sensation of weakness in whole limb/lack of muscle control in whole limb
Numbness	Numbness not localized and with nonsegmental distribution
Phantom swelling sensation	Sensation of swollen limb in the absence of visual evidence of edema or swelling
Phantom swelling enhancement	Phantom swelling sensations increase when patient closes eyes
Phantom swelling diminishment	Phantom swelling sensations decrease when viewing affected limb
Phantom stiffness	Sensation of joint stiffness in the absence of objective signs of decreased mobility
Dyskinesthesia	Sensation of clumsiness or less aware of where limbs are in space
Impaired tactile localization	Increased two-point discrimination in the affected region
Sleeping difficulties	Difficulty falling asleep/unrefreshed sleep
Cognitive deficits	Poor concentration, short-term memory disturbance/brain fog
Altered perception of affected body part	Perception that body part is smaller or larger than normal/inability to feel the affected part of the body without visual or tactile input

unclear whether manual therapists recognize the process of central sensitization in patients[81] and in many cases it remains an 'unrelated' theoretical concept that is unlikely to be present in a person presenting with musculoskeletal pain. Here, data strongly suggest that sensory hypersensitivity influences the outcome of physical therapy for people with chronic whiplash disorders, in which group those with widespread hyperalgesia show least improvement.[79]

Smart and colleagues, who in their comprehensive set of studies investigating pain classification worked through the research processes described in the previous sections, identified key symptoms and signs associated with central sensitization in patients with low back pain. Here, they found three symptoms and one sign that predicted central sensitization in people with low back pain (Table 6.6).[80]

In addition to the above classifications, Nijs and colleagues describe additional signs and symptoms often seen in patients with central sensitization (Table 6.7).[82] However, while not required for classification, descriptions of these findings are informative in helping to clarify the presence of central sensitization in people presenting with CP disorders.

Clinical reasoning and chronic pain

Models of clinical reasoning in manual therapeutic settings were traditionally similar to those of physicians and chiefly concerned with a hypothetico-deductive diagnosis.[83] This analytical reasoning model states that truth or reality (knowledge) is objective and measurable. Here, observation and examination produce a result that can be validated against available standards and are thus diagnostic and predictive.[84] For example, in cases of chronic low back or neck pain a manual therapist may attribute symptoms to incorrect heavy lifting practices or poor workplace posture, with treatment involving only a 'hands-on' muscle and/or joint treatment. Therapists may attempt to validate somatic tissues and nerves as a definite source of pain and advise patients to reduce physical exercise and thus increase the chances of patients becoming fear-avoidant.[85]

Importantly, manual therapists' attitudes towards chronic musculoskeletal pain are now changing and they are more aware of biopsychosocial beliefs, helping to inform more appropriate diagnoses and management strategies. Additionally, an advance in our understanding of the neurophysiological basis of pain now helps assessment, treatment, and prognoses for people with CP. Moreover, this mechanism-based approach has been expanded by integrating our knowledge concerning the physiology of stress with the biopsychosocial model of pain and perceived disability.[66] Smart and Doody promisingly show that experienced musculoskeletal physiotherapists show a dynamic, multidimensional reasoning ability based on five reasoning-based categories: (1) biomedical, (2) psychosocial, (3) pain mechanisms, (4) chronicity, and (5) pain severity. Concerning nonspecific low back pain, Josephson and colleagues show that physiotherapists' clinical reasoning reflect the view that intervention was related to case complexity, with more environmental factors being related to very complex cases.[86]

Summary

Pain is a subjective state, and thus its evaluation depends on what the patient says and does in response to pain. While listening to the patient's reporting of pain is important, relying solely on this and standard medical evaluation can be unreliable. The initial assessments of pain intensity, pain affect, and pain quality is important to the initial assessment of people presenting with CP. Administering self-reporting measures is considered by clinicians and researchers as the most direct way to access these pain domains.[10] However, it is often difficult to select the most appropriate approach, one that is adequately inclusive but effective. It is important when selecting measurement tools that they should be valid, reliable, and, importantly, responsive: that is they are sensitive to change over a course of treatment. Given the numerous psychosocial and behavioral factors that affect subjective reporting of pain, the use of validated measures is essential for successful pain management.

Chapter 6

Critical information can be gathered from the case history, observation of patient behavior, and physical examination to help identify the underlying mechanisms of CP. Here, as opposed to diagnosing patients based on etiologies, it is probably more relevant to identify in individual patients what mechanism(s) operates to produce the subjective experience. This information can then be used to determine the most suitable management plan.

Manual therapists see pain conditions from many different diagnostic categories (e.g., osteoarthritis, fibromyalgia, chronic low back pain); in some, pain may be due to peripheral nociceptive input while others may have pain symptoms reflective of peripheral or central sensitization or multiple mechanisms. Thus, according to Woolf, a good starting point is to understand what mechanisms can potentially produce pain.

References

1. Dansie EJ, Turk DC. Assessment of patients with chronic pain. British Journal of Anaesthesia. 2013;111(1):19–25.

2. Kumar SP, Saha S. Mechanism-based classification of pain for physical therapy management in palliative care: a clinical commentary. Indian Journal of Palliative Care. 2011;17(1):80–6.

3. McCracken LM. 'Attention' to pain in persons with chronic pain: a behavioral approach. Behavior Therapy. 1997;28(2):271–84.

4. Holroyd KA, Malinoski P, Davis MK, Lipchik GL. The three dimensions of headache impact: pain, disability and affective distress. Pain. 1999;83(3):571–8.

5. Breivik H, Collett B, Ventafridda V, Cohen R, Gallacher D. Survey of chronic pain in Europe: prevalence, impact on daily life, and treatment. European Journal of Pain. 2006;10(4):287–333.

6. Hooten W, Timming R, Belgrade M, Gaul J, Goertz M, et al. Assessment and management of chronic pain. 6th ed. Bloomington, Minnesota: Institute for Clinical Systems Improvement; 2013.

7. Pasero C, McCaffery M. Pain assessment and pharmacologic management. St Louis: Mosby; 2011.

8. C de C Williams A. Chronic pain investigation. In: Lindsey S, Powell G, editors. Handbook of clinical adult psychology. 3rd ed. London: Routledge; 2007. p. 689–707.

9. Turk DC, Melzack R. The measurement of pain and the assessment of people experiencing pain. In: Turk DC, Melzack R, editors. Handbook of pain assessment. 2nd ed. New York: Guilford Press; 2011.

10. Jensen MP, Karoly P. Self-reporting scales and procedures for assessing pain in adults. In: Turk DC, Melzack R, editors. Handbook of pain assessment 2nd ed. New York: Guilford Press; 2011. p. 19–44.

11. Turk DC, Robinson J. Assessments of patients with chronic pain. In: Turk DC, Melzack R, editors. Handbook of pain assessment. 2nd ed. New York: Guilford Press; 2011. p. 188–210.

12. Blyth FM, March LM, Nicholas MK, Cousins MJ. Chronic pain, work performance and litigation. Pain. 2003;103(1–2):41–7.

13. de CWAC, Davies HT, Chadury Y. Simple pain rating scales hide complex idiosyncratic meanings. Pain. 2000;85(3):457–63.

14. Riffenburgh RH. Chapter 2 - Planning analysis: what do i do with my data? Statistics in medicine, 3rd ed. San Diego: Academic Press; 2012. p. 27–63.

15. Vaughan L. Statistical methods for the information professional. 2nd ed. Bryans J, editor: Information Today; 2003.

16. Aaron LA, Mancl L, Turner JA, Sawchuk CN, Klein KM. Reasons for missing interviews in the daily electronic assessment of pain, mood, and stress. Pain. 2004;109(3):389–98.

17. Williamson A, Hoggart B. Pain: a review of three commonly used pain rating scales. Journal of Clinical Nursing. 2005;14(7):798–804.

18. Ogon M, Krismer M, Sollner W, Kantner-Rumplmair W, Lampe A. Chronic low back pain measurement with visual analogue scales in different settings. Pain. 1996;64(3):425–8.

19. Aun C, Lam YM, Collett B. Evaluation of the use of visual analogue scale in Chinese patients. Pain. 1986;25(2):215–21.

20. Price DD, Staud R, Robinson ME. How should we use the visual analogue scale (VAS) in rehabilitation outcomes? II: Visual analogue scales as ratio scales: an alternative to the view. Journal of Rehabilitation Medicine. 2012;44(9):800–4.

21. Thomee R, Grimby G, Wright BD, Linacre JM. Rasch analysis of visual analog scale measurements before and after treatment of patellofemoral pain syndrome in women. Scandinavian Journal of Rehabilitation Medicine. 1995;27(3):145–51.

22. Price DD, McGrath PA, Rafii A, Buckingham B. The validation of visual analogue scales as ratio scale measures for chronic and experimental pain. Pain. 1983;17(1):45–56.

23. Price DD, Bush FM, Long S, Harkins SW. A comparison of pain measurement characteristics of mechanical visual analogue and simple numerical rating scales. Pain. 1994;56(2):217–26.

24. Price DD, Harkins SW. Combined use of experimental pain and visual analogue scales in providing standardized measurement of clinical pain. Clinical Journal of Pain. 1987;3(1):1–8.

25. Price DD, Patel R, Robinson ME, Staud R. Characteristics of electronic visual analogue and numerical scales for ratings of experimental pain in healthy

subjects and fibromyalgia patients. Pain. 2008;140(1):158–66.

26. Joyce CR, Zutshi DW, Hrubes V, Mason RM. Comparison of fixed interval and visual analogue scales for rating chronic pain. European Journal of Clinical Pharmacology. 1975;8(6):415–20.

27. Dijkers M. Comparing quantification of pain severity by verbal rating and numeric rating scales. Journal of Spinal Cord Medicine. 2010;33(3):232–42.

28. Aicher B, Peil H, Peil B, Diener H-C. Pain measurement: visual analogue scale (VAS) and verbal rating scale (VRS) in clinical trials with OTC analgesics in headache. Cephalalgia. 2012;32(3):185–97.

29. Wong DL, Baker CM. Pain in children: comparison of assessment scales. Oklahoma Nurse. 1988;33(1):8.

30. Kim EJ, Buschmann MT. Reliability and validity of the Faces Pain Scale with older adults. International Journal of Nursing Studies. 2006;43(4):447–56.

31. Bijur PE, Silver W, Gallagher EJ. Reliability of the visual analog scale for measurement of acute pain. Academic Emergency Medicine. 2001;8(12):1153–7.

32. Rosier EM, Iadarola MJ, Coghill RC. Reproducibility of pain measurement and pain perception. Pain. 2002;98(1–2):205–16.

33. Farrar JT, Young JP, Jr., LaMoreaux L, Werth JL, Poole RM. Clinical importance of changes in chronic pain intensity measured on an 11-point numerical pain rating scale. Pain. 2001;94(2):149–58.

34. Boonstra AM, Schiphorst Preuper HR, Reneman MF, Posthumus JB, Stewart RE. Reliability and validity of the visual analogue scale for disability in patients with chronic musculoskeletal pain. International Journal of Rehabilitation Research. 2008;31(2):165–9.

35. Childs JD, Piva SR, Fritz JM. Responsiveness of the numeric pain rating scale in patients with low back pain. Spine. 2005;30(11):1331–4.

36. Bech RD, Lauritsen J, Ovesen O, Overgaard S. The verbal rating scale is reliable for assessment of postoperative pain in hip fracture patients. Pain Research and Treatment. 2015;2015:7.

37. Brunelli C, Zecca E, Martini C, Campa T, Fagnoni E, Bagnasco M, et al. Comparison of numerical and verbal rating scales to measure pain exacerbations in patients with chronic cancer pain. Health and Quality of Life Outcomes. 2010;8(1):1–8.

38. Ferreira-Valente MA, Pais-Ribeiro JL, Jensen MP. Validity of four pain intensity rating scales. Pain. 2011;152(10):2399–404.

39. Huber A, Suman AL, Rendo CA, Biasi G, Marcolongo R, Carli G. Dimensions of 'unidimensional' ratings of pain and emotions in patients with chronic musculoskeletal pain. Pain. 2007;130(3):216–24.

40. Menezes Costa LdC, Maher CG, McAuley JH, Costa LOP. Systematic review of cross-cultural adaptations of McGill Pain Questionnaire reveals a paucity of clinimetric testing. Journal of Clinical Epidemiology. 2009;62(9):934–43.

41. Katz J, Melzack R. The McGill Pain Questionnaire. In: Melzack R, Turk DC, editors. Handbook of pain assessment. 3rd ed. New York: Guilford Press; 2011.

42. Breivik H, Borchgrevink PC, Allen SM, Rosseland LA, Romundstad L, Breivik Hals EK, et al. Assessment of pain. British Journal of Anaesthesia. 2008;101(1):17–24.

43. Jensen MP, Karoly P. Self-report scales and procedures for assessing pain in adults. In Turk DC, Melzack R. Handbook of pain assessment. 3rd ed. New York: Guildford Press; 2001. ch. 2.

44. Smart KM, Blake C, Staines A, Doody C. The discriminative validity of 'nociceptive,' 'peripheral neuropathic,' and 'central sensitization' as mechanisms-based classifications of musculoskeletal pain. Clinical Journal of Pain. 2011;27(8):655–63.

45. Jensen MP, Gammaitoni AR, Olaleye DO, Oleka N, Nalamachu SR, Galer BS. The pain quality assessment scale: assessment of pain quality in carpal tunnel syndrome. Journal of Pain. 2006;7(11):823–32.

46. Smart KM, Blake C, Staines A, Doody C. Clinical indicators of 'nociceptive', 'peripheral neuropathic' and 'central' mechanisms of musculoskeletal pain. A Delphi survey of expert clinicians. Manual Therapy. 2010;15(1):80–7.

47. Bennett M. The LANSS Pain Scale: the Leeds assessment of neuropathic symptoms and signs. Pain. 2001;92(1–2):147–57.

48. Bennett MI, Smith BH, Torrance N, Potter J. The S-LANSS score for identifying pain of predominantly neuropathic origin: validation for use in clinical and postal research. Journal of Pain. 2005;6(3):149–58.

49. Galer BS, Jensen MP. Development and preliminary validation of a pain measure specific to neuropathic pain: the Neuropathic Pain Scale. Neurology. 1997;48(2):332–8.

50. Boureau F, Doubrere JF, Luu M. Study of verbal description in neuropathic pain. Pain. 1990;42(2):145–52.

51. Bouhassira D, Attal N, Alchaar H, Boureau F, Brochet B, Bruxelle J, et al. Comparison of pain syndromes associated with nervous or somatic lesions and development of a new neuropathic pain diagnostic questionnaire (DN4). Pain. 2005;114(1–2):29–36.

52. Ware JE, Jr., Sherbourne CD. The MOS 36-item short-form health survey (SF-36). I.Conceptual framework and item selection. Medical Care. 1992;30(6):473–83.

53. Stratford PW, Binkley JM. A comparison study of the back pain functional scale and Roland Morris Questionnaire. North American Orthopaedic Rehabilitation Research Network. Journal of Rheumatology. 2000;27(8):1928–36.

54. Jamison RN, Edwards RR. Integrating pain management in clinical practice. Journal of Clinical Psychology in Medical Settings. 2012;19(1):49–64.

55. Wood BM, Nicholas MK, Blyth F, Asghari A, Gibson S. The utility of the short version of the Depression Anxiety Stress Scales (DASS-21) in elderly patients with persistent pain: does age make a difference? Pain Medicine (Malden, Mass). 2010;11(12):1780–90.

56. Morley S, Williams AC, Black S. A confirmatory factor analysis of the Beck Depression Inventory in chronic pain. Pain. 2002;99(1–2):289–98.

57. Jackson-Koku G. Beck Depression Inventory. Occupational Medicine. 2016;66(2):174–5.

58. Jensen MP, Karoly P. Control beliefs, coping efforts, and adjustment to chronic pain. Journal of Consulting and Clinical Psychology. 1991;59(3):431–8.

59. Denison E, Asenlof P, Lindberg P. Self-efficacy, fear avoidance, and pain intensity as predictors of disability in subacute and chronic musculoskeletal pain patients in primary health care. Pain. 2004;111(3):245–52.

60. Costa Lda C, Maher CG, McAuley JH, Hancock MJ, Smeets RJ. Self-efficacy is more important than fear of movement in mediating the relationship between pain and disability in chronic low back pain. European Journal of Pain. 2011;15(2):213–9.

61. Sullivan MJL, Bishop SR, Pivik J. The Pain Catastrophizing Scale: development and validation. Psychological Assessment. 1995;7(4):524–32.

62. Waddell G, Newton M, Henderson I, Somerville D, Main CJ. A Fear-Avoidance Beliefs Questionnaire (FABQ) and the role of fear-avoidance beliefs in chronic low back pain and disability. Pain. 1993;52(2):157–68.

63. Asghari A, Nicholas MK. Pain self-efficacy beliefs and pain behaviour. A prospective study. Pain. 2001;94(1):85–100.

64. Siddall PJ, Duggan AW. Towards a mechanisms-based approach to pain medicine. Anesthesia and Analgesia. 2004;99(2):455–6.

65. Smart K, Doody C. Mechanisms-based clinical reasoning of pain by experienced musculoskeletal physiotherapists. Physiotherapy. 2006;92(3):171–8.

66. Smart K, Doody C. The clinical reasoning of pain by experienced musculoskeletal physiotherapists. Manual Therapy. 2007;12(1):40–9.

67. Jones M. Clinical reasoning and pain. Manual Therapy. 1995;1(1):17–24.

68. Scholz J, Mannion RJ, Hord DE, Griffin RS, Rawal B, Zheng H, et al. A novel tool for the assessment of pain: validation in low back pain. PLoS Med. 2009;6(4):e1000047.

69. Schafer A, Hall T, Briffa K. Classification of low back-related leg pain – a proposed patho-mechanism-based approach. Manual Therapy. 2009;14(2):222–30.

70. Smart KM, Blake C, Staines A, Thacker M, Doody C. Mechanisms-based classifications of musculoskeletal pain: part 3 of 3: symptoms and signs of nociceptive pain in patients with low back (+/- leg) pain. Manual Therapy. 2012;17(4):352–7.

71. Clauw DJ. Diagnosing and treating chronic musculoskeletal pain based on the underlying mechanism(s). Best Practice and Research Clinical Rheumatology. 2015;29(1):6–19.

72. Treede RD, Jensen TS, Campbell JN, Cruccu G, Dostrovsky JO, Griffin JW, et al. Neuropathic pain: redefinition and a grading system for clinical and research purposes. Neurology. 2008;70(18):1630–5.

73. Woolf CJ. Dissecting out mechanisms responsible for peripheral neuropathic pain: implications for diagnosis and therapy. Life Sciences. 2004;74(21):2605–10.

74. Bouhassira D, Lantéri-Minet M, Attal N, Laurent B, Touboul C. Prevalence of chronic pain with neuropathic characteristics in the general population. Pain. 2008;136(3):380–7.

75. Freynhagen R, Baron R, Gockel U, Tolle TR. painDETECT: a new screening questionnaire to identify neuropathic components in patients with back pain. Current Medical Research and Opinion. 2006;22(10):1911–20.

76. Topp KS, Boyd BS. Structure and biomechanics of peripheral nerves: nerve responses to physical stresses and implications for physical therapist practice. Physical Therapy. 2006;86(1):92–109.

77. Smart KM, Blake C, Staines A, Thacker M, Doody C. Mechanisms-based classifications of musculoskeletal pain: part 2 of 3: symptoms and signs of peripheral neuropathic pain in patients with low back (+/- leg) pain. Manual Therapy. 2012;17(4):345–51.

78. Staud R, Craggs JG, Robinson ME, Perlstein WM, Price DD. Brain activity related to temporal summation of C-fiber evoked pain. Pain. 2007;129(1–2):130–42.

79. Nijs J, Van Houdenhove B, Oostendorp RAB. Recognition of central sensitization in patients with musculoskeletal pain: application of pain neurophysiology in manual therapy practice. Manual Therapy. 2010;15(2):135–41.

80. Smart KM, Blake C, Staines A, Thacker M, Doody C. Mechanisms-based classifications of musculoskeletal pain: part 1 of 3: symptoms and signs of central sensitisation in patients with low back (+/- leg) pain. Manual Therapy. 2012;17(4):336–44.

81. Woolf CJ. Central sensitization: implications for the diagnosis and treatment of pain. Pain. 2011;152(3 Suppl):S2–15.

82. Nijs J, Torres-Cueco R, van Wilgen CP, Girbes EL, Struyf F, Roussel N, et al. Applying modern pain neuroscience in clinical practice: criteria for the classification of central sensitization pain. Pain Physician. 2014;17(5):447–57.

83. Payton OD. Clinical reasoning process in physical therapy. Physical Therapy. 1985;65(6):924–8.

84. Edwards I, Jones M, Carr J, Braunack-Mayer A, Jensen GM. Clinical reasoning strategies in physical therapy. Physical Therapy. 2004;84(4):312–30; discussion 31–5.

85. Nijs J, Roussel N, Paul van Wilgen C, Köke A, Smeets R. Thinking beyond muscles and joints: therapists' and patients' attitudes and beliefs regarding chronic musculoskeletal pain are key to applying effective treatment. Manual Therapy. 2013;18(2):96–102.

86. Josephson I, Bülow P, Hedberg B. Physiotherapists' clinical reasoning about patients with non-specific low back pain, as described by the International Classification of Functioning, Disability and Health. Disability and Rehabilitation. 2011;33(22–23):2217–28.

Efficacy of manual therapy for chronic musculoskeletal pain

Introduction

Nonpharmacological treatments have become a common and essential part of managing people with chronic pain (CP). However, practitioners and patients alike continue to consider CP as a prolonged form of acute pain, and the attraction of a cure has delayed the implementation of more appropriate multidisciplinary approaches. As discussed in previous chapters, CP develops as a result of many factors. First, CP progresses as a result of changes in nociceptive function due to local tissue damage from injury, to disease, or to damage to the peripheral and/or central nervous system presently not demonstrable using current diagnostic procedures.[1] Second, the level and extent of CP is determined largely by a person's unique genotype, early life history, the effects of environmental and socioeconomic influences, and psychological factors. Thus, to treat people with CP requires a practitioner to both understand and recognize all these factors. Although CP disorders are classified on the basis of anatomical location, cause (e.g., nociceptive, neuropathic) and body systems,[2,3] there is substantial overlap concerning underlying pathological mechanisms for most pain conditions for which, presently, for the most part, there are no cures. Thus, like other chronic problems such as diabetes mellitus and hypertension, ongoing management is essential, not only from health care professionals but also from patients themselves.[4]

In addition to accepted pharmacological treatments, a growing number of non-pharmacological therapies now show noteworthy efficacy in the management of CP conditions. Practitioners should be familiar with such approaches, categorized as behavioral, cognitive, integrative, educational, and physical therapies, so that they can offer a flexible approach to CP that is both manageable and worthwhile for the patient. A comprehensive review of the effectiveness of all these treatments for specific pain conditions is beyond the scope of this chapter, which focuses on manual therapy, therapeutic exercise, and acupuncture. To convey what are considered the most efficacious of treatment approaches, systematic search protocols were used to locate relevant articles for review in this chapter.

Levels of evidence and clinical studies

Modern day health care relies not only on individual clinical skills, but additionally on the best information on the effectiveness of each intervention available to practitioners, patients, and policy makers. Evidence-based approaches rely on global, unbiased, and independently reviewed information that may help to improve patient care. The quality or the strength of evidence is determined by the methods used to minimize bias within study design.[7] Therefore, evidence is ranked to assign a level of proof for the results found in clinical trials and other research studies. Before the efficacy of physical therapy is reviewed, a brief outline of evidence-based practice, especially relating to therapeutic intervention, is presented below.

Evidence hierarchy

Evidence-based practice hierarchies rank study types based on the rigor (strength and accuracy) of their methods: the higher up the hierarchy, the more rigorous the methodology and thus the less likely to be affected by bias. For the purpose of this chapter, intervention and prognostic study design are briefly reviewed. Table 7.1 shows a simplified table for levels of evidence. For a more detailed classification, the Centre for Evidence-Based Medicine webpage is recommended.[5]

Systematic reviews and meta-analyses

Systematic reviews and meta-analyses lie at the top of most hierarchies, while expert opinion and anecdotal evidence lie at the bottom. Meta-analysis is a method allowing results of multiple studies to be combined

Chapter 7

Table 7.1: A simplified table for hierarchical levels of evidence[6]

Level of evidence	Type of study
1a	• Meta-analyses and systematic reviews of (homogenous) RCTs
1b	• Individual RCTs (with narrow confidence intervals)
2a	• Systematic reviews of (homogenous) cohort studies of 'exposed' and 'unexposed' subjects
2b	• Individual cohort studies/low quality RCTs
3a	• Systematic reviews of (homogenous) case-control studies
3b	• Individual case-control studies
4	• Case series/low quality cohort or case-control studies
5	• Expert opinion based on non-systematic reviews/mechanistic studies

to increase statistical power to identify real effects. Systematic reviews, with or without meta-analysis, are considered to show the best evidence for all types of research question as they are based on the findings of multiple studies with the most rigorous methods found in systematic searches of literature databases (filtered information). Because critical appraisal of studies has been completed by more than one reviewer, it not only saves the reader time but also provides a more conclusive answer than a single clinical study. However, it should be noted that such reviews can take years to complete and thus can be outdated by more recent evidence. Additionally, it should be noted that a large, methodologically rigorous RCT may show more conclusive evidence than a systematic review of smaller, less rigorous randomized controlled trials (RCTs).[7]

Primary studies

If an up-to-date, well-designed systematic review is not available, primary studies (original research) may help to answer a clinical question. However, this type of information is unfiltered and data have not been synthesized, and thus are more difficult to interpret and apply to clinical practice. Manual therapists are usually interested in studies that involve treatment interventions, identification of risk factors for injury/ disease, and prognosis of clinical conditions.[8] In each case, a variety of available study designs may be used to help answer a given research question. Often, however, the choices of research methods are governed by available resources, such as equipment, expertise in data collection, data analysis, and subject availability. For example, RCTs are most appropriate for studying the effect of an intervention (therapeutic studies) in experimental environments because of unbiased distributions of confounding factors and blinding of subjects to evaluators. However, RCTs are expensive both in time and money, and may also be prone to volunteer bias.[9] Concerning the effect of therapy over time (prognostic studies), highest evidence is gained from prospective cohort studies where all patients enroll at the same point in their disease and where over 80% (of enrolled patients) follow up at the same time point.[5] However, while subjects can be matched with disease time points, gender, age, etc., randomization is not possible and blinding of evaluators is difficult. Moreover, hidden variables that may further confound results, such as a subject history of drug use or smoking, may not be known to evaluators.[9]

Efficacy and evidence for physical therapies

There are a number of physical treatments used to manage chronic musculoskeletal pain. These include manual therapies, exercise, acupuncture, electrotherapy, and thermal modalities. However, although different therapies are advocated by different groups of practitioners, it is increasingly evident that many physical therapists are adopting more evidence-based approaches to chronic pain management.[10] Thus, the aim of this section is to provide current evidence for the efficacy for each of the above therapeutic categories. Additionally, given the variation in quality of evidence, the following sections will focus on results mainly from systematic reviews and meta-analyses. It should also be noted that many different pain and disability measures (see previous chapter) are used between studies, thus showing an apparent lack of homogeneity in findings between studies. This chapter reviews studies discussing or using only validated outcome measures. A review of the multitude of therapeutic approaches used by physical therapists is beyond the scope of this chapter. Thus, this chapter will focus on manual therapy, therapeutic exercise, and acupuncture as these therapeutic approaches are described as the most commonly used within manual therapeutic settings. However, other modalities such as electrotherapy (e.g., transcutaneous electrical nerve stimulation, interferential therapies) and thermal treatments (e.g., superficial and deep tissue heating, ultrasound, and cryotherapy) may be briefly discussed in chapters reviewing pain disorders. For more in-depth discussion of these treatment modalities, please refer to Wright and Sluka,[10] Clar, et al.,[11] and Chang et al.[12]

Manual therapy

Manual therapy techniques are intended to promote movement and relieve pain in musculoskeletal structures.[10] Techniques such as joint manipulation and mobilization are aimed at moving joints in specific directions and at different speeds in order to restore movement. Active and passive muscle stretching is also used to improve muscle activation and function,[13] while soft tissue techniques are aimed at mobilizing skin, underlying muscle, and connective tissue. Within manual therapy, most research has focused on joint mobilization, manipulation, and massage, with studies showing varying degrees of methodological rigor and treatment efficacy. The most common classification of manual therapies is based on the distinction between massage, passive movement, mobilization, and manipulative techniques, as shown in Figure 7.1.

Chronic low back pain

Mobilization and manipulative techniques are most commonly applied to people complaining of low back pain and thus this is the most extensively researched. Studies show that manipulation techniques reduce pain intensity, decrease functional disability, and increase spinal mobility.[14–17] However, although these improvements are generally observed at one month follow-up, there is virtually no difference when compared to sham therapies or continued improvement at one year follow-up. Concerning mobilization techniques, studies show similar findings. For example, muscle energy technique[18,19] and posteroanterior mobilization[20] are shown to significantly improve lumbar range of motion over the short term while

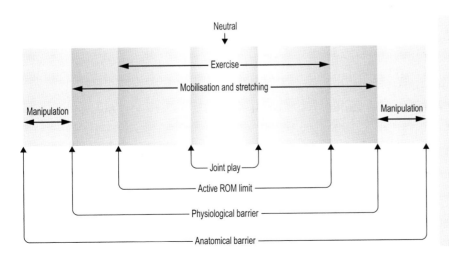

Figure 7.1

The presumed barriers to joint motion and the position and/or range of motion where manual therapy and exercise are performed

also increasing function and decreasing disability in patients with acute low back pain.[21] Overall, evidence suggests that multidisciplinary treatments involving both manipulation and mobilization techniques are more effective than general physical therapy, home exercise, and general practice medical care alone for reducing long-term disability.[22] However, while these individual techniques are effective for improvements in objective functional measurement of chronic low back pain, exercise still provides the longest interval of relief.[23] Currently, systematic review data show a mixture of findings. First, there is moderate to strong evidence for the benefit of manipulation over sham treatments for pain, function and quality of life in the short-term. Second, moderate evidence shows combinations of manipulation, mobilization, soft tissue techniques, and exercise for pain, function, and quality of life both short and long term are more beneficial than exercise alone, 'back school,' or usual medical care. Third, there is limited evidence showing the benefit of mobilization and soft tissue techniques combined with exercise compared to usual medical care.[24]

Meta-analyses generally show moderate efficacy for a range of techniques including high-velocity low amplitude (HLVA) manipulation, low-velocity low-amplitude (LVLA) oscillation, and massage techniques. However, an overall lack of studies with a low risk of bias prevents any strong recommendations regarding spinal manipulation.[25] Additionally, van Middelkoop and co-workers state that most RCTs show methodological deficiencies due mostly to heterogeneity of sampled populations, interventions outcome measures, and comparison groups.[26] More encouragingly, in a recent meta-analysis, Franke and colleagues show moderate-quality evidence that osteopathic manipulative treatment improves pain and functional status in patients with nonspecific low back pain.[26a] These meta-analyses also show manual techniques to be mostly effective in the short term for chronic non-specific low back pain (less than three weeks).

Concerning soft tissue technique, systematic reviews also show short-term benefits for the treatment of chronic low back pain.[27] However, like mobilization and manipulative techniques, the qualities

of studies reviewed are again poor. For example, two systematic reviews identified trials that focused on the efficacy of massage for chronic low back pain. Here, results showed that although massage showed similar short-term benefits compared to mobilization techniques, there was significant heterogeneity due to differences in interventions, differences in control groups, and duration of intervention.[28,29]

Chronic neck pain

The effects of manipulative and mobilization techniques for neck pain have also been examined using systematic reviews and meta-analysis. Similar to chronic low back pain, these techniques have been shown to provide short-term relief for both chronic neck and shoulder pain, especially in combination with advice and exercise.[30,31] Interestingly, in a smaller study, Gemmell and Miller compared the effectiveness of (1) specific segmental HVLA, (2) segmental mobilization, and (3) the Activator® instrument that delivered an HVLA within normal physiological ranges of the segments manipulated.[32] Although all treatments showed reduced disability and improved quality of life at 12-month follow up, sample sizes were small and thus it is uncertain if these treatment effects were true or simply due to chance.

In two Cochrane reviews, moderate quality evidence also suggests that multiple sessions of cervical manipulation and mobilization show similar effects on pain, function, and patient satisfaction at immediate follow-up.[33,34] The same reviews located only a few low-quality studies that support thoracic manipulation for pain reduction and increased function in chronic neck pain. Given the paucity and quality of studies relating to the manual treatment of neck and shoulder pain and the potential for positive outcomes, there is a need for better quality studies that should address: (1) treatment dose comparisons between manipulation and mobilization; (2) intermediate and long-term follow-up changes in pain severity, functional disability, and quality of life; and (3) the effectiveness of manipulative and mobilization techniques in the thoracic spine for chronic neck and shoulder pain.

The efficacy of soft tissue massage techniques for neck pain remains uncertain. Although Chinese massage, strain/counterstrain techniques when compared to no treatment,[35] and placebo[36] show significant improvement in subjects with chronic neck pain, levels of evidence are low.[37] Given these findings and the fact that assessed outcomes at immediate post-treatment are not adequate to assess clinical change, currently no recommendations can be made concerning the effectiveness of soft tissue massage techniques for chronic neck pain.

Chronic headaches

Despite the common occurrence of chronic cervicogenic and tension-type headaches, there are surprisingly very few recommendations concerning the efficacy of manual therapy techniques. This is due mainly to the lack of randomization, the lack of blinded evaluators, and inadequate statistical analysis.[38] However, although inconclusive, data show that spinal manipulation relieves cervicogenic and tension-type headaches. One systematic review found that of nine RCTs accepted for review, six suggested that spinal manipulation was more effective than physical therapy, gentle massage, drug therapy, or no intervention.[39] However, the remaining three studies show no differences in pain relief compared to placebo manipulation, physical therapy, massage, or waiting list controls. Due to a lack of methodological rigor, a similar review accepted only six studies from 55 potentially relevant articles.[40] Selected studies assessed different techniques such as spinal manipulation, classic massage, soft tissue massage, Cyriax mobilization, manual traction, and craniosacral techniques. Although, there is limited evidence for the effectiveness of soft tissue techniques, overall, results showed no rigorous evidence for other manual therapy techniques for reducing pain intensity in tension-type headaches. The authors in their discussion suggest that the aim of soft tissue techniques is to correct mechanical stress caused by myofascial tissue conditions, and thus they may be the effective choice. However, given that systematic reviews identify so few RCTs, and the potential for the use of manual therapy techniques, there is a clear need for well-designed RCTs evaluating the effectiveness of specific types of manual therapy techniques for both cervicogenic and tension-type headaches.

Chronic shoulder pain

Generally, studies investigating the effect of manual therapy in painful shoulder conditions examine a variety of techniques including manipulation, joint mobilization with and without other modes of passive therapy, and exercise.[11] Concerning rotator cuff disorders, there is moderate evidence from existing systematic reviews to suggest that manipulation and mobilization in conjunction with multimodal exercise show positive treatment outcomes compared to manipulation and mobilization alone.[41,42] However, the use of manipulation and mobilization alone only shows better outcomes when compared to no treatment. Furthermore, a recent Cochrane database study reviewing over 60 studies shows manual therapy and exercise to be similar in effect to glucocorticoid injection and subacromial decompression surgery.[43] These findings are substantiated by Dickens and colleagues, who showed that 26% of patients diagnosed with subacromial impingement that had failed three steroid injections into the subacromial space avoided surgery using mobilization techniques and exercises.[44] Regarding soft tissue techniques for painful shoulder conditions only a few studies exist. However, a systematic review of manual therapy for rotator cuff tendinopathy showed only one study investigating the effect of deep friction massage compared to therapeutic ultrasound. In this RCT, the authors reported patients receiving massage therapy showed lower pain at rest and greater active abduction range of motion. Unfortunately, however, they further state that these changes were not clinically significant.[45]

Some authors suggest that mobilization and manipulation techniques in combination with exercise including proprioceptive retraining are shown to be beneficial for adhesive capsulitis.[41,46] Studies have investigated a number of manual techniques that include HVLA, end-of-range mobilization, and mid-range mobilization in conjunction with or without movement of the shoulder girdle.[41] However, two recent systematic reviews show that these treatments are less effective than glucocorticoid injection in the short term while also showing a number of adverse reactions.[43,47] Encouragingly, however, Page and colleagues, in their Cochrane review of 32 studies, suggest that manual therapy and exercise do provide greater patient-reported treatment success in active range of motion. Nevertheless, due to low standards of methodological rigor, they go on to suggest high-quality RCTs are required to (1) compare combinations of manual therapy and exercise versus placebo or no intervention and (2) establish the benefits and harms of these forms of rehabilitation that reflect actual practice.[48]

Temporomandibular disorders

Temporomandibular disorders (TMD) are conditions that affect the temporomandibular joint, the masticatory muscles, and related structures.[49] Manual therapy has been used for many years for the treatment of such conditions; however, evidence regarding their effectiveness is outdated. Recently, two systematic reviews (same research group) examined the quality of RCTs investigating the effectiveness of manual therapy and exercise compared to more standard treatments.[50,51] The first review investigated the effectiveness of manual therapy for the management of pain and limited range of motion in people with signs and symptoms of TMD where seven of the eight RCTs included were of high methodological quality. Results encouragingly showed that myofascial release and massage techniques to the masticatory muscles were equally as effective as toxin botulinum injections[52] and more effective than controls. Equally, although upper cervical manipulation and mobilization techniques[53] were more effective than controls, thoracic manipulative techniques were not.[54]

The same group later reviewed the effectiveness of manual therapy and therapeutic exercise for TMD. Although they included 48 studies, evidence was considered low due to many RCTs showing unclear or high risk of bias.[51] Examples of the studies included in this review examined the effectiveness of posture correction and TMDs,[55] general jaw exercises combined with neck exercises,[56] intraoral myofascial therapy,[57] and jaw and neck exercises alone.[58] Overall, their results showed that manual therapy alone or in combination with both active and passive exercises of the jaw or cervical spine showed favorable outcomes.

Fibromyalgia

Clar and colleagues identified three systematic reviews evaluating manual therapy in patients with fibromyalgia.[11] While all three reviews showed significant improvement in most of the recognized tender points, these improvements were not maintained over time. In the same year, another systematic review identified 10 quantitative and qualitative studies assessing the effectiveness of different styles of massage therapy in fibromyalgia. Overall, they found that most styles of massage consistently improved quality of life. Although of low level evidence, narrative review data results nevertheless show that the effects of manual lymphatic drainage may be superior to connective tissue massage, while Swedish massage is shown to have little or no effect.[59] Additionally, while evidence is limited, results are favorable for the effectiveness of chiropractic manipulation,[60] craniosacral therapy,[61] and massage therapies[62] for fibromyalgia.

Summary

Although manual therapies for musculoskeletal disorders appear to be effective, the effect of these treatments on musculoskeletal pain generally lack methodical rigor and mostly show short-acting positive effects. Given the findings reviewed in this section, the efficacy of manual therapy would greatly benefit from studies that investigate single interventions on homogenous subject groups, for example the sampling of age- and gender-matched subject and comparison groups. Moreover, methodological rigor can be further increased by sampling subject groups with the same pain condition from the same population. Unhelpfully, previous studies have also used a wide range of self-reporting measures to gain data regarding levels of pain and disability, producing potentially different findings. Table 7.2 summarizes evidence for manual therapy and chronic low back pain, chronic neck pain, chronic headaches, chronic shoulder pain, temporomandibular disorders, and fibromyalgia.

Therapeutic exercise

Therapeutic exercise is used extensively in the management of a wide-range of musculoskeletal disorders.

Table 7.2: Evidence summary for manual therapy and chronic low back pain, chronic neck pain, chronic headaches, chronic shoulder pain, temporomandibular disorders, and fibromyalgia

Manual therapy	Evidence level	Outcome
Chronic low back pain		
Spinal mobilization alone	Moderate to high	Positive
Spinal manipulation alone	Moderate	Positive in short term
Soft tissue techniques alone	Poor to moderate	Positive in short term
Manual therapy–exercise combination	Moderate	Positive in short and long term
Chronic neck pain		
Cervical mobilization and manipulation combination	Moderate	Positive in short term
Thoracic manipulation	Poor to moderate	Positive in short term
Soft tissue techniques alone	Poor	Positive in short term
Chronic cervicogenic/tension headache		
Spinal manipulation	Poor	Unclear
Soft tissue technique	Poor	Positive
Mobilization	Poor	Unclear
Chronic shoulder pain (rotator cuff disorders)		
Mobilization and manipulation	Poor-moderate	Positive
Manual therapy–exercise combination	Moderate	Positive
Soft tissue technique	Poor	Unclear
Chronic shoulder pain (adhesive capsulitis)		
Mobilization and mobilization (mid and end ROM)	Moderate	Unclear-positive
Manual therapy-exercise combination	Moderate	Positive
Temporomandibular disorders		
Massage and myofascial release	Moderate to high	Positive
Manual therapy–exercise combination	Moderate	Positive
Fibromyalgia		
Massage and myofascial release	Poor to moderate	Positive

Clinical trials and systematic reviews repeatedly show high levels of evidence for the effectiveness of exercise for people with CP.[63–65] As described throughout this book, CP conditions are strongly associated with altered pain modulation, with research further showing that exercise helps to modulate pain perception and suppression, resulting in hyperalgesic effects.[63,66] Here, evidence suggests that exercise stimulates the release of endogenous opioids (endorphins) that are associated with changes in both mood and pain sensitivity (Figure 7.2).[67] Research also shows that the effect of exercise on muscle fibers, the cardiovascular system and the suppression of inflammatory mediators all influence similar brain mechanisms and neurotransmitters associated with descending inhibitory pain pathways.[68–71]

Many different forms of exercise have been used in the management of chronic musculoskeletal pain conditions. These include varying levels of aerobic exercise, strengthening exercise, mobility training, and specific re-activation and re-education exercise programs.[10] Types of aerobic exercise studied include stationary running, cycling, and step exercises. Strengthening exercises involve both isometric resistance in which the angle of the joint does not change (static contraction) and dynamic resistance, where muscle contraction does produce joint movement.[68] Mobility training includes yoga and various stretching exercises while re-activation training includes disciplines such as Pilates exercises. The following sections review the evidence for the above types of exercise.

Aerobic exercise

Aerobic exercise is shown to reduce pain severity in both healthy and older adults in experimental conditions.[29,68,69,72] Meta-analysis of the general hypoalgesic effects of exercise show that the overall effect of aerobic exercise moderately correlates with

Figure 7.2
Mechanisms underlying the effect of therapeutic exercise for chronic pain conditions

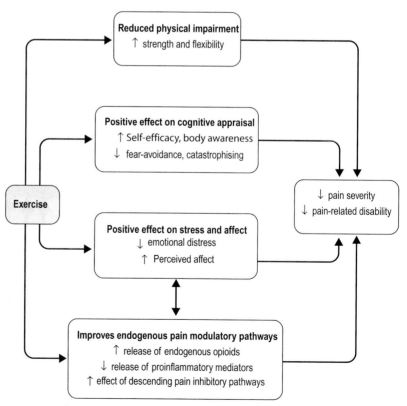

improvements in pain reduction.[68] However, these changes in pain perception generally last only up to 30 minutes.[73,74] Generally, analyses from the review show that the strongest reductions in pain perception were gained using moderate to high intensity exercises, while experimental studies using pressure pain stimuli show consistently more hyperalgesic effects compared to those using thermal stimulation. Unfortunately, nearly all studies investigating aerobic exercise use either healthy adults or subjects who are active or inactive rather than using people suffering from CP. Surprisingly, there have been very few studies investigating the effects of aerobic exercise on CP subjects. Of the studies located, two trials found that submaximal bicycle exercise had pain reducing effects on pressure pain thresholds in multiple body regions.[75,76] Thus, while at present evidence is weak, there is much potential for further research in this area.

Isometric exercise

Decreased muscle strength in patients with CP may be related to pain-induced inhibition of motor systems in addition to structural changes in muscle mass.[77,78] Such findings suggest that strengthening exercises should encourage morphological changes in muscles. In healthy adults, the effect of isometric exercise on the perception of pain is strong for both thresholds and intensity taken during and/or after exercise, regardless of site, intensity or duration of muscle contraction.[68] Interestingly, studies also show that hypoalgesic effects are increased with low to moderate intensity muscle contractions that are held for a longer duration. For example, the greatest changes in pain threshold and intensity follow low intensity contraction to failure (between five and nine minutes) compared to high intensity contractions held for three to five seconds.[79] Mechanisms for this response are thought to be due to the fact that when active motor units fatigue, higher threshold motor units become progressively recruited to maintain the necessary force.

Concerning studies in CP patients, local isometric exercises are shown to be of benefit for people with chronic low back pain,[80] neck pain,[81] and cervicogenic

headaches,[82] with increased levels of muscle activity being correlated with the degree of pain relief. Interestingly there are differences in the effect of isometric exercise between subjects with specific pain disorders (shoulder myalgia) and those with widespread pain (fibromyalgia).[83] Here, Lannersten and colleagues showed that distal (quadriceps) but not local (infraspinatus) contractions decreased shoulder pain intensities while subjects with fibromyalgia showed no changes in levels of pain for all contractions. These results suggest that exercising non-painful areas of the body will have beneficial effects. However, these findings interestingly highlight the lack of endogenous pain inhibition in people suffering widespread pain conditions.

Stretching exercise

Most studies investigate stretching not as a single treatment, but as part of a general exercise therapy routine.[84] Here, stretching has been shown to be most beneficial for chronic low back pain when incorporated into supervised exercise programs that also involve muscle strengthening exercises.[12,85] Only one systematic review examining the efficacy of stretching for people with chronic pain was found. Here, Barros and colleagues investigated the effects of muscle stretching exercises for people with fibromyalgia. While only four studies were accepted, they all showed that stretching exercises, regardless of type, reduced levels of pain.[86] However, as with many other studies, methodological rigor, interventions, parameters used and follow-up varied widely.

Several studies investigate the effects of yoga on chronic pain conditions. Recently, a systematic review evaluating the use of yoga for chronic low back pain found that yoga is effective in reducing pain as well as improving physical and mental function, with benefits lasting several months.[87] However, one of the studies included shows that although yoga is more effective than a self-care book, it is no more effective than general stretching.[88] These results are corroborated by Holtzman and Beggs who, in their meta-analysis of RCTs, found yoga to be consistently beneficial for people suffering chronic low back pain, but only in the short term.[89] Additionally, the authors also warn of methodological concerns that need to be addressed, especially the need for an active control group such as general stretching.

Concerning chronic neck pain, results from low-evidence articles generally suggest that stretching alone and/or with other exercise modalities may not change pain intensity or improve function immediately or at short-term follow-up.[82] However, Häkkinen and colleagues compared the effectiveness of a 12-month home-based combined strength and stretching program against stretching alone, randomized in two groups.[90] While there were no significant differences in improvements in both neck pain and disability between programs, they did find effects on neck pain to be encouraging. However, as with many program-based regimens, there was low adherence to training in both groups.

Dynamic resistance exercise

Dynamic strengthening exercises are aimed at improving neuromuscular control, strength, and endurance of muscles that are key to maintaining spinal and trunk stability.[91] While lumbar spinal stability relies in part on passive support such as ligaments and connective tissues of skeletal muscles, active contractions of muscles play a leading role. The central nervous system also has a significant role in spinal and trunk stability. By responding to sensations produced by muscles and passive soft tissue structures, the central nervous system controls motor coordination and thus governs physical actions to maintain stability.[92] These muscles include the transverse abdominis, lumbar multifidus, internal oblique, and quadratus lumborum.[93] First, the lumbar multifidus attach to each lumbar vertebral segment and the transverse abdominis and thus initiate a co-contraction mechanism.[94] Subsequent abdominal draw-in provides spinal segmental stability. Second, other more shallow core muscles (rectus abdominis, internal/external oblique muscles, erector spinae, quadratus lumborum, and hip muscle groups) also enable spinal control due to their attachments to the spine and thoracic ribs, and legs.[95]

Very few studies have examined the effectiveness of dynamic resistance exercise in people with chronic pain. Of these, only one has systematically reviewed their efficacy among chronic low back pain patients. Chang and colleagues identified only four articles suitable for review, each of which examined four core strength training exercises (trunk balance, stabilization, and motor control exercises), all of which were compared to more common resistance training such as straight leg raises, push-ups, and sit ups.[94] They found that while all core strength training exercises alleviated chronic low back pain, those focusing on the deep core muscles (transverse abdominis and lumbar multifidus) were most effective. Importantly, such programs have also been shown to have a positive effect on patients with low back pain due to spondylolisthesis and spondylolysis.[96] Interestingly, Ekstrom and colleagues aimed to determine which muscles were activated by dynamic resistance exercises so practitioners can have a better idea about the effect specific exercises have on muscle stabilization. Using surface EMG analysis they showed that dynamic resistance exercises such as unilateral bridge and quadruped extremity lifts significantly activate gluteus medius, gluteus maximus, and external oblique muscles.[95]

Summary

Currently, exercise therapy has been demonstrated to be effective at moderately decreasing levels of pain and levels of disability in people with chronic pain. Hayden and colleagues in their meta-analysis suggest the supervised, individually designed programs are the most effective, with stretching and muscle strengthening exercises being the most effective, especially for chronic low back pain.[84] Currently, it is thought that exercise in all forms is sufficient to activate endogenous pain inhibitory mechanisms in both animals and humans, especially opioid systems via the pituitary and hypothalamus.[10] For example, both swimming and running produce opioid-induced analgesia that is reversed by the administration of naloxone (an opioid receptor antagonist).[97,98] Interestingly, increases in beta-endorphins in peripheral circulation

Table 7.3: Evidence summary for aerobic, isometric, stretching, and dynamic resistance exercises in people with chronic pain

Therapeutic exercise	Evidence level	Outcome
Aerobic exercise High intensity	None	None
Moderate intensity	Weak	Unclear
Isometric exercise		
Moderate intensity – long duration	Moderate	Positive (CLBP, CNP, CH)
High intensity – short duration	Moderate	Unclear
Stretching exercise General muscle	Moderate	Positive (FMS)
stretches Yoga	Moderate	Positive in short term
Dynamic resistance exercise		Positive (CLBP, spondylolisthesis,
Motor control/stabilization	Moderate	spondylolysis)

are associated with both increased lactate concentrations and duration of exercise.[99] However, while evidence is strong, mechanisms of endogenous analgesia are relatively complex, with the exact type of analgesic mechanism possibly depending on the type of exercise stressor. Table 7.3 summarizes evidence for aerobic, isometric, stretching and dynamic resistance exercises in people with CP.

CLBP – chronic low back pain; CNP – chronic neck pain; CH – chronic headache; FMS – fibromyalgia

Acupuncture

Acupuncture is a treatment based on the theories of Traditional Chinese Medicine, in which its effect on pain-related disorders has been recognized from the earliest texts right up to present-day research.[100] A recent review estimated that 3.5 million American adults receive acupuncture treatment each year, with the number increasing each year over a recent 10 year period.[101] Currently, people receive acupuncture for CP conditions because of the low perceived effectiveness of conventional medical treatments.[102,103] However, while acupuncture is considered to have physiological effects relevant to analgesia,[104] there is no accepted mechanism by which it could produce long-lasting effects on CP. There are a number of methods of stimulating anatomical points in

acupuncture, such as needle insertion, with or without manipulation, and the application of surface pressure and electrical stimulation of inserted needles.[105] Of these, the use of thin metal needles that penetrate the skin and which are manually manipulated is by far the most extensively researched. Like other forms of non-pharmacological treatment approaches to musculoskeletal pain, acupuncture is thought to activate endogenous opioid analgesia in humans and animals. Blockade of opioid receptors in limbic system and descending pain pathway nuclei with naloxone in animals is shown to prevent analgesia.[10] Interestingly, animals made tolerant to mu- and delta-opioid agonists are only tolerant to 2 Hz but not 100 Hz electroacupuncture, whereas animals made tolerant to kappa-opioid are also tolerant to 100 Hz.[106] These results suggest that manual acupuncture and low-frequency and high-frequency types of electroacupuncture stimulation activate different analgesic opioid mechanisms.

While systematic reviews consistently show acupuncture to be effective for short-term pain relief in several CP conditions, such as low back pain, osteoarthritis, and chronic headache,[107] the long-term effects of acupuncture are less certain. For example, studies show decreases in pain at between 6- and 12-month follow-up for chronic headache[108] and osteoarthritis of the knee.[109] Concerning meta-analysis of chronic headaches across eight RCTs, Davis and colleagues found that subjects showed 1.34 fewer headache days per month and a 3.74 point decrease in pain intensity (VAS).[110] However, these findings were not significantly different to reports from subjects in sham groups. Generally, the effect of acupuncture on chronic low back pain is less conclusive, with some studies showing significant pain relief in the short-term[111] and others showing it to be only more effective than no or sham treatment.[112] However, as for nearly all therapies reviewed in this chapter, more effort is needed to improve both internal and external validity of primary studies. Concerning neck pain and neck pain with radicular symptoms, meta-analyses also show mixed results, with moderate evidence suggesting that acupuncture is more effective than sham treatments immediately and at short-term follow-up.[113]

Issues surrounding sham acupuncture

Typically, RCTs set sham treatments as a control to investigate the specific effects of a test treatment. However, 'sham acupuncture' is more difficult and expensive to set up. Sham acupuncture uses needles with blunt tips without skin penetration or 'minimal acupuncture' where needles are inserted either superficially or away from studied acupuncture points.[111] Non-penetrating needles retract into the clinician's hand rather than penetrating the skin. Here, the pressure of the needle felt by the patient is very similar. Additionally, RCTs also use non-needle sham controls, including inactivated laser and transcutaneous electrical nerve stimulation devices.[114] However, findings from research using sham acupuncture show that neither non-penetration nor minimal penetration models are physiologically inert because 'touching' the skin may also elicit an emotional or hormonal response, and activate afferent nerve fibers and changes in limbic system function.[111] Thus, these sham treatments may partially or fully represent the effects of actual needles.

Summary

There is good evidence from experimental studies to suggest that manual therapy, therapeutic exercise, and acupuncture can be effective in the treatment of chronic musculoskeletal pain. However, findings from this area of research so far have not been acceptably replicated in clinical studies. Importantly, the effectiveness of treatments may show changes in endogenous analgesia; however, these changes are most often short-lasting and modest, due in part to other exogenous and endogenous confounding factors, such as altered mood and cognition also associated with the maintenance of CP. Additionally, clinical trials in most cases lack the rigor to show strong evidence concerning the efficacy of treatment, due in part to the heterogeneity of sampling, investigated treatments, and multiple outcome measures, as well as inadequate randomization and blinding procedures. Currently, therapeutic exercise stands out as a form of therapy best suited to the treatment of CP, not due to stronger research methods but to homogeneity in the prescription of exercises. However, it should also be recognized that by tightening homogeneity in sample selection, outcome measures, and intervention-type, manual therapy and acupuncture have a significant role in the treatment of CP. Thus, by sampling subject groups with the same pain disorder, from the same population, at the same time-point in the condition, applying the same treatments and using the same outcome measures, evidence will become much clearer as to how and what we can best use to manage people suffering CP.

References

1. Turk DC, Wilson HD, Cahana A. Treatment of chronic non-cancer pain. Lancet. 2011;377(9784):2226–35.

2. Treede R-D, Rief W, Barke A, Aziz Q, Bennett MI, Benoliel R, et al. A classification of chronic pain for ICD-11. Pain. 2015;156(6):1003–7.

3. Merskey H, Bogduk N, editors. Classification of Chronic Pain. 2nd ed. (revised). Seattle, WA: IASP Press; 2012.

4. Turk DC, McCarberg B. Non-pharmacological treatments for chronic pain: a disease management context. Disease Management and Health Outcomes. 2006;13(1):19–30.

5. Centre for Evidence-Based Medicine. Oxford Centre for Evidence-based Medicine – Levels of Evidence Oxford: University of Oxford; 2009 [Available from: http://www.cebm.net/oxford-centre-evidence-based-medicine-levels-evidence-march-2009/].

6. Guyatt GH, Sackett DL, Cook DJ. Users' guides to the medical literature. II. How to use an article about therapy or prevention. A. Are the results of the study valid? Evidence-Based Medicine Working Group. Jama. 1993;270(21):2598–601.

7. Liamputtong P. Research methods in health: foundations for evidence-based practice. Melbourne: Oxford University Press; 2013.

8. McNair P, Lewis G. Levels of evidence in medicine. International Journal of Sports Physical Therapy. 2012;7(5):474–81.

9. Centre for Evidence-Based Medicine. Study Designs Cambridge: CEBM; 2016 [Available from: http://www.cebm.net/study-designs/].

10. Wright A, Sluka KA. Nonpharmacological treatments for musculoskeletal pain. Clinical Journal of Pain. 2001;17(1):33–46.

11. Clar C, Tsertsvadze A, Court R, Hundt GL, Clarke A, Sutcliffe P. Clinical effectiveness of manual therapy for the management of musculoskeletal and non-musculoskeletal conditions: systematic review and update of UK evidence report. Chiropractic and Manual Therapies. 2014;22:12.

12. Chang KL, Fillingim R, Hurley RW, Schmidt S. Chronic pain management: nonpharmacological therapies for chronic pain. FP Essentials. 2015;432:21–6.

13. Bokarius AV, Bokarius V. Evidence-based review of manual therapy efficacy in treatment of chronic musculoskeletal pain. Pain Practice. 2010;10(5):451–8.

14. Triano JJ, McGregor M, Hondras MA, Brennan PC. Manipulative therapy versus education programs in chronic low back pain. Spine. 1995;20(8):948–55.

15. Mohseni-Bandpei MA, Critchley J, Staunton T, Richardson B. A prospective randomised controlled trial of spinal manipulation and ultrasound in the treatment of chronic low back pain. Physiotherapy. 2006;92(1):34–42.

16. Licciardone JC, Stoll ST, Fulda KG, Russo DP, Siu J, Winn W, et al. Osteopathic manipulative treatment for chronic low back pain: a randomized controlled trial. Spine. 2003;28(13):1355–62.

17. Sims-Williams H, Jayson MI, Young SM, Baddeley H, Collins E. Controlled trial of mobilisation and manipulation for patients with low back pain in general practice. British Medical Journal. 1978;2(6148):1338–40.

18. Schenk RJ, MacDiarmid A, Rousselle J. The effects of muscle energy technique on lumbar range of motion. Journal of Manual and Manipulative Therapy. 1997;5(4):179–83.

19. Selkow NM, Grindstaff TL, Cross KM, Pugh K, Hertel J, Saliba S. Short-term effect of muscle energy technique on pain in individuals with non-specific lumbopelvic pain: a pilot study. Journal of Manual and Manipulative Therapy. 2009;17(1):E14–E8.

20. Goodsell M, Lee M, Latimer J. Short-term effects of lumbar posteroanterior mobilization in individuals with low-back pain. Journal of Manipulative and Physiological Therapeutics. 2000;23(5):332–42.

21. Wilson E, Payton O, Donegan-Shoaf L, Dec K. Muscle energy technique in patients with acute low back pain: a pilot clinical trial. Journal of Orthopaedic and Sports Physical Therapy. 2003;33(9):502–12.

22. Bronfort G, Haas M, Evans RL, Bouter LM. Efficacy of spinal manipulation and mobilization for low back pain and neck pain: a systematic review and best evidence synthesis. Spine Journal. 2004;4(3):335–56.

23. Timm KE. A randomized-control study of active and passive treatments for chronic low back pain following L5 laminectomy. Journal of Orthopaedic and Sports Physical Therapy. 1994;20(6):276–86.

24. Hidalgo B, Detrembleur C, Hall T, Mahaudens P, Nielens H. The efficacy of manual therapy and exercise for different stages of non-specific low back pain: an update of systematic reviews. Journal of Manual andManipulative Therapy. 2014;22(2):59–74.

25. Rubinstein SM, van Middelkoop M, Kuijpers T, Ostelo R, Verhagen AP, de Boer MR, et al. A systematic review on the effectiveness of complementary and alternative medicine for chronic non-specific low-back pain. European Spine Journal. 2010;19(8):1213–28.

26. van Middelkoop M, Rubinstein SM, Kuijpers T, Verhagen AP, Ostelo R, Koes BW, et al. A systematic review on the effectiveness of physical and rehabilitation interventions for chronic non-specific low back pain. European Spine Journal. 2011;20(1):19–39.

26a. Franke H, Franke JD, Fryer G. Osteopathic manipulative treatment for nonspecific low back pain: a systematic review and meta-analysis. BMC Musculoskelet Disord. 2014 Aug 30;15:286

27. Kumar S, Beaton K, Hughes T. The effectiveness of massage therapy for the treatment of nonspecific low back pain: a systematic review of systematic reviews. International Journal of General Medicine. 2013;6:733–41.

28. Furlan AD, Yazdi F, Tsertsvadze A, Gross A, Van Tulder M, Santaguida L, et al. A systematic review and meta-analysis of

efficacy, cost-effectiveness, and safety of selected complementary and alternative medicine for neck and low-back pain. Evidence Based Complementary and Alternative Medicine. 2012;2012:953139.

29. van Middelkoop M, Rubinstein SM, Kuijpers T, Verhagen AP, Ostelo R, Koes BW, et al. A systematic review on the effectiveness of physical and rehabilitation interventions for chronic non-specific low back pain. European Spine Journal. 2011;20(1):19–39.

30. Miller J, Gross A, D'Sylva J, Burnie SJ, Goldsmith CH, Graham N, et al. Manual therapy and exercise for neck pain: a systematic review. Manual Therapy. 2010;15(4):334–54.

31. Gross AR, Goldsmith C, Hoving JL, Haines T, Peloso P, Aker P, et al. Conservative management of mechanical neck disorders: a systematic review. Journal of Rheumatology. 2007;34(5):1083–102.

32. Gemmell H, Miller P. Relative effectiveness and adverse effects of cervical manipulation, mobilisation and the activator instrument in patients with sub-acute non-specific neck pain: results from a stopped randomised trial. Chiropractic and Osteopathy. 2010;18:20.

33. Gross A, Miller J, D'Sylva J, Burnie SJ, Goldsmith CH, Graham N, et al. Manipulation or mobilisation for neck pain: a Cochrane review. Manual Therapy. 2010;15(4):315–33.

34. Gross A, Langevin P, Burnie SJ, Bedard-Brochu MS, Empey B, Dugas E, et al. Manipulation and mobilisation for neck pain contrasted against an inactive control or another active treatment. Cochrane Database of Systematic Reviews. 2015(9):Cd004249.

35. Cen SY, Loy SF, Sletten EG, McLaine A. The effect of traditional Chinese therapeutic massage on individuals with neck pain. Clinical Acupuncture and Oriental Medicine. 2003;4(2–3):88–93.

36. Blikstad A, Gemmell H. Immediate effect of activator trigger point therapy

and myofascial band therapy on non-specific neck pain in patients with upper trapezius trigger points compared to sham ultrasound: a randomised controlled trial. Clinical Chiropractic. 2008;11(1):23–9.

37. Patel KC, Gross A, Graham N, Goldsmith CH, Ezzo J, Morien A, et al. Massage for mechanical neck disorders. Cochrane Database of Systematic Reviews. 2012(9):Cd004871.

38. Wanderley D, Lemos A, Carvalho L, Oliveira D. Manual therapies for pain relief in patients with headache: a systematic review. Reviews in the Neurociences. 2015;23(1):89–96.

39. Posadzki P, Ernst E. Spinal manipulations for cervicogenic headaches: a systematic review of randomized clinical trials. Headache. 2011;51(7):1132–9.

40. Fernandez-de-Las-Penas C, Alonso-Blanco C, Cuadrado ML, Miangolarra JC, Barriga FJ, Pareja JA. Are manual therapies effective in reducing pain from tension-type headache?: a systematic review. Clinical Journal of Pain. 2006;22(3):278–85.

41. Brantingham JW, Cassa TK, Bonnefin D, Jensen M, Globe G, Hicks M, et al. Manipulative therapy for shoulder pain and disorders: expansion of a systematic review. Journal of Manipulative and Physiological Therapeutics. 2011;34(5):314–46.

42. Desjardins-Charbonneau A, Roy JS, Dionne CE, Fremont P, MacDermid JC, Desmeules F. The efficacy of manual therapy for rotator cuff tendinopathy: a systematic review and meta-analysis. Journal of Orthopaedic and Sports Physical Therapy. 2015;45(5):330–50.

43. Page MJ, Green S, McBain B, Surace SJ, Deitch J, Lyttle N, et al. Manual therapy and exercise for rotator cuff disease. Cochrane Database of Systematic Reviews. 2016;6:Cd012224.

44. Dickens VA, Williams JL, Bhamra MS. Role of physiotherapy in the treatment of subacromial impingement syndrome:

a prospective study. Physiotherapy. 2005;91(3):159–64.

45. Bansal K, Padamkumar S. A comparative study between the efficacy of therapeutic ultrasound and soft tissue massage (deep friction massage) in supraspinatus tendinitis. Indian Journal of Physiotherapy and Occupational Therapy. 2011;5:80–4.

46. Vermeulen HM, Rozing PM, Obermann WR, le Cessie S, Vliet Vlieland TP. Comparison of high-grade and low-grade mobilization techniques in the management of adhesive capsulitis of the shoulder: randomized controlled trial. Physical Therapy. 2006;86(3):355–68.

47. Maund E, Craig D, Suekarran S, Neilson A, Wright K, Brealey S, et al. Management of frozen shoulder: a systematic review and cost-effectiveness analysis. Health Technology Assessment. 2012;16(11):1–264.

48. Page MJ, Green S, Kramer S, Johnston RV, McBain B, Chau M, et al. Manual therapy and exercise for adhesive capsulitis (frozen shoulder). Cochrane Database of Systematic Reviews. 2014(8):Cd011275.

49. Di Fabio RP. Physical therapy for patients with TMD: a descriptive study of treatment, disability, and health status. Journal of Orofacial Pain. 1998;12(2):124–35.

50. Calixtre LB, Moreira RF, Franchini GH, Alburquerque-Sendin F, Oliveira AB. Manual therapy for the management of pain and limited range of motion in subjects with signs and symptoms of temporomandibular disorder: a systematic review of randomised controlled trials. Journal of Oral Rehabilitation. 2015;42(11):847–61.

51. Armijo-Olivo S, Pitance L, Singh V, Neto F, Thie N, Michelotti A. Effectiveness of manual therapy and therapeutic exercise for temporomandibular disorders: systematic review and meta-analysis. Physical Therapy. 2016;96(1):9–25.

52. Guarda-Nardini L, Stecco A, Stecco C, Masiero S, Manfredini D. Myofascial pain of the jaw muscles: comparison of

short-term effectiveness of botulinum toxin injections and fascial manipulation technique. Cranio. 2012;30(2):95–102.

53. La Touche R, Paris-Alemany A, Mannheimer JS, Angulo-Diaz-Parreno S, Bishop MD, Lopez-Valverde-Centeno A, et al. Does mobilization of the upper cervical spine affect pain sensitivity and autonomic nervous system function in patients with cervico-craniofacial pain?: A randomized-controlled trial. Clinical Journal of Pain. 2013;29(3):205–15.

54. Packer AC, Pires PF, Dibai-Filho AV, Rodrigues-Bigaton D. Effects of upper thoracic manipulation on pressure pain sensitivity in women with temporomandibular disorder: a randomized, double-blind, clinical trial. American Journal of Physical Medicine and Rehabilitationj. 2014;93(2):160–8.

55. Wright EF, Domenech MA, Fischer JR, Jr. Usefulness of posture training for patients with temporomandibular disorders. Journal of the American Dental Association. 2000;131(2):202–10.

56. Kraaijenga S, van der Molen L, van Tinteren H, Hilgers F, Smeele L. Treatment of myogenic temporomandibular disorder: a prospective randomized clinical trial, comparing a mechanical stretching device (TheraBite(R)) with standard physical therapy exercise. Cranio. 2014;32(3):208–16.

57. Kalamir A, Pollard H, Vitiello A, Bonello R. Intra-oral myofascial therapy for chronic myogenous temporomandibular disorders: a randomized, controlled pilot study. Journal of Manual and Manipulative Therapy. 2010;18(3):139–46.

58. Diracoglu D, Saral IB, Keklik B, Kurt H, Emekli U, Ozcakar L, et al. Arthrocentesis versus nonsurgical methods in the treatment of temporomandibular disc displacement without reduction. Oral Surgery, Oral Medicine, Oral Pathology, Oral Radiology and Endodontics. 2009;108(1):3–8.

59. Yuan SL, Matsutani LA, Marques AP. Effectiveness of different styles of massage therapy in fibromyalgia: a systematic review and meta-analysis. Manual Therapy. 2015;20(2):257–64.

60. Schneider M, Vernon H, Ko G, Lawson G, Perera J. Chiropractic management of fibromyalgia syndrome: a systematic review of the literature. Journal of Manipulative and Physiological Therapeutics. 2009;32(1):25–40.

61. Castro-Sánchez AM, Matarán-Peñarrocha GA, Sánchez-Labraca N, Quesada-Rubio JM, Granero-Molina J, Moreno-Lorenzo C. A randomized controlled trial investigating the effects of craniosacral therapy on pain and heart rate variability in fibromyalgia patients. Clinical Rehabilitation. 2011;25(1):25–35.

62. Li Y-h, Wang F-y, Feng C-q, Yang X-f, Sun Y-h. Massage therapy for fibromyalgia: a systematic review and meta-analysis of randomized controlled trials. PLOS ONE. 2014;9(2):e89304.

63. Kawi J, Lukkahatai N, Inouye J, Thomason D, Connelly K. Effects of exercise on select biomarkers and associated outcomes in chronic pain conditions: systematic review. Biological Research For Nursing. 2016;18(2):147–59.

64. Nijs J, Lluch Girbés E, Lundberg M, Malfliet A, Sterling M. Exercise therapy for chronic musculoskeletal pain: innovation by altering pain memories. Manual Therapy. 2015;20(1):216–20.

65. Patti A, Bianco A, Paoli A, Messina G, Montalto MA, Bellafiore M, et al. Effects of Pilates exercise programs in people with chronic low back pain: a systematic review. Medicine (Baltimore). 2015;94(4):e383.

66. Khan J, Benavent V, Korczeniewska OA, Benoliel R, Eliav E. Exercise-induced hypoalgesia profile in rats predicts neuropathic pain intensity induced by sciatic nerve constriction injury. Journal of Pain. 2014;15(11):1179–89.

67. Bement MKH, Sluka KA. Low-intensity exercise reverses chronic muscle pain in the rat in a naloxone-dependent manner. Archives of Physical Medicine and Rehabilitation. 2005;86(9):1736–40.

68. Naugle KM, Fillingim RB, Riley JL. A meta-analytic review of the hypoalgesic effects of exercise. Journal of Pain. 2012;13(12):1139–50.

69. Naugle KM, Naugle KE, Fillingim RB, Samuels B, Riley JL, 3rd. Intensity thresholds for aerobic exercise-induced hypoalgesia. Medicine and Science in Sports and Exercise. 2014;46(4):817–25.

70. Naugle KM, Naugle KE, Riley JL, 3rd. Reduced modulation of pain in older adults after isometric and aerobic exercise. Journal of Pain. 2016;17(6):719–28.

71. Peake JM, Della Gatta P, Suzuki K, Nieman DC. Cytokine expression and secretion by skeletal muscle cells: regulatory mechanisms and exercise effects. Exercise Immunology Review. 2015;21:8–25.

72. Vaegter HB, Handberg G, Jorgensen MN, Kinly A, Graven-Nielsen T. Aerobic exercise and cold pressor test induce hypoalgesia in active and inactive men and women. Pain Medicine. 2015;16(5):923–33.

73. Koltyn KF, Garvin AW, Gardiner RL, Nelson TF. Perception of pain following aerobic exercise. Medicine and Science in Sports Exercise. 1996;28(11):1418–21.

74. Ruble SB, Hoffman MD, Shepanski MA, Valic Z, Buckwalter JB, Clifford PS. Thermal pain perception after aerobic exercise. Archives of Physical Medicine and Rehabilitation. 2005;86(5):1019–23.

75. Meeus M, Roussel NA, Truijen S, Nijs J. Reduced pressure pain thresholds in response to exercise in chronic fatigue syndrome but not in chronic low back pain: an experimental study. Journal of Rehabilitation Medicine. 2010;42(9):884–90.

76. Hoffman MD, Shepanski MA, Mackenzie SP, Clifford PS. Experimentally induced pain perception is acutely reduced by aerobic exercise in people with chronic low back pain. Journal of Rehabilitation Research and Development. 2005;42(2):183–90.

77. Larsson SE, Bengtsson A, Bodegard L, Henriksson KG, Larsson J. Muscle

changes in work-related chronic myalgia. Acta Orthopaedica Scandinavica. 1988;59(5):552–6.

78. Ylinen J, Takala EP, Kautiainen H, Nykanen M, Hakkinen A, Pohjolainen T, et al. Association of neck pain, disability and neck pain during maximal effort with neck muscle strength and range of movement in women with chronic non-specific neck pain. European Journal of Pain. 2004;8(5):473–8.

79. Hoeger Bement MK, Rasiarmos RL, DiCapo JM, Lewis A, Keller ML, Harkins AL, et al. The role of the menstrual cycle phase in pain perception before and after an isometric fatiguing contraction. European Journal of Applied Physiology. 2009;106(1):105–12.

80. Rhyu H-S, Park H-K, Park J-S, Park H-S. The effects of isometric exercise types on pain and muscle activity in patients with low back pain. Journal of Exercise Rehabilitation. 2015;11(4):211–4.

81. Khan M, Soomro RR, Ali SS. The effectiveness of isometric exercises as compared to general exercises in the management of chronic non-specific neck pain. Pakistani Journal of Pharmaceutical Sciences. 2014;27(5 Suppl):1719–22.

82. Gross A, Kay T, Paquin J, et al. Exercise for neck pain. Cochrane Database of Systematic Reviews. 2015(1).

83. Lannersten L, Kosek E. Dysfunction of endogenous pain inhibition during exercise with painful muscles in patients with shoulder myalgia and fibromyalgia. Pain. 2010;151(1):77–86.

84. Hayden JA, van Tulder MW, Tomlinson G. Systematic review: strategies for using exercise therapy to improve outcomes in chronic low back pain. Annals of Internal Medicine. 2005;142(9):776–85.

85. Hayden JA, van Tulder MW, Tomlinson G. Systematic review: strategies for using exercise therapy to improve outcomes in chronic low back pain. Annals of Internal Medicine. 2005;142(9):776–85.

86. Lorena SBd, Lima MdCCd, Ranzolin A, Duarte ÂLBP. Effects of muscle stretching exercises in the treatment of fibromyalgia: a systematic review. Revista Brasileira de Reumatologia (English edition). 2015;55(2):167–73.

87. Chang DG, Holt JA, Sklar M, Groessl EJ. Yoga as a treatment for chronic low back pain: a systematic review of the literature. Journal of Orthopedics and Rheumatology. 2016;3(1):1–8.

88. Sherman KJ, Cherkin DC, Wellman RD, Cook AJ, Hawkes RJ, Delaney K, et al. A randomized trial comparing yoga, stretching, and a self-care book for chronic low back pain. Archives of Internal Medicine. 2011;171(22):2019–26.

89. Holtzman S, Beggs RT. Yoga for chronic low back pain: a meta-analysis of randomized controlled trials. Pain Research and Management. 2013;18(5):267–72.

90. Hakkinen A, Kautiainen H, Hannonen P, Ylinen J. Strength training and stretching versus stretching only in the treatment of patients with chronic neck pain: a randomized one-year follow-up study. Clinical Rehabilitation. 2008;22(7):592–600.

91. Moon HJ, Choi KH, Kim DH, Kim HJ, Cho YK, Lee KH, et al. Effect of lumbar stabilization and dynamic lumbar strengthening exercises in patients with chronic low back pain. Annals of Rehabilitation Medicine. 2013;37(1):110–7.

92. Akbari A, Khorashadi S, Abdi G. The effect of motor control exercises versus conventional exercises on lumbar local stabilizing muscles thickness: a randomized controlled trial in patients with chronic low back pain. ZUMS Journal. 2008;16(62):1–16.

93. Huang J-T, Chen H-Y, Hong C-Z, Lin M-T, Chou L-W, Chen H-S, et al. Lumbar facet injection for the treatment of chronic piriformis myofascial pain syndrome: 52 case studies. Patient Preference and Adherence. 2014;8:1105–11.

94. Chang W-D, Lin H-Y, Lai P-T. Core strength training for patients with chronic low back pain. Journal of Physical Therapy Science. 2015;27(3):619–22.

95. Ekstrom RA, Donatelli RA, Carp KC. Electromyographic analysis of core trunk, hip, and thigh muscles during 9 rehabilitation exercises. Journal of Orthopaedic and Sports Physical Therapy. 2007;37(12):754–62.

96. O'Sullivan PB, Phyty GD, Twomey LT, Allison GT. Evaluation of specific stabilizing exercise in the treatment of chronic low back pain with radiologic diagnosis of spondylolysis or spondylolisthesis. Spine. 1997;22(24):2959–67.

97. Shyu BC, Andersson SA, Thoren P. Endorphin mediated increase in pain threshold induced by long-lasting exercise in rats. Life Sciences. 1982;30(10):833–40.

98. Nijs J, Kosek E, Van Oosterwijck J, Meeus M. Dysfunctional endogenous analgesia during exercise in patients with chronic pain: to exercise or not to exercise? Pain Physician. 2012;15(3 Suppl):Es205–13.

99. Schwarz L, Kindermann W. Changes in beta-endorphin levels in response to aerobic and anaerobic exercise. Sports Medicine. 1992;13(1):25–36.

100. Leung L. Neurophysiological basis of acupuncture-induced analgesia – an updated review. Journal of Acupuncture and Meridian Studies. 2012;5(6):261–70.

101. Clarke TC, Black LI, Stussman BJ, Barnes PM, Nahin RL. Trends in the use of complementary health approaches among adults: United States, 2002–2012. National Health Statistics Reports. 2015(79):1–16.

102. Austin S, Ramamonjiarivelo Z, Qu H, Ellis-Griffith G. Acupuncture use in the United States: who, where, why, and at what price? Health Marketing Quarterly. 2015;32(2):113–28.

103. Sherman KJ, Cherkin DC, Eisenberg DM, Erro J, Hrbek A, Deyo RA. The practice of acupuncture: who are the providers and what do they do? Annals of Family Medicine. 2005;3(2):151–8.

104. Lin JG, Chen WL. Acupuncture analgesia: a review of its mechanisms of actions. American Journal of Chinese Medicine. 2008;36(4):635–45.

105. Thomas D-A, Maslin B, Legler A, Springer E, Asgerally A, Vadivelu N. Role of alternative therapies for chronic pain syndromes. Current Pain and Headache Reports. 2016;20(5):1–7.

106. Chen XH, Han JS. Analgesia induced by electroacupuncture of different frequencies is mediated by different types of opioid receptors: another cross-tolerance study. Behavioural Brain Research. 1992;47(2):143–9.

107. Ambrosio EM, Bloor K, MacPherson H. Costs and consequences of acupuncture as a treatment for chronic pain: a systematic review of economic evaluations conducted alongside randomised controlled trials.

Complementary Therapies in Medicine. 2012;20(5):364–74.

108. Sun Y, Gan TJ. Acupuncture for the management of chronic headache: a systematic review. Anesthesia and Analgesia. 2008;107(6):2038–47.

109. White A, Foster NE, Cummings M, Barlas P. Acupuncture treatment for chronic knee pain: a systematic review. Rheumatology (Oxford). 2007;46(3):384–90.

110. Davis MA, Kononowech RW, Rolin SA, Spierings EL. Acupuncture for tension-type headache: a meta-analysis of randomized, controlled trials. Journal of Pain. 2008;9(8):667–77.

111. Liu L, Skinner M, McDonough S, Mabire L, Baxter GD. Acupuncture for low back pain: an overview of systematic reviews. Evidence-based Complementary

and Alternative Medicine: eCAM. 2015;2015:328196.

112. Furlan AD, van Tulder M, Cherkin D, Tsukayama H, Lao L, Koes B, et al. Acupuncture and dry-needling for low back pain: an updated systematic review within the framework of the Cochrane collaboration. Spine. 2005;30(8):944–63.

113. Vickers AJ, Cronin AM, Maschino AC, Lewith G, MacPherson H, Foster NE, et al. Acupuncture for chronic pain: individual patient data meta-analysis. Archives of Internal Medicine. 2012;172(19):1444–53.

114. MacPherson H, Vertosick E, Lewith G, Linde K, Sherman KJ, Witt CM, et al. Influence of control group on effect size in trials of acupuncture for chronic pain: a secondary analysis of an individual patient data meta-analysis. PLoS ONE. 2014;9(4):e93739.

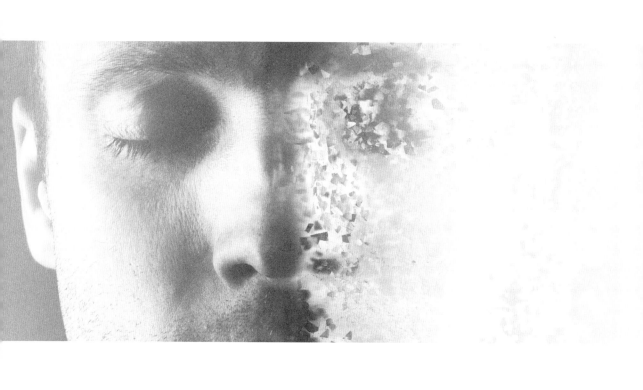

SECTION 3
Clinical presentations of chronic pain

Introduction

Non-malignant musculoskeletal pain is a major cause of disability worldwide and is the most common reason people seek medical attention.[1,2] A recent epidemiological study shows that chronic musculoskeletal pain affects between 14% and 47% of the general population, with risk factors including age, gender, smoking, low education, low physical activity, and sleep disorders.[3] Musculoskeletal pain can be caused by many conditions, including a variety of low back pain conditions, fibromyalgia, osteoarthritis, tendinopathies, muscle overuse/damage, and bone fracture, as well as inflammatory joint disorders such as rheumatoid arthritis. The quality of pain associated with muscles and joints differs from injuries to the skin. Tissue damage to these deeper structures causes more diffuse, non-localized pain which is difficult to differentiate; pain may be originating from tendons, ligaments, or bones as well as from joints and their capsules.[4] Additionally, musculoskeletal pain often refers to distant somatic structures. In contrast, pain from cutaneous structures is specifically localized, sharp, stabbing, or burning.[5] However, mechanisms of musculoskeletal pain change depending on the chronicity of the condition.

As musculoskeletal pain transitions from an acute to a more chronic presentation, further sensory abnormalities occur, such as the spread of local pain and subsequently, widespread hyperalgesia. Evidence suggests that both the intensity of ongoing pain and its duration determine the amount of generalized muscle hyperalgesia.[2,6] This spread of pain and increases in severity over time reflect progressive sensitization both peripherally and centrally. As previously described, hyperalgesia or indeed allodynia are terms used to describe an increased response to a previously noxious or a non-noxious stimulus respectively. Additionally, musculoskeletal pain is further associated with spontaneous pain behaviors such as the protecting or guarding of a joint.[5] Thus, although studies suggest manual therapy as an effective treatment of musculoskeletal pain, the mechanisms through which it exerts its effects are not established in more chronic conditions.[7] The treatments of common musculoskeletal conditions are reviewed in Chapter 7. This chapter will review the epidemiology, peripheral and central mechanisms of musculoskeletal pain, clinical perspectives on musculoskeletal conditions, and testing protocols for CP conditions.

Epidemiology of musculoskeletal pain

Prevalence

It is difficult to report accurately the prevalence of chronic musculoskeletal pain due to marked differences in reported prevalence between studies.[3,8] For example, reports of low back pain range from 8% to 44%, depending on the study and the type of pain condition investigated, while the prevalence of chronic widespread pain ranges between 14% and 25%.[8] These discrepancies are thought to be due to differences in time intervals where new cases are reported (incidence) and different methods of investigation. Generally speaking, there are two methods for collection of epidemiological data, those being Health Interview Surveys (face to face, phone, postal) and Health Examination Surveys (clinical attendance).[3] Although the survey approach is cheaper, simpler, and faster, participants are often unable to differentiate between pain or pain-related signs such as peripheral edema and/or reduced range of motion. Additionally, in this setting the term 'chronic' is difficult to determine accurately, due to different definitions describing duration and the actual recall of duration by participants. Chronic musculoskeletal pain is most commonly reported among adults, with almost 50% reporting low back pain; approximately 30% shoulder pain; and 20% widespread pain.[8] However, there is significant variation between different countries. For example, community-based studies show prevalence rates in Sweden at 17%, 38% in Portugal,[9] 30% in Finland,[10] and 41% in the USA.[11] Additionally, people with chronic widespread pain present with increased levels of disability and decreased rates of observed pathology compared to those with regional pain conditions. Although the level and extent of disability remains to be acknowledged, affective, emotional, and cognitive dysfunction are shown to be significantly higher in this chronic pain group,[12] suggesting disability to be perceived.

Risk factors

Several sociodemographic factors are associated with both regional and widespread musculoskeletal pain.[3] For example, physical exposure to different types of occupation (static postures, repetitive tasks, heavy load lifting, and vibration) and psychological conditions related to work (high demands, no influence on work situation, and no support). It should be noted that physical and psychological factors appear to be equally important; however, it is uncertain whether these factors contribute specifically to regional or to widespread pain conditions.[13] Furthermore, the presence of widespread pain is a not only a risk factor for decreased physical activity but also for excess mortality, as those with long-term pain inactivity are more prone to cardiovascular disease.[14] Importantly, it should also be noted that the spreading of pain from local pain to widespread pain occurs in a large proportion of the general population.[15] For example, a systematic review including nearly 5000 subjects found that female sex, higher age, a family history of pain, and the presence of mood disorders are reported to be risk factors for the likelihood for the transition from local musculoskeletal pain to chronic widespread pain.

As reviewed in Chapter 4, additional risk factors include low education, social isolation, low family income, mood, anxiety, and sleep disorders, being widowed, as well as being a recent immigrant.[3] However, musculoskeletal pain is most often attributed to occupation. Although limited evidence exists regarding occupational causes, work-related factors are thought to be multifactorial and include workplace characteristics such as physical load (e.g., repetitive movements, hand force exertion), work environment (e.g., poor layout, lighting, noise levels), work organization (e.g., time deadlines, lack of support, job insecurity), and other psychosocial factors.[16] Recent European Agency for Safety and Health at Work findings show musculoskeletal pain conditions to be the most prevalent and most serious health problem in the past 12 months (Figure 8.1).

Mechanisms of musculoskeletal pain

Although pathological mechanisms of musculoskeletal injury are relatively well understood, CP arising from musculoskeletal tissue remains a mystery. Additionally, even if many clinical features are consistent with tissue disturbance (i.e., pain is localized, persistent, and specifically associated with tissue loading), many others are not. Here, investigation results do not correlate with the severity of pain and disability, while painless musculoskeletal tissue can be catastrophically degenerated. Thus, what causes musculoskeletal tissues to be painful? This section briefly reviews current evidence for mechanisms of pathology and nociceptive mechanisms in musculoskeletal tissues. For more detailed information please refer to *Fundamentals of Musculoskeletal Pain*.[17]

Features of skeletal muscle pain

Compared to localized cutaneous pain, muscle pain is more diffuse. These differences are thought to be due to (1) larger receptive fields for single nociceptive fibers and (2) a lower innervation density of muscle tissue.[18] Animal studies show cutaneous nociceptors to have receptive fields between 2 mm^2 (cats) and 6–32 mm^2 (rabbits).[18] Owing to the subcutaneous location of muscle tissue, the measurement of muscle nociceptor receptive fields is difficult to determine. However, studies investigating more receptive fields

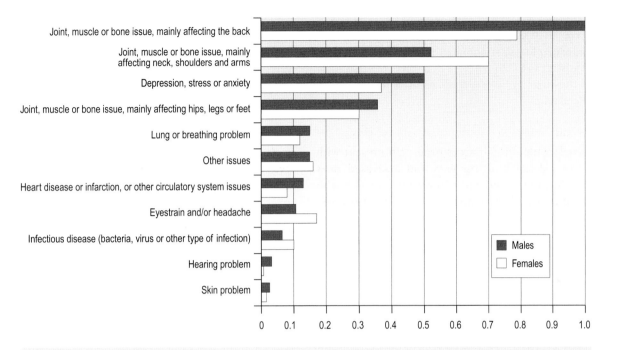

Figure 8.1

The relative occurrence of work-related health issues indicated as most serious in the previous 12 months in the European Union by sex. The value of '0' reflects a work-related health issue as least often reported while '1' reflects a work-related health issue most often reported

on superficial muscle surfaces report areas up to and more than 1 cm^2.[19] There are also subjective differences between muscle and cutaneous pain. For example, the character of muscle pain is often described as cramping or tearing while cutaneous pain is described as stabbing or burning.[20] Additionally, pain originating in muscle tissue tends to be referred more often than pain from cutaneous tissue. Thus, one cannot assume that mechanisms of cutaneous pain are shared by those relating to muscle pain.[20]

Skeletal muscle nociceptors do not respond to everyday stimuli such as normal contractions or stretching within a normal range. These muscles are innervated by large myelinated fibers, thinly myelinated (e.g., Aδ) and unmyelinated (C) afferent fibers that have non-specialized terminal endings which can respond to noxious mechanical and chemical stimuli.[21] Muscle nociceptors can be activated by strong mechanical

stimuli (trauma, mechanical overloading. and local inflammatory mediators), which, if prolonged, can lead to central sensitization and subsequent pain symptoms such as hyperalgesia and allodynia. Generally, research shows that thinly myelinated and unmyelinated fibers innervating skeletal muscle have high mechanical thresholds and slowly adapting responses (e.g., static or dynamic stretch) that are consistent with the role of mechanical nociception.[22] These fibers respond to several inflammatory mediators, such as bradykinin, 5-HT, and to prostaglandin E2 (PGE2), as well as to innocuous and noxious thermal stimuli (40–50°C). Thinly myelinated and unmyelinated fibers innervating skeletal muscle act, in effect, as polymodal nociceptors.[22] It should also be noted that interactions occur between neurotransmitters and locally released inflammatory mediators where both stimulating and sensitizing substances are released together.[23] For example, an injection of bradykinin and serotonin into the temporalis muscle in human subjects caused more severe pain compared to each stimulant alone.[24] Additionally, the same authors showed that prostaglandin E2 significantly increased the effect of bradykinin on the discharge rate of muscle nociceptive receptors (Figure 8.2).[25]

Experimentally, muscle pain can be elicited by intense pressure (pressure cuff), noxious chemical stimuli (capsaicin, hypertonic saline), intramuscular electrical stimulation, or local ischemia (tourniquet).[21] Ischemic pain is a common form of muscle pain that can be experienced during exercise (ischemic contractions). In animal studies, several factors, including the number of contractions, the amount of force, and the duration, augment the build-up of algesic mediators such as bradykinin and calcitonin that contribute to ischemic pain.[19] Surprisingly, however, in these types of studies, lactate was not seen to induce this type of ischemic pain. In similar ischemic pain studies with human subjects, 'muscle pain' does not originate exclusively from muscle tissue, but additionally, from skin, periosteum, and connective tissue.[21] Here, as described in Chapter 1, neurotransmitters (e.g., substance P) released on the activation of nociceptive nerve endings initiate vasodilatation, local edema, and thus further activation of local and adjacent nociceptors over a prolonged period. Several authors suggest that this vicious circle may contribute to the formation of trigger points.[26–28]

Mechanisms of chronic muscle pain

Prolonged pathophysiological change in muscle tissue both sensitizes and increases innervation densities of nociceptors to muscle tissue with neuropeptide-containing (e.g., substance P and bradykinin) nerve endings.[23] Several animal studies that show inflammation to muscle tissue for approximately two weeks correlate strongly with increases in innervation density, especially substance P and reduced pain thresholds (hyperalgesia). Importantly, increases in neuronal impulses

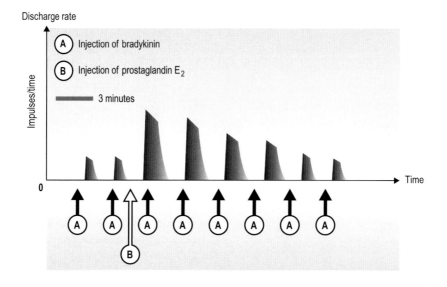

Figure 8.2

Sensitization by PGE2 of C fiber muscle receptors to bradykinin. Bradykinin was injected into skeletal muscle every 3 minutes and the responses of muscle receptors recorded. After the second response an additional injection of PGE2 was given. Mense states that although PGE2 did not excite the receptor, it did sensitize it to subsequent injections of bradykinin (Mense 1981)[25]

from muscle nociceptors to the spinal cord increase the excitability of dorsal horn neurons more so than from cutaneous nociceptors.[29] In addition, persistent input from muscle nociceptors also leads to increases in the number of dorsal horn neurons being activated. This occurs mostly due to the effect of glutamate on NMDA (N-methyl-D-aspartate) receptors and substance P on NK1 (neurokinin 1) receptors in the spinal cord, as described in Chapters 1 and 2. Increased excitability in dorsal horn neurons (due to tenderness to pressure and pain on movement or exercise) is considered to be the main cause of allodynia and hyperalgesia in people with chronic muscle pain.[20] It is because of these changes in the spinal cord that people presenting with chronic muscle pain are difficult to treat. It should be noted that the same changes in the dorsal horn are responsible for the persistence of pain in other musculoskeletal tissues reviewed in the following sections.

Muscle-induced referred pain

Chronic pain from muscles is more likely to refer to adjacent and distal body regions compared to pain arising from cutaneous tissue.[20] Recent evidence shows that referred pain from muscle tissue is due to dorsal horn and brainstem neurons receiving convergent inputs from various sources, and thus cortical regions in the brain cannot accurately identify the actual tissues that are causing pain.[30] Mense suggests that this is due to persistent excitation of dorsal horn neurons innervating body regions beyond the site of the original muscle lesion (Figure 8.3). Thus, central hyperexcitability is thought to modulate the onset of referred pain. Here, animal studies show recordings from dorsal neurons with a receptive field found in the bicep femoris muscle also show new receptive fields in the tibialis anterior muscle after the application of noxious stimuli to the tibialis anterior muscle.[30]

Features of tendon pain

Tendon pain is confusing for both clinicians and researchers. Unlike skeletal muscle pain, the mechanisms underlying tendinous pain are poorly understood. Painful rotator cuff and Achilles

tendinopathies are common examples which are typically resistant to many forms of treatment.[31] People of different ages can present with varying degrees of tendon-related pain and disability, and while some recover quickly using simple interventions, others fail to recover using a range of treatments. The lack of general consensus among practitioners, a wide range of treatments, and the lack of correlation between pain

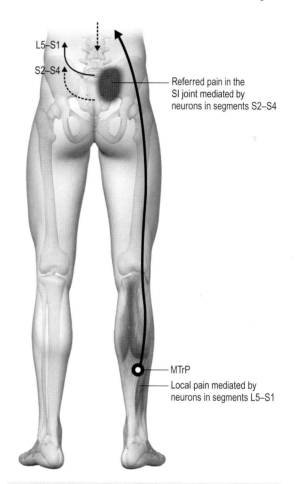

L5–S1
S2–S4

Referred pain in the
SI joint mediated by
neurons in segments S2–S4

MTrP
Local pain mediated by
neurons in segments L5–S1

Figure 8.3

Pain referred from a myofascial trigger point in the soleus muscle to the sacroiliac joint. Nociceptive input from the trigger point arrives at the dorsal horn at L5–S1. However, due to the spread of spinal excitation, adjacent segments (S2–4) become activated[20]

and tendon pathology supports this lack of knowledge. For example, despite biopsy studies showing the absence of inflammatory involvement in many tendinopathies, anti-inflammatory agents are currently most often prescribed for treatment.[32] Generally, tendinopathy occurs in loaded tendons due to overuse, decreased exercise tolerance, and reduced capacity to sustain repeated tensile loading,[33] causing disruption and disorder in the cellular matrix of tendon tissue.[34] Interestingly, although mid-tendon and bony insertion morphology differ in normal states, they appear indistinguishable in pathological states.[35] However, studies show that exercises specific for mid-tendon or the bony insertion provide improved treatment responses, due probably to the loading profiles of each tendon.[33]

Previously, tendon pathology has been described as being either degenerative or failed healing, neither of which explain the heterogeneity of both presentation and reaction to treatment. Recently, however, a simple three-stage pathology model has

been developed that includes reactive tendinopathy, tendon disrepair (failed healing), and degenerative tendinopathy where pain can occur along a continuum.[33] Here, Cook and colleagues propose a model that involves a continuum of transition from normal through to degenerative tendinopathy. This model further describes the potential for reversibility of injury early, but not later (degenerative phase), in this continuum (Figure 8.4).

Concerning nociceptive characteristics, animal studies show tendons and their sheaths have more dense innervations of both Aδ and C afferent fibers compared to associated muscles.[19,36] However, innervation studies show that compared to tendinous connective tissues and local vasculature, tendinous tissues receive limited innervation.[34] Acute or repetitive trauma to tendons results in many changes in tendon structure, in which cell activation and proliferations lead to collagen disorganization, increased levels of proteoglycans, fibril separation, and neovascularization.[37] Sympathetic nerve endings are

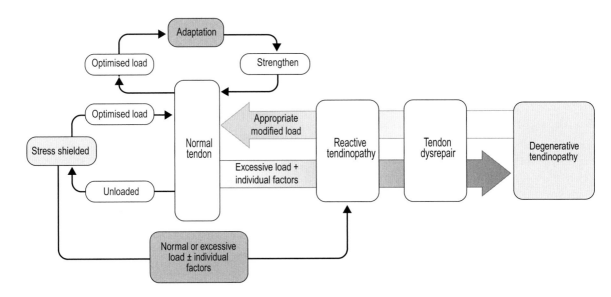

Figure 8.4

Cook and colleagues' model proposing a continuum from normal tendon tissue state through to degenerative tendinopathy, highlighting the potential for reversibility early in the process

also found in all tendinous and associated connective tissues.[38] Studies show that sympathetic nervous system markers become significantly increased in abnormal tenocytes of painful tendons.[39] Although these changes in structure and function are the most likely cause of increased nociception, the loss of collagen integrity does not correlate with the severity of tendon pain.

Peripheral mechanisms of chronic tendinopathy

As described above, chronic tendon pain, especially in the Achilles and patella, is very common; however, the exact cause of chronic tendon pain is largely unknown. There appears to be multifactorial processes involving a wide range of exogenous and endogenous factors driven mostly by longstanding overloading of tendon tissue, age, decreased arterial blood flow, increases in neuropeptide release, and impaired tenocyte metabolism.[40] As in other musculoskeletal tissues, inflammatory mediators such as TNFα and substance P contribute significantly to chronic tendon pain. However, TNFα is specifically implicated in chronic tendinopathies where it has been shown to be activated by mechanotransduction and is also involved in changes in matrix structure.[41] TNFα is further responsible for increased firing of Aδ and C fibers that, if persistent, leads to localized sensitization. Additionally, endogenously released substance P from tenocytes not only causes local vasodilatation and protein extravasation, but also local cell proliferation of tenocytes themselves.[42] New nerve growth has also been shown in tendinopathies, especially in the Achilles tendon.[40] Given the above findings, it is not surprising that nearly all studies investigating chronic tendinopathies show thickening of tendon fibers, loss of fascicle organization, degeneration of collagen and hyalin, intratendonous calcification, and micro-tears.[40]

Features of bone pain

While not as well studied as muscle and tendon pain, chronic pain in the skeleton occurs in a wide and diverse set of pain-related conditions. A major reason for this is because the skeleton provides structural support, movement, protection of internal organs, mineral and growth factor storage/release, and the genesis and maturation of blood cells.[43] Not surprisingly, the prevalence of skeletal pain is shown to increase with age[44] and body mass.[45] Bone pain is associated with bony pathology, including bone marrow edema, osteomyelitis, and fracture. However, skeletal pain is mostly associated with metastatic bone pain or cancer-induced bone pain, which are complex and involve background pain, spontaneous pain, and movement-evoked pain.[46] However, this book only refers to chronic non-malignant/non-infectious pain. For further information on cancer pain please refer to Falk and colleagues.[46]

Sensory neurons supplying bone tissue are shown to innervate the periosteum and marrow cavity and are most associated with nociception (Figure 8.5).[47] Due to ease of access for experimental investigation, periosteal nociception has received greatest attention. Here, neurophysiological studies show that contrary to the rich variety of sensory receptors in cutaneous tissue, the skeleton is innervated mostly by thinly myelinated Aδ fibers and surprisingly receive few larger Aβ or, more surprisingly, unmyelinated C fibers.[48] Several studies show that differences in distribution of sensory nerves between cutaneous and skeletal tissues occur during perinatal and postnatal development.[43] Concerning bone marrow innervation, little is known about the activity of sensory neurons. For example, although the marrow cavity shows nociceptive innervation, it is not clear if single neurons respond to mechanical, chemical, or thermal stimuli or if they respond to multiple types of stimuli (e.g., polymodal nociceptors).[47]

Bone pain occurs due to activation or sensitization of nociceptive afferents by either direct mechanical injury (e.g., fracture) or the release of algesic substances from bone or joints (inflammatory joint disease). Concerning fractures, distortion of mechanoreceptors gives rise to immediate stabbing, sharp pain transmitted by Aδ fibers. However, when the fracture is stabilized, the stabbing pain recedes and is

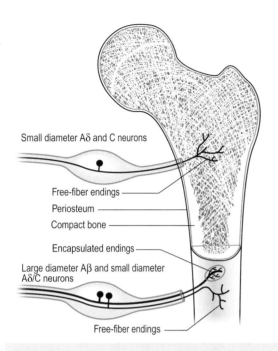

Small diameter Aδ and C neurons

Free-fiber endings

Periosteum

Compact bone

Encapsulated endings

Large diameter Aβ and small diameter Aδ/C neurons

Free-fiber endings

Figure 8.5

A schematic diagram showing sensory neurons that innervate bones. Primary afferent neurons innervating bone marrow and periosteum are mostly thinly myelinated and unmyelinated Aδ and C fibers however, larger Aβ fibers exist in the periosteum

replaced by dull aching pain conveyed by C fibers in the periosteum, bony tissue, and marrow.[43] Ongoing release of algesic factors (e.g., bradykinin, PGE2, TNFα) from the fractured bone cells is responsible for the continued activation and sensitization of nociceptive afferents.[49] Similar pain mechanisms occur with injury or degeneration of articular cartilage during trauma or osteoarthritis. Here algesic substances activate Aδ fibers and C fibers in the synovium and subchondral bone. Thus, when sensitized, normally non-noxious loading and movement of a joint are perceived as painful.[43]

Peripheral mechanisms of chronic bone pain

Concerning chronic bone pain, virtually all existing literature refers to mechanisms of cancer-induced bone pain. Evidence regarding chronic non-cancer skeletal

pain relates to the mechanisms of osteoarthritis, which are reviewed in the following section. However, an interesting but mostly unexplored mechanism relates to pathological sprouting and neuroma formation from sensory and sympathetic fibers innervating bone, due mostly to the sustained release of nerve growth factor (NGF).[43] Although most animal studies show ectopic neuronal sprouting in a variety of primary and secondary bone cancers, several noncancer examples have been observed. Here, sensory neuron growth has been shown in human chronic discogenic pain with neuronal sprouting into avascular areas of the intervertebral disc (Figure 8.6).[50,51] However, while likely, it is not reported in such cases if this growth of sensory innervation spreads to adjacent bony tissue. Nevertheless, such *de novo* neuronal growth has been observed around bone fracture sites in animals that are similar to those of bone cancer, again driven by continued release of NGF released by inflammatory cells.[43]

Features of joint pain

One of the most common forms of CP sensation people experience is related to the condition of joints. Although injuries, infections, and systemic diseases often produce acute arthralgias, the most common cause of joint pain is osteoarthritis.[52] In osteoarthritis, which is common worldwide, pain comes from nociceptive receptors in disrupted superficial bone and soft tissue joint structures.[53] Although degeneration of articular cartilage and narrowing of the joint space are obvious disease traits, associations between the level of physical damage and joint pain are weak. In joint disorders, pain most often occurs during exercise or during daily activities. Primary afferents innervating joint tissue respond mostly to mechanical stimuli. However, as reviewed in Chapter 1, joint tissues also have populations of silent nociceptors which only respond after ongoing sensitization by inflammatory mediators.[52] Mechanoreceptors are activated by noxious stimuli such as overstretching of a joint, while polymodal receptors respond to noxious thermal and chemical stimuli from the presence of inflammatory mediators. Joint innervation is highly specific. Here, the joint capsule, ligaments, periosteum, subchondral bone and menisci are innervated by myelinated (Aβ), thinly myelinated (Aδ) and unmyelinated C fibers. Alternatively, the synovial membrane is only supplied by C fibers, while the articular cartilage is aneuronal.[54,55] Although Aα and Aβ fibers respond mostly to innocuous light pressure, the majority of Aδ fibers and all C fibers respond to noxious stimuli. Like all other musculoskeletal tissues, responsiveness is heightened (sensitization) by the release of NGF and inflammatory mediators such as bradykinin and PGE2.[56] Thus, peripherally mediated joint pain is relieved by nonsteroidal anti-inflammatory medication and selective cyclooxygenase (COX)-2 enzyme inhibitors that block PGE2 synthesis.

Mechanical factors of joint pain

Diarthroidal joints are encapsulated by a fibrous capsule that contains synovial fluid. Following an injurious or inflammatory event, synovial blood vessels become permeable to plasma proteins that leak out of the vasculature and effuse into the joint space.[57] Because the joint is enclosed, this effusion causes an increase in intraarticular pressure. In normal synovial joints, intraarticular pressure is sub-atmospheric

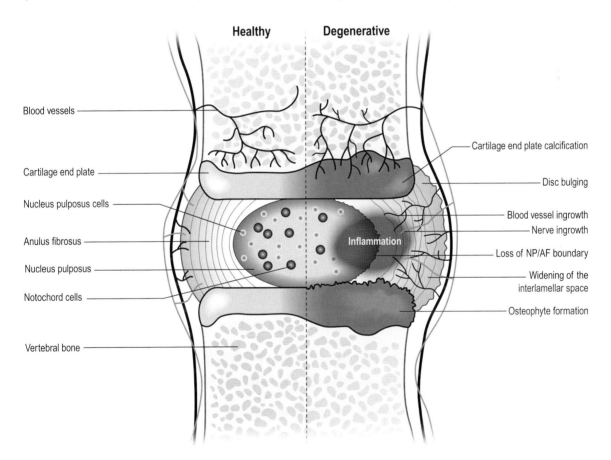

Figure 8.6

A schematic diagram showing comparisons between a healthy intervertebral disc and a degenerative disc. There is increased inflammation and blood vessel and neuronal in-growth into previously aneuronal and vascular tissue Nucleus pulposis (NP), annulus fibrosus (AF)

(-2 to -10 mmHg).[58] However, in conditions such as rheumatoid arthritis, synovial fluid volume can increase to a point where intraarticular pressure rises to approximately supra-atmospheric pressures of over 20 mmHg.[59] Here, there is a linear correlation between increases in joint pressure and pain intensity in subjects with osteoarthritis.[60] Conversely, aspiration of traumatic joint hematomas significantly decreases pain severity of subjects presenting with radial head fractures.[61]

Acute and repetitive joint injuries are responsible for damage to soft tissue joint structures. For example, cumulative research shows that joint instability due to ligament injuries, periarticular muscle weakness, or joint hypermobility leads to abnormal joint loading.[62,63] Additionally, chronic instability due to poor joint healing mechanisms of ligaments also leads to focal erosion of articular surfaces and therefore contributes to joint degeneration.[64] Changes in joint cartilage associated with osteoarthritis include degenerative changes in the cartilage matrix resulting in cartilage surface fibrillation, cleft formation, and loss of volume.[65] Although cartilage is aneural, chondrocytes when degraded produce a host of inflammatory mediators, including cytokines and prostanoids, that further drive cartilage damage and adjacent tissue changes, thus establishing a vicious circle leading to the progression of joint degeneration.[66]

Peripheral mechanisms of chronic joint pain

Like other types of musculoskeletal tissue, continued inflammation sensitizes primary afferent neurons in joint-related tissues. Here, sensitization causes normally high-threshold nociceptors to respond to lower threshold stimuli such as light pressure and 'within range' movements of the joints. Additionally, prolonged inflammation of joint tissue produces reduced thresholds to pressure and joint movement in Aβ and Aδ low threshold non-nociceptive mechanoreceptors.[67] Because these fibers are not chemosensitive, it is thought that they respond to increases in pressure due to intracapsular swelling and other mechanical factors.[68] Importantly, concerning joint tissue, normally silent mechanically insensitive receptors become responsive to mechanical stimulation of the joint which further contributes to nociceptive input to the spinal cord. Given that silent nociceptors are reported to be found only in joints within the musculoskeletal system, it is the recruitment of these fibers that significantly increases input to the spinal cord. Thus, under persistent inflammatory or joint disease conditions, normal joint movement and other usually non-painful stimuli activate the nociceptive system.[67] Many chemical factors have been shown to sensitize joint nociceptors for mechanical stimuli. For example, PGE2 is shown to be a key mediator in osteoarthritis models. Increases in the excitability of ion channels expressed on primary afferent C fibers is due mostly to the expression of COX enzymes both at C fiber peripheral terminals and the spinal cord during arthritis.[69] Additionally, cytokines such as TNFα and interleukins 1 and 6 are also major contributors, especially in rheumatoid arthritis.[52] They contribute significantly to factors such as bone resorption and osteoblast maturation while contributing to the onset of mechanical allodynia.[70]

Central mechanisms of chronic musculoskeletal pain

Expanded receptive fields and referred pain

Chronic musculoskeletal pain conditions often present with expanded local receptive fields (area of pain) and/or referred pain that are maintained by central mechanisms (Figure 8.7).[53] Concerning the expansion of receptive fields, animal studies show that the opening of previously inactive synapses in the dorsal horn due to persistent nociceptive input initiate the activation of post-synaptic NMDA and NK1 receptors.[2] Hoheisal and colleagues showed that within two hours of the induction of a noxious stimulus in animals (induced myositis), a local anesthetic block can prevent the development of central sensitization. Importantly, however, if the block is applied after two hours, central sensitization will then occur.[71] These findings highlight the importance of early and effective analgesic treatment in preventing the development of central hyperexcitability.[2] Although referred pain is defined as being felt in a different body region from the primary source of pain (site of nociceptive stimulation), it is unclear if mechanisms differ to that of changes in local receptive fields (local spread). Here, referred pain has also been defined as a 'new receptive field' due to central hyperexcitability.[72]

In human experimental studies, results are mixed, and while some studies have shown referred hyperalgesia in distal sites,[30,73] others have not.[74] Thus, referred musculoskeletal pain is most likely a combination of central processing and peripheral input, as referred pain can be induced in limbs with complete sensory loss due to anesthetic block[75] or spinal injury,[76] suggesting more supraspinal influences. Although research into increased receptive fields in CP conditions is not advanced, many patients with,

for example, fibromyalgia experience stronger pain intensity and larger referred pain areas compared to healthy controls.[77] Interestingly, referred pain, muscle hyperalgesia, and temporal summation are reduced by the NMDA-receptor antagonist in fibromyalgia patients.[78] These results further suggest a link between central hyperexcitability and mechanisms of hyperalgesia and referred pain. However, it is not known if these mechanisms are related to other CP conditions. Importantly, practitioners should also be aware that a central sensitization process may not be present at the beginning of treatment but may become apparent during the course of treatment and rehabilitation.[79] It is also important to note that manual therapy itself can add to ongoing physical and emotional stressors, further increasing sensitization mechanisms. Thus, signs and symptoms discussed above can provide clues to the transition from acute to chronic pain mechanisms

Acute localized pain

Chronic widespread pain

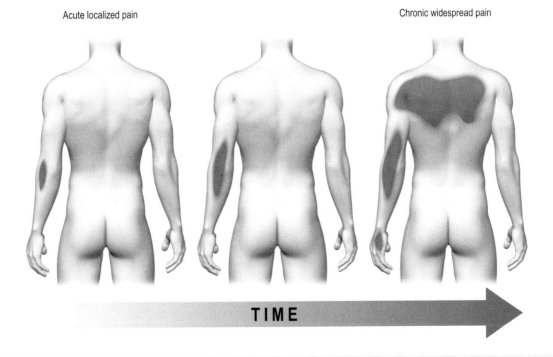

TIME

Figure 8.7
Figures showing how localized musculoskeletal pain (work-related arm pain) may spread to adjacent areas over time due to central mechanisms related to increases in receptive fields and referred pain

at initial presentation, during treatment, and in fol-low-up consultations.

Descending pain modulation

Descending control of nociceptive neuronal excitability in the spinal cord in CP conditions originates in the cerebral cortex, thalamus, and brainstem (Chapter 3). From a musculoskeletal perspective, levels of descending pain control have been examined using different forms of exercise in both healthy individuals and people with chronic pain. Concerning healthy individuals, changes in descending pain modulation are shown following both and isometric muscle contractions[80] and aerobic exercise.[81] Research shows both moderate and vigorous aerobic exercise to produce hypoalgesic effects (increased pressure pain thresholds), suggestive of descending pathways.[82] The same research group, using the parallel test protocols, showed similar findings using isometric muscle contractions in the form of hand grip exercises.[83] Recent findings suggest that descending inhibition is diminished, or in many cases reversed, in people with CP where it becomes facilitatory, following persistent peripheral nociception. For example, patients with fibromyalgia show increased pressure pain thresholds in multiple body sites including the upper trapezius following isometric muscle contractions (shoulder abductions) compared to healthy controls (pain increases only shown in upper trapezius), suggesting a shift from descending inhibition towards facilitation.[84]

Another area of descending inhibitory influence explored in clinical studies involving people with musculoskeletal pain is diffuse noxious inhibitory control (DNIC). In this spinobulbo-spinal pathway, there is a reduction in pain in response to a conditioning noxious stimulus outside the area of pain (Chapter 3).[85] This inhibitory pathway is serotonergic and inhibits the activity of wide dynamic range (WDR) nociceptive neurons in the dorsal horn. Inefficient DNIC-like mechanisms are shown in many chronic musculoskeletal pain conditions such as fibromyalgia,[86] chronic tension headaches,[87] and chronic low back pain.[88]

Clinical indicators of chronic musculoskeletal pain

The implication of muscle and joint pain depends largely on the etiology and the subjective associations. For example, muscle pain after physical exercise may bring a sense of pleasure as a sign of a good or improved performance whereas musculoskeletal pain due to disease can bring considerable physical suffering associated with psychological distress. Very often, it is not possible to differentiate where pain originates. For example, inflammatory or degenerative changes within a joint will also affect surrounding musculoskeletal structures such as tendons, muscles, and other connective tissue structures. Additionally, as reviewed in the previous section, further complications occur with the spread of pain both locally and distally due to peripheral and central hyperexcitability. Thus, there is considerable overlap in the clinical presentation of pain in different musculoskeletal pain conditions, which confuses practitioners and complicates diagnosis.

Causative factors

Although strenuous or unaccustomed work/exercise may cause simple muscle pain, repetitive occupational strain is more often associated with chronic musculoskeletal pain. Most notably, there is strong evidence showing that repetitive heavy lifting, driving, and vibration are associated with the onset and maintenance of occupational back and neck pain.[89-91] Additionally, people working on assembly lines or as machine operators frequently present with neck, shoulder, and elbow pain.[92-94] For example, holding a muscle or joint in a fixed position or repeatedly moving a muscle, usually with loading, for prolonged periods does not allow the muscle to completely recover or relax between contractions. Here, as little as 10–20% of maximal voluntary contraction may be sufficient to occlude microcirculation in muscles, thus leading to localized ischemia.[23] However, single traumatic events such as whiplash injury or other physical trauma may also lead to CP. Although, there is strong evidence showing the effect of psychological impact of such events on the maintenance of CP, there are also physical causal relationships. For example, whiplash injury has been shown to cause damage to discs by shear forces and to facet joints by compression and/or stretching, even without significant tissue failure.[95] Furthermore, prolonged excitability of primary afferent nociceptors in these and associated muscle tissue due to ongoing inflammation are also shown to initiate central sensitization mechanisms.[96]

Similarly, joint diseases, both inflammatory and degenerative, are accompanied by dysfunction, pain, and varying degrees of disability.[97] Although biomechanical factors including degenerative changes or those following joint injury are common causes of joint pain, the prevalence of joint pain and osteoarthritis is increasing with obesity. Additionally, inflammatory mediators released from a joint may decrease muscle efficiency and activate trigger points in adjacent muscles, while degenerative changes or injury to a joint may alter loading of muscles, again causing muscle pain.[97] For example, abnormal loading characteristics of weight-bearing joint osteoarthritis are reflected in local muscle impairment.[98] Here, systematic review data shows the extent of such muscle impairment associated with knee osteoarthritis where significant impairment of quadriceps, hamstrings, and hip muscles results not only in reported loss in physical function but also significant levels of muscle pain.[99]

Diagnostic considerations

Chronic musculoskeletal pain conditions tend to be widespread and diffuse in nature. Unfortunately, the specific etiology of chronic musculoskeletal pain is unclear, and there is often no obvious cause such as injury or infection.[100] People presenting with these chronic symptoms frequently use health care resources mostly without any significant improvement and therefore become frustrated. Thus, when patients present with chronic pain, they are generally concerned with (1) what is wrong and (2) what can be done about it. Thus, if patients leave a consultation without these answers, they will remain frustrated.[101]

Although specific conditions such as tendonitis are relatively straightforward to diagnose, more generalized musculoskeletal pain is less so. Practitioners should therefore consider the flag system in order to identify any significant underlying conditions that contribute to or maintain the pain. Although imaging studies and laboratory tests are essential for serious and specific occult pathology, they are seldom indicated or useful for chronic musculoskeletal pain.[101] Walsh and colleagues suggest that practitioners should explore all options where pain is both adequately and conservatively controlled. However, in more anatomically specific CP presentations, such as low back pain, there are other specific red flag symptoms to be aware of. These include fever, unexpected weight loss, a history of cancer, novel neurological deficit, or discrete changes in the character of pain, as well as the emergence of other symptoms in the presence of pain.

While establishing a diagnosis is important to the management of CP, over-diagnosis often leads to delays in management. Importantly, an accurate pain mechanism diagnosis is better than an inaccurate specific anatomical diagnosis. With the exception of conditions such as lateral epicondylitis or subacromial bursitis, the precise drivers of pain are not identifiable using general diagnostic practice. Even though diagnoses such as sacroiliac joint dysfunction or segmental misalignment are often used to describe a potential source of pain, an exact cause of pain cannot be found in approximately 85% of patients with chronic low back pain.[102] For example, continuing with the example of low back pain, an imaging study in people with no pain showed that only 36% had normal discs while the remainder had varying degrees of disc pathology. That is not to say that disc pathology does not cause back pain, but that pain is multifactorial and it is not clear if positive findings are predictive for the onset of chronic pain.

Quantitative sensory testing (QST)

Quantitative sensory testing (QST) (Figure 8.8) is a psychophysiological, noninvasive testing approach in which stimuli are quantified using a pain rating

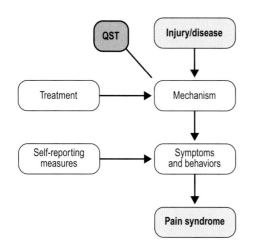

Figure 8.8

A diagram showing proposed relationships between causative factors, pain mechanisms, clinical symptoms and pain syndromes where QST is able to detect features of chronic pain mechanisms

scale to measure pain perception. Pain hypersensitivity can be elicited by threshold tests that evaluate the least amount of sensory input needed to experience pain.[103,104] Thus, by using different sensory inputs (e.g., mechanical pressure, thermal), it is possible to assess sensory processing in both large and small afferent fibers innervating musculoskeletal tissue. Recent evidence shows that QST is useful in differential diagnosis including the detection of hypersensitivity and other more structural causes of pain.[103] For example, QST is able to differentiate people with neck pain due to neural contribution from those with purely mechanical signs and symptoms.[105] Additionally, in a systematic review, Suokas and colleagues found that mechanical pressure QST showed good reliability in differentiating people with osteoarthritis from healthy controls. Their findings also show that lower pressure pain thresholds in affected sites suggest peripheral sensitization while

lower pain thresholds at remote sites represent central sensitization.[106]

QST responses have also been found to predict responses to different types of pain treatments. For example, the use of conditioned pain modulation (test and conditioning stimuli) predicts the response to nonsteroidal anti-inflammatory medication in patients with knee osteoarthritis.[107] In other CP conditions, electrical stimulation predicts the analgesic effect of pregabalin in patients with chronic pancreatitis,[108] while conditioned pain modulation predicts duloxetine efficacy in people with painful diabetic peripheral neuropathy.[109] QST equipment is expensive, cumbersome, and not applicable to 'bedside examinations', and evaluations have been developed but not as yet standardized. However, Cruz-Almeida and Fillingim suggest inexpensive equipment that with further reliability studies may be useful as a future form bedside QST[110] (Table 8.1).

Summary

Chronic musculoskeletal pain is challenging to treat and has a huge socioeconomic impact. Looking at musculoskeletal pain in isolation is considered too narrow a focus since patients presenting with chronic widespread pain are equally likely to consult for other, non-pain, symptoms such as fatigue, poor sleep, and affective disorders. Chronic musculoskeletal pain is also driven by non-musculoskeletal mechanisms such as central sensitization and altered descending modulation where symptoms are typified by widespread hyperalgesia and allodynia. Effective management is therefore markedly different from that of acute musculoskeletal pain. Although not straightforward, implementing current understanding of central sensitization during clinical evaluation, manual therapists can apply management protocols more relevant to neuropathophysiological processing.

Table 8.1: Proposed inexpensive bedside quantitative sensory testing (QST) equipment for use in clinical settings (Cruz-Almeida & Fillingim 2014)[110]

Stimulus type	Afferents	Central pathways	Possible bedside QST
Thermal			
Cold (25°C)	Aδ	Spinothalamic	Cold and warm metallic rollers or test tubes
Warmth (41°C)	C	Spinothalamic	
Heat pain (>45°C)	Aδ, C	Spinothalamic	
Cold pain (<5°C)	Aδ, C	Spinothalamic	
Mechanical			
Static light touch	Aβ	Dorsal column	Cotton swab
Vibration	Aβ	Dorsal column	Tuning fork
Brushing	Aβ	Dorsal columns	Brush
Pinprick	Aδ, C	Spinothalamic	Pin
Blunt pressure	Aδ, C	Spinothalamic	Examiner's thumb

References

1. Breivik H, Borchgrevink PC, Allen SM, Rosseland LA, Romundstad L, Breivik Hals EK, et al. Assessment of pain. British Journal of Anaesthesia. 2008;101(1):17–24.

2. Arendt-Nielsen L, Graven-Nielsen T. Translational musculoskeletal pain research. Best Practice and Research Clinical Rheumatology. 2011;25(2):209–26.

3. Cimmino MA, Ferrone C, Cutolo M. Epidemiology of chronic musculoskeletal pain. Best Practice and Research Clinical Rheumatology. 2011;25(2):173–83.

4. IASP. Assessment of musculoskeletal pain: experimental and clinical. Seattle: IASP Press; 2009. p. 2.

5. Sluka KA. Pain mechanisms involved in musculoskeletal disorders. Journal of Orthopaedic and Sports Physical Therapy. 1996;24(4):240–54.

6. Fernandez-de-Las-Penas C, Ge HY, Arendt-Nielsen L, Cuadrado ML, Pareja JA. The local and referred pain from myofascial trigger points in the temporalis muscle contributes to pain profile in chronic tension-type headache. Clinical Journal of Pain. 2007;23(9):786–92.

7. Bialosky JE, Bishop MD, Price DD, Robinson ME, George SZ. The mechanisms of manual therapy in the treatment of musculoskeletal pain: a comprehensive model. Manual Therapy. 2009;14(5):531–8.

8. McBeth J, Jones K. Epidemiology of chronic musculoskeletal pain. Best Practice and Research Clinical Rheumatology. 2007;21(3):403–25.

9. Elliott AM, Smith BH, Hannaford PC, Smith WC, Chambers WA. The course of chronic pain in the community: results of a 4-year follow-up study. Pain. 2002;99(1–2):299–307.

10. Mäkelä M, Heliövaara M, Sainio P, Knekt P, Impivaara O, Aromaa A. Shoulder joint impairment among Finns aged 30 years or over: prevalence, risk factors and co-morbidity. Rheumatology. 1999;38(7):656–62.

11. Von Korff M, Dworkin SF, Le Resche L, Kruger A. An epidemiologic comparison of pain complaints. Pain. 1988;32(2):173–83.

12. Bushnell MC, Čeko M, Low LA. Cognitive and emotional control of pain and its disruption in chronic pain. Nature Reviews Neuroscience. 2013;14(7):502–11.

13. Herin F, Vezina M, Thaon I, Soulat JM, Paris C. Predictive risk factors for chronic regional and multisite musculoskeletal pain: a 5-year prospective study in a working population. Pain. 2014;155(5):937–43.

14. Andersson HI. Increased mortality among individuals with chronic widespread pain relates to lifestyle factors: a prospective population-based study. Disability and Rehabilitation. 2009;31(24):1980–7.

15. Larsson B, Björk J, Börsbo B, Gerdle B. A systematic review of risk factors associated with transitioning from regional musculoskeletal pain to chronic widespread

pain. European Journal of Pain. 2012;16(8):1084–93.

16. European Agency for Safety and Health at Work. Hazards and risks leading to work-related neck and upper limb disorders (WRULDs). Bilbao: Facts and Figures; 2010.

17. Graven-Nielsen T, Nielsen L, Mense S. Fundamentals of musculoskeletal pain. Seattle: IASP Press; 2008.

18. Mense S, Hoheisel U. Morphology and functional types of muscle nociceptors. In: Nielsen T, Nielsen L, Mense S, editors. Fundamentals of musculoskeletal pain. Seattle: IASP Press; 2008.

19. Mense S, Meyer H. Different types of slowly conducting afferent units in cat skeletal muscle and tendon. Journal of Physiology. 1985;363:403–17.

20. Mense S. Muscle pain: mechanisms and clinical significance. Deutsches Arzteblatt International. 2008;105(12):214–9.

21. Graven-Nielsen T, Mense S. The peripheral apparatus of muscle pain: evidence from animal and human studies. Clinical Journal of Pain. 2001;17(1):2–10.

22. Cairns B. Physiological properties of thin-fiber muscle afferents: excitation and modulatory effects. In: Nielsen T, Nielsen L, Mense S, editors. Fundamentals of musculoskeletal pain. Seattle,: IASP Press; 2008.

23. Mense S. Peripheral mechanisms of muscle pain: response behavior of muscle nociceptors and factors eliciting local muscle pain. In: Mense S, Gerwin DR, editors. Muscle pain: understanding the mechanisms. Berlin, Heidelberg: Springer; 2010. p. 49–103.

24. Jensen K, Tuxen C, Pedersen-Bjergaard U, Jansen I, Edvinsson L, Olesen J. Pain and tenderness in human temporal muscle induced by bradykinin and 5-hydroxytryptamine. Peptides. 1990;11(6):1127–32.

25. Mense S. Sensitization of group IV muscle receptors to bradykinin by 5-hydroxytryptamine and prostaglandin E2. Brain Research. 1981;225(1):95–105.

26. Simons DG. New views of myofascial trigger points: etiology and diagnosis. Archives of Physical Medicine and Rehabilitation. 2008;89(1):157–9.

27. Shah JP, Danoff JV, Desai MJ, Parikh S, Nakamura LY, Phillips TM, et al. Biochemicals associated with pain and inflammation are elevated in sites near to and remote from active myofascial trigger points. Archives of Physical Medicine and Rehabilitation. 2008;89(1):16–23.

28. Ge HY, Monterde S, Graven-Nielsen T, Arendt-Nielsen L. Latent myofascial trigger points are associated with an increased intramuscular electromyographic activity during synergistic muscle activation. Journal of Pain. 2014;15(2):181–7.

29. Wall PD, Woolf CJ. Muscle but not cutaneous C-afferent input produces prolonged increases in the excitability of the flexion reflex in the rat. Journal of Physiology. 1984;356:443–58.

30. Arendt-Nielsen L, Svensson P. Referred muscle pain: basic and clinical findings. Clinical Journal of Pain. 2001;17(1):11–9.

31. Slater H, Gibson W, Graven-Nielsen T. Sensory responses to mechanically and chemically induced tendon pain in healthy subjects. European Journal of Pain. 2011;15(2):146–52.

32. Alfredson H, Lorentzon R. Chronic tendon pain: no signs of chemical inflammation but high concentrations of the neurotransmitter glutamate. Implications for treatment? Current Drug Targets. 2002;3(1):43–54.

33. Cook JL, Purdam CR. Is tendon pathology a continuum? A pathology model to explain the clinical presentation of load-induced tendinopathy. British Journal of Sports Medicine. 2009;43(6):409–16.

34. Rio E, Moseley L, Purdam C, Samiric T, Kidgell D, Pearce AJ, et al. The pain of tendinopathy: physiological or pathophysiological? Sports Medicine. 2014;44(1):9–23.

35. Tan SC, Chan O. Achilles and patellar tendinopathy: current understanding of pathophysiology and management.

Disability and Rehabilitation. 2008;30(20–22):1608–15.

36. Andres KH, von During M, Schmidt RF. Sensory innervation of the Achilles tendon by group III and IV afferent fibers. Anatomy and Embryology. 1985;172(2):145–56.

37. Cook JL, Feller JA, Bonar SF, Khan KM. Abnormal tenocyte morphology is more prevalent than collagen disruption in asymptomatic athletes' patellar tendons. Journal of Orthopaedic Research. 2004;22(2):334–8.

38. Jewson JL, Lambert GW, Storr M, Gaida JE. The sympathetic nervous system and tendinopathy: a systematic review. Sports Medicine. 2015;45(5):727–43.

39. Danielson P, Alfredson H, Forsgren S. Studies on the importance of sympathetic innervation, adrenergic receptors, and a possible local catecholamine production in the development of patellar tendinopathy (tendinosis) in man. Microscopy Research and Technique. 2007;70(4):310–24.

40. Fredberg U, Stengaard-Pedersen K. Chronic tendinopathy tissue pathology, pain mechanisms, and etiology with a special focus on inflammation. Scandinavian Journal of Medicine and Science in Sports. 2008;18(1):3–15.

41. Gaida JE, Bagge J, Purdam C, Cook J, Alfredson H, Forsgren S. Evidence of the TNF-alpha system in the human Achilles tendon: expression of TNF-alpha and TNF receptor at both protein and mRNA levels in the tenocytes. Cells Tissues Organs. 2012;196(4):339–52.

42. Backman LJ, Fong G, Andersson G, Scott A, Danielson P. Substance P is a mechanoresponsive, autocrine regulator of human tenocyte proliferation. PLoS one. 2011;6(11):e27209.

43. Mantyh PW. The neurobiology of skeletal pain. European Journal of Neuroscience. 2014;39(3):508–19.

44. Seeman E. Pathogenesis of bone fragility in women and men. Lancet. 2002;359(9320):1841–50.

45. Seaman DR. Body mass index and musculoskeletal pain: is there a connection? Chiropractic and Manual Therapies. 2013;21:15.

46. Falk S, Bannister K, Dickenson AH. Cancer pain physiology. British Journal of Pain. 2014;8(4):154–62.

47. Nencini S, Ivanusic JJ. The physiology of bone pain. How much do we really know? Frontiers in Physiology. 2016;7(157).

48. Jimenez-Andrade JM, Bloom AP, Mantyh WG, Koewler NJ, Freeman KT, Delong D, et al. Capsaicin-sensitive sensory nerve fibers contribute to the generation and maintenance of skeletal fracture pain. Neuroscience. 2009;162(4):1244–54.

49. Inglis JJ, Nissim A, Lees DM, Hunt SP, Chernajovsky Y, Kidd BL. The differential contribution of tumour necrosis factor to thermal and mechanical hyperalgesia during chronic inflammation. Arthritis Research and Therapy. 2005;7(4):R807–R16.

50. Freemont AJ, Watkins A, Le Maitre C, Baird P, Jeziorska M, Knight MT, et al. Nerve growth factor expression and innervation of the painful intervertebral disc. Journal of Pathology. 2002;197(3):286–92.

51. Risbud MV, Shapiro IM. Notochordal cells in the adult intervertebral disc: new perspective on an old question. Critical Reviews in Eukaryotic Gene Expression. 2011;21(1):29–41.

52. Nagy I, Lukacs KV, Urban L. Mechanisms underlying joint pain. Drug Discovery Today: Disease Mechanisms. 2006;3(3):357–63.

53. Arendt-Nielsen L, Fernandez-de-Las-Penas C, Graven-Nielsen T. Basic aspects of musculoskeletal pain: from acute to chronic pain. Journal of Manual and Manipulative Therapy. 2011;19(4):186–93.

54. Grubb BD. Activation of sensory neurons in the arthritic joint. Novartis Foundation Symposium. 2004;260:28–36; discussion 48, 100–4, 277–9.

55. Alzaharani A, Bali K, Gudena R, Railton P, Ponjevic D, Matyas JR, et al. The innervation of the human acetabular labrum and hip joint: an anatomic study. BMC Musculoskeletal Disorders. 2014;15(1):1–8.

56. Lewin GR, Rueff A, Mendell LM. Peripheral and central mechanisms of NGF-induced hyperalgesia. European Journal of Neuroscience. 1994;6(12):1903–12.

57. McDougall JJ. Arthritis and pain. Neurogenic origin of joint pain. Arthritis Research and Therapy. 2006;8(6):220.

58. Guyton AC. Interstitial fluid presure. II. Pressure-volume curves of interstitial space. Circulation Research. 1965;16:452–60.

59. Jayson MI, St Dixon AJ. Intra-articular pressure in rheumatoid arthritis of the knee. I. Pressure changes during passive joint distension. Annals of the Rheumatic Diseases. 1970;29(3):261–5.

60. Goddard NJ, Gosling PT. Intra-articular fluid pressure and pain in osteoarthritis of the hip. Journal of Bone and Joint Surgery British volume. 1988;70(1):52–5.

61. Ditsios KT, Stavridis SI, Christodoulou AG. The effect of haematoma aspiration on intra-articular pressure and pain relief following Mason I radial head fractures. Injury. 42(4):362–5.

62. Hurley MV. The role of muscle weakness in the pathogenesis of osteoarthritis. Rheumatic Disease Clinics. 25(2):283–98.

63. Scheper MC, de Vries JE, Verbunt J, Engelbert RHH. Chronic pain in hypermobility syndrome and Ehlers–Danlos syndrome (hypermobility type): it is a challenge. Journal of Pain Research. 2015;8:591–601.

64. McDaniel WJJ, Dameron TBJ. The untreated anterior cruciate ligament rupture. Clinical Orthopaedics and Related Research. 1983;172:158–63.

65. Dieppe PA, Lohmander LS. Pathogenesis and management of pain in osteoarthritis. Lancet. 2005;365(9463):965–73.

66. Houard X, Goldring MB, Berenbaum F. Homeostatic mechanisms in articular cartilage and role of inflammation in osteoarthritis. Current Rheumatology Reports. 2013;15(11):375.

67. Schaible H-G, Ebersberger A, Von Banchet GS. Mechanisms of pain in arthritis. Annals of the New York Academy of Sciences. 2002;966(1):343–54.

68. Schaible H-G, Richter F, Ebersberger A, Boettger MK, Vanegas H, Natura G, et al. Joint pain. Experimental Brain Research. 2009;196(1):153–62.

69. England S, Bevan S, Docherty RJ. PGE2 modulates the tetrodotoxin-resistant sodium current in neonatal rat dorsal root ganglion neurones via the cyclic AMP-protein kinase A cascade. Journal of Physiology. 1996;495(2):429–40.

70. Nanes MS. Tumor necrosis factor-alpha: molecular and cellular mechanisms in skeletal pathology. Gene. 2003;321:1–15.

71. Hoheisel U, Sardy M, Mense S. Experiments on the nature of the signal that induces spinal neuroplastic changes following a peripheral lesion. European Journal of Pain. 1997;1(4):243–59.

72. Sessle BJ, Hu JW, Amano N, Zhong G. Convergence of cutaneous, tooth pulp, visceral, neck and muscle afferents onto nociceptive and non-nociceptive neurones in trigeminal subnucleus caudalis (medullary dorsal horn) and its implications for referred pain. Pain. 1986;27(2):219–35.

73. Feinstein B, Langton JN, Jameson RM, Schiller F. Experiments on pain referred from deep somatic tissues. Journal of Bone and Joint Surgery American volume. 1954;36-a(5):981–97.

74. Graven-Nielsen T, Arendt-Nielsen L, Svensson P, Jensen TS. Stimulus-response functions in areas with experimentally induced referred muscle pain – a psychophysical study. Brain Research. 1997;744(1):121–8.

75. Laursen RJ, Graven-Nielsen T, Jensen TS, Arendt-Nielsen L. The effect of compression and regional anaesthetic

block on referred pain intensity in humans. Pain. 1999;80(1–2):257–63.

76. Soler MD, Kumru H, Vidal J, Pelayo R, Tormos JM, Fregni F, et al. Referred sensations and neuropathic pain following spinal cord injury. Pain. 2010;150(1):192–8.

77. Arendt-Nielsen L, Graven-Nielsen T. Central sensitization in fibromyalgia and other musculoskeletal disorders. Current Pain and Headache Reports. 2003;7(5):355–61.

78. Graven-Nielsen T, Aspegren Kendall S, Henriksson KG, Bengtsson M, Sörensen J, Johnson A, et al. Ketamine reduces muscle pain, temporal summation, and referred pain in fibromyalgia patients. Pain. 2000;85(3):483–91.

79. Nijs J, Van Houdenhove B, Oostendorp RAB. Recognition of central sensitization in patients with musculoskeletal pain: application of pain neurophysiology in manual therapy practice. Manual Therapy. 2010;15(2):135–41.

80. Koltyn KF, Brellenthin AG, Cook DB, Sehgal N, Hillard C. Mechanisms of exercise-induced hypoalgesia. Journal of Pain. 2014;15(12):1294–304.

81. Naugle KM, Naugle KE, Fillingim RB, Samuels B, Riley JL, 3rd. Intensity thresholds for aerobic exercise-induced hypoalgesia. Medicine and Science in Sports and Exercise. 2014;46(4):817–25.

82. Naugle KM, Naugle KE, Fillingim RB, Samuels B, Riley JL. Intensity thresholds for aerobic exercise-induced hypoalgesia. Medicine and Science in Sports and Exercise. 2014;46(4):817–25.

83. Naugle KM, Naugle KE, Fillingim RB, Riley JL. Isometric exercise as a test of pain modulation: Effects of experimental pain test, psychological variables, and sex. Pain Medicine (Malden, Mass). 2014;15(4):692–701.

84. Ge HY, Nie H, Graven-Nielsen T, Danneskiold-Samsoe B, Arendt-Nielsen L. Descending pain modulation and its interaction with peripheral sensitization following sustained isometric muscle contraction in fibromyalgia. European Journal of Pain. 2012;16(2):196–203.

85. Arendt-Nielsen L, Sluka KA, Nie HL. Experimental muscle pain impairs descending inhibition. Pain. 2008;140(3):465–71.

86. Staud R, Robinson ME, Vierck CJ, Jr., Price DD. Diffuse noxious inhibitory controls (DNIC) attenuate temporal summation of second pain in normal males but not in normal females or fibromyalgia patients. Pain. 2003;101(1–2):167–74.

87. Bezov D, Ashina S, Jensen R, Bendtsen L. Pain perception studies in tension-type headache. Headache. 2011;51(2):262–71.

88. Corrêa JB, Costa LOP, de Oliveira NTB, Sluka KA, Liebano RE. Central sensitization and changes in conditioned pain modulation in people with chronic nonspecific low back pain: a case–control study. Experimental Brain Research. 2015;233(8):2391–9.

89. Hayden JA, Chou R, Hogg-Johnson S, Bombardier C. Systematic reviews of low back pain prognosis had variable methods and results: guidance for future prognosis reviews. Journal of Clinical Epidemiology. 2009;62(8):781–96.e1.

90. Al-Otaibi ST. Prevention of occupational back pain. Journal of Family and Community Medicine. 2015;22(2):73–7.

91. Palmer KT, Walker-Bone K, Griffin MJ, Syddall H, Pannett B, Coggon D, et al. Prevalence and occupational associations of neck pain in the British population. Scandinavian Journal Work, Environment and Health. 2001;27(1):49–56.

92. Kaergaard A, Andersen J. Musculoskeletal disorders of the neck and shoulders in female sewing machine operators: prevalence, incidence, and prognosis. Occupational and Environmental Medicine. 2000;57(8):528–34.

93. Piligian G, Herbert R, Hearns M, Dropkin J, Landsbergis P, Cherniack M. Evaluation and management of chronic work-related musculoskeletal disorders of the distal upper extremity. American Journal of Industrial Medicine. 2000;37(1):75–93.

94. Mani L, Gerr F. Work-related upper extremity musculoskeletal disorders. Primary Care: Clinics in Office Practice. 2000;27(4):845–64.

95. Davis CG. Mechanisms of chronic pain from whiplash injury. Journal of Forensic and Legal Medicine. 2013;20(2):74–85.

96. Van Oosterwijck J, Nijs J, Meeus M, Paul L. Evidence for central sensitization in chronic whiplash: a systematic literature review. European Journal of Pain. 2013;17(3):299–312.

97. Bliddal H, Curatolo M. Clinical manifestations of muscle and joint pain. In: Graven-Nielsen T, Arendt-Nielsen L, Mense S, editors. Fundamentals of musculoskeletal pain. Seattle: IASP Press; 2008. p. 327–43.

98. Maly MR. Abnormal and cumulative loading in knee osteoarthritis. Current Opinion in Rheumatology. 2008;20(5):547–52.

99. Alnahdi AH, Zeni JA, Snyder-Mackler L. Muscle impairments in patients with knee osteoarthritis. Sports Health. 2012;4(4):284–92.

100. Carlson H, Carlson N. An overview of the management of persistent musculoskeletal pain. Therapeutic Advances in Musculoskeletal Disease. 2011;3(2):91–9.

101. Walsh NE, Brooks P, Hazes JM, Walsh RM, Dreinhofer K, Woolf AD, et al. Standards of care for acute and chronic musculoskeletal pain: the Bone and Joint Decade (2000–2010). Archives of Physical Medicine and Rehabilitation. 2008;89(9):1830–45.

102. Carlson H, Carlson N. An overview of the management of persistent musculoskeletal pain. Therapeutic Advances in Musculoskeletal Disease. 2011;3(2):91–9.

103. Uddin Z, MacDermid JC. Quantitative sensory testing in chronic musculoskeletal pain. Pain Medicine (Malden, Mass). 2016;17(9):1694–703.

104. Arendt-Nielsen L, Yarnitsky D. Experimental and clinical applications of quantitative sensory testing applied to skin, muscles and viscera. Journal of Pain. 2009;10(6):556–72.

105. Uddin Z, MacDermid JC, Galea V, Gross AR, Pierrynowski MR. The current perception threshold test differentiates categories of mechanical neck disorder. Journal of Orthopaedic and Sports Physical Therapy. 2014;44(7):532–40, c1.

106. Suokas AK, Walsh DA, McWilliams DF, Condon L, Moreton B, Wylde V, et al. Quantitative sensory testing in painful osteoarthritis: a systematic review and meta-analysis. Osteoarthritis Cartilage. 2012;20(10):1075–85.

107. Edwards RR, Dolman AJ, Michna E, Katz JN, Nedeljkovic SS, Janfaza D, et al. Changes in pain sensitivity and pain modulation during oral opioid treatment: the impact of negative affect. Pain Medicine. 2016;17(10):1882–91.

108. Olesen SS, Graversen C, Bouwense SA, van Goor H, Wilder-Smith OH, Drewes AM. Quantitative sensory testing predicts pregabalin efficacy in painful chronic pancreatitis. PloS one. 2013;8(3):e57963.

109. Yarnitsky D, Granot M, Nahman-Averbuch H, Khamaisi M, Granovsky Y. Conditioned pain modulation predicts duloxetine efficacy in painful diabetic neuropathy. Pain. 2012;153(6):1193–8.

110. Cruz-Almeida Y, Fillingim RB. Can quantitative sensory testing move us closer to mechanism-based pain management? Pain Medicine. 2014;15(1):61–72.

Introduction

Nociceptive pain is an essential warning function of the peripheral and central nervous systems that signals potential or actual tissue damage. However, pain may also arise due to altered activity within the somatosensory system without sufficient stimulation of its peripheral nerve endings. Thus, neuropathic pain is defined as pain directly due to lesions or disease affecting the somatosensory system.[1] Given this definition, there are numerous diseases that may be responsible for the onset and maintenance of neuropathic pain. Examples include autoimmune diseases (e.g., multiple sclerosis), metabolic diseases (e.g., diabetic peripheral neuropathy), infection (e.g., postherpetic neuralgia due to shingles), vascular disease (e.g., stroke), trauma, and cancer.[2] It is now recognized that specific signs and symptoms are associated with involved structures and pathophysiological mechanisms in the nociceptive system.

However, a classification based on disease alone is often inadequate. For example, different 'neuropathic' conditions often share the same clinical presentation (e.g., postherpetic neuralgia and painful diabetic neuropathy). Alternatively, different signs and symptoms may occur in the same disease, for example, spontaneous pain paroxysms and stimulus-evoked hyperalgesia in postherpetic neuralgia.[3] Additionally, pain due to other syndromes such as complex regional pain syndrome (CRPS) is also classified as being neuropathic in nature.[4] Although the International Association for the Study of Pain (IASP) defines neuropathic pain as pain initiated or caused by a primary lesion or dysfunction in the nervous system, there are issues surrounding diagnostic specificity and anatomical accuracy.[1] First, Treede and colleagues suggest that neuropathic pain needs to be distinguished from pain due to sensitization of the nociceptive system that results in secondary neuroplastic changes. Second, neuropathic pain should also be distinguished from musculoskeletal pain that occurs secondarily in the course of neurological disorders such as multiple sclerosis.[1,5] Thus, questions arise when considering neuropathic pain as a single 'global' entity as opposed to symptoms that reflect many different pathological conditions.

The aim of this chapter is to review and describe the epidemiology and impact of neuropathic pain, pathophysiological mechanisms, signs and symptoms, and the evaluation and treatment of neuropathic pain in clinical settings.

Epidemiology

Prevalence and incidence

Neuropathic pain brings substantial costs to patients and their families in terms of pain and suffering, health care expenses, and quality of life as well as lost productivity and career disability.[6] Estimates for the prevalence of neuropathic pain are well-established with studies showing approximately 8% of adults presently having pain with neuropathic characteristics.[7] However, when considering the presence of neuropathic pain in specific conditions, prevalence and incidence rates are much higher. For example, in the UK, 26% of people with diabetes are shown to have peripheral neuropathic pain.[8] In this context it is important to note that the incidence of diabetes in the general population is estimated to be due to rise from 2.8% to 4.4% by 2030.[7] In other studies, the prevalence of peripheral diabetic neuropathy varies between 8% and 20% in people with type 2 diabetes.[9] Concerning other neuropathic pain conditions, 8% of people diagnosed with herpes zoster develop postherpetic neuralgia,[10] while approximately 35% of people infected with HIV have neuropathic pain.[11] Furthermore, around 37% of people with chronic low back pain present with a major neuropathic pain component.[12] Neuropathic pain is also a significant consequence of chemotherapy treatment in people with cancer.[13] The prevalence of neuropathic pain has also been examined in a number of countries as a single entity. Here, data show prevalence rates of 8.2% in the UK,[14] while in France, Bouhassira and co-workers found a prevalence rate of 6.9%.[15]

Neuropathic pain is also responsible for significant direct and indirect costs to patients and to their families and employers in terms of pain suffering, health care expenditure, reduced quality of life, and absence from work. For example, patients with either postherpetic neuralgia or peripheral diabetic neuropathy have significant costs for diagnostic procedures, medications, and other interventional treatments compared to patients with herpes zoster and diabetes mellitus without neuropathic pain.[16]

Risk factors

Factors associated with the onset and maintenance of neuropathic pain include physical occupation, female gender, old age, unemployed, manual work, and lower socioeconomic status.[9,17] However, the majority of data are cross-sectional and thus it is difficult to determine associations between cause and effect. Although poor psychological and social status are associated with the chance of developing neuropathic pain, data are limited. Additionally, there are several modifiable factors regarding neuropathic pain in conditions such as peripheral

diabetic neuropathy,[18] postherpetic neuropathy,[19] and postsurgical pain.[20] Psychological interventions are shown to improve the general health of patients with neuropathic pain;[21,22] however, more longitudinal studies are needed to confirm these observations.

There are more obvious risk factors associated with more common causes of neuropathic pain. For example, risk factors associated with peripheral diabetic neuropathy include smoking, obesity, hypertension, and hypercholesterolemia.[23,24] Alternatively, risk factors for postherpetic neuralgia are more likely to be due to older age, female gender, greater rash severity and greater acute pain severity.[9,19] In this case, early awareness and treatment of shingles symptoms is essential for reducing the occurrence and/or severity of neuropathic pain. Concerning patients with HIV, several epidemiological studies show that the risk of peripheral neuropathy is increased by older age, a history of diabetes mellitus, a high CD4 count (T-lymphocyte cell count), and the use of protease inhibitors (antiviral drugs widely used in the treatment of HIV/AIDS).[25,26]

Types of neuropathic pain

Neuropathic pain differs from other pain conditions in which pain is generated by dysfunction of

Table 9.1: Common causes of neuropathic pain

Classification	Cause/type	Presentation
Traumatic	Surgery, Spinal cord injury, Amputation	Focal
Entrapment	Spinal stenosis, Carpal/tarsal tunnel syndromes, Chronic radiculopathy	Focal
Vascular	Ischemic peripheral neuropathy, Brain infarction	Focal/multifocal
Metabolic	Diabetes mellitus, Hypothyroidism, Porphyria	Generalized
Immune-related	Multiple sclerosis, Guillain–Barré syndrome, Rheumatoid arthritis	Generalized/multifocal
Infectious	HIV, Infectious mononucleosis, Postherpetic neuralgia	Generalized Focal/multifocal
Cancer-related	Compressive, Infiltrative	Focal/multifocal
Complex neuropathic pain disorders	Complex regional pain syndrome	Focal/multifocal

non-neural tissues. There are numerous traumatic, entrapment, metabolic, autoimmune, infectious, and cancerous causes of neuropathic pain, some common examples of which are shown in Table 9.1.

Chronic neuropathic pain is a common presentation in clinical practice and, as noted in Table 9.1, neuropathic pain syndromes are heterogeneous conditions that cannot be described by a single etiology or specific lesion.[3] Additionally, people present with focal (e.g., surgery and trauma), multifocal (e.g., ischemic and inflammatory), or generalized (e.g., HIV and hypothyroidism) nerve lesions. Clinically, neuropathic pain is challenging because of several important factors:[6]

- Most neuropathic pain conditions are associated with several pathophysiological mechanisms.

- Different disease states may mechanistically generate the same neuropathic pain syndrome.

- Presenting signs and symptoms and clinical testing may differ with a specific neuropathic pain syndrome.

For example, postherpetic neuralgia, a complication of shingles and a good example of how infection can lead to pain, has been found to have at least three different mechanisms for pain, infectious, inflammatory, and ischemic, that are due to both central and peripheral nerve damage.[6] Moreover, each mechanism is associated with different symptoms, with some patients presenting with severe pain in an area of significant sensory loss while others may present with allodynia and no sensory loss. And not only do people present with different symptoms, they may also respond differently to the same treatment.

In another example, CRPS, a set of painful symptoms, which develops after trauma such as fractures, dislocations, rheumatoid arthritis, and other musculoskeletal comorbidities, is clinically characterized by allodynia, hyperalgesia, abnormal skin color, abnormal sudomotor activity, localized edema, and motor and trophic disturbances.[27]

Although the mechanisms of CRPS are not clearly understood, it is likely that immobility may be an independent factor, as Terkelsen and colleagues showed that immobilizing limbs in healthy volunteers produced similar sensory abnormalities to those found in people diagnosed with CRPS.[28] Interestingly, although people with CRPS present with symptoms of painful neuropathies, no observable nerve lesions are evident.[29] However, experimental findings from animal studies show that pain hypersensitivity symptoms are likely due to peripheral and central sensitization processes, while sympathetic symptoms are thought to be due to interaction of sympathetic fibers with afferent neurons located within the skin.[30,31]

Symptoms of neuropathic pain

Patients presenting with neuropathic pain show distinct positive and negative sensory symptoms, which may occur in various combinations.[3] Negative symptoms include deficits in tactile hypoesthesia, thermal hypoesthesia, pinprick hypoalgesia, and reductions or losses in vibration sense. Although these symptoms are troublesome, they are not painful. Positive symptoms include abnormal sensations such as paresthesias (tingling or pricking) and dysesthesia (abnormal unpleasant sensation felt when touched). Neuropathic-type pain is classified as hyperalgesic or allodynic and may be either dynamic (with movement across sensitized skin surface) or static (applied pressure) (Table 9.2). Additionally, cold and heat hyperalgesia and allodynia may also be evoked by normally mildly painful or non-painful warm and cold stimuli. These positive symptoms can also occur as 'spontaneous' pain (occurring in the absence of stimulus) or as 'stimulus-evoked' pain, occurring either statically (e.g., applied pressure) or dynamically (movement-induced).

Spontaneous pain

Spontaneous pain occurs without provocation. This type of pain can arise at any time without warning and is due to spontaneous activity in nociceptive afferent neurons. Spontaneous pain is most often described as brief but

Table 9.2: Definitions of symptoms of hyperalgesia and allodynia (adapted from Baron 2006[3] and Jensen et al. 2014[4])

Symptom	Definition	Response
Negative		
Hypoesthesia	Reduced sensation to non-painful stimuli	Reduced sensation/numbness
Thermal hypoesthesia	Reduced sensation to cold and heat stimuli	Reduced sensation
Hypoalgesia	Reduced sensation to painful stimuli	Reduced sensation and numbness
Positive – stimulus-evoked		
Mechanical static (superficial)	Pain from normally non-painful static pressure on the skin	Dull pain in damaged/sensitized primary afferent nerve endings
Mechanical static (deep)	Pain from pressure from normally non-painful finger pressure on underlying tissues	Dull pain in damaged area
Mechanical dynamic	Pain from normally non-painful moving (stroking, brushing) stimuli on the skin	Sharp pain across the site of primary affected area but spreads to adjacent secondarily affected tissues
Thermally-evoked stimuli		
Cold	Pain from normally non-painful cold stimuli (<20°C)	Burning pain sensation in damaged/sensitized primary afferent nerve endings
Heat	Pain from normally non-painful heat stimuli (>40°C)	Burning pain sensation in damaged/sensitized primary afferent nerve endings
Spontaneous pain		
Paresthesia	Non-painful pricking/skin crawling sensations	Reduced sensation
Paroxysmal pain	Short-lasting shooting/electric-type pain	

acute episodes of stabbing, shooting, and/or electrical pain as well as altered sensation such as pins and needles. Such ectopic discharges are a result of increased depolarization at injured sites on the nerve fiber. However, lesions of sensory or mixed peripheral nerves with a cutaneous branch also lead to sensory loss in associated innervation regions. Thus, in addition to spontaneous pain, other negative sensory signs may include deficits in mechanical and vibratory stimuli that indicate damage to large myelinated fibers or the dorsal columns and loss of nociceptive noxious and thermal perception.[32] These are primary examples for the co-occurrence of both nociceptive and neuropathic mechanisms. Additionally,

central inhibitory circuits may be impaired within the dorsal horn or the brainstem, or both.

Hyperalgesia

Hyperalgesia refers to an increased pain response to a painful stimulus such as a pinprick (Figure 9.1). Hyperalgesic responses can occur from both altered peripheral and altered central nociceptive mechanisms. Peripherally, injury produces ongoing pain and two types of hyperalgesia. Primary hyperalgesia occurs at the site of tissue injury (e.g., mechanical trauma, burn) and is mediated by inflammatory mediators such as bradykinin and substance P that sensitize

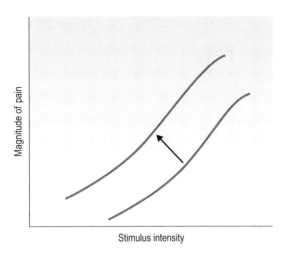

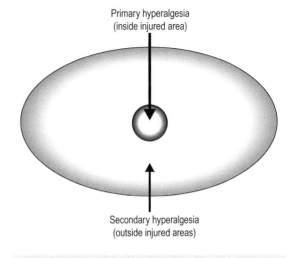

Figure 9.1

This pain intensity (*y* axis) – stimulus intensity (*x* axis) graph shows hyperalgesic responses to stimuli shift to the left when thresholds become lower due to tissue injury (Meyer et al. 2005)

Figure 9.2

Shows a cutaneous area of primary hyperalgesia at an injury site. This is surrounded by an area of secondary hyperalgesia that develops in tissue adjacent the site of injury

primary Aδ and C fiber nociceptive nerve endings. Secondary hyperalgesia occurs in non-injured tissue surrounding an injury site and is thought be centrally mediated (Figure 9.2). Additionally, secondary hyperalgesia is characterized by an increased pain response to mechanical (especially light touch), but not heat stimuli in people with neuropathic pain (e.g., shingles).[33,34] Another peripheral mechanism for stimulus-evoked hyperalgesia occurs in the presence of a neuroma, a disorganized mass of nervous tissue surrounded by scar and/or connective tissue.[6] Neuromas normally arise at the proximal end of injured nerves where regenerative axon sprouts commonly show extreme mechanical sensitivity.[35] After injury, voltage-gated sodium channels (VGSCs) accumulate in the axon at the neuroma site, resulting in areas of hyperexcitability and spontaneous action potential discharge.[36]

Allodynia

Allodynia is evoked by continued peripheral simulation of nociceptor terminals in the periphery (overstimulation) and by the action of low-threshold myelinated Aβ on sensitized central nervous system.[37] Central sensitization mechanisms cause reductions in threshold for both myelinated (low threshold, non-nociceptive) fibers and thinly and non-myelinated nociceptive fibers. Concerning mechanical allodynia, even gentle stimuli, such as stroking or the bending of body hair, can evoke intense pain. Levels of allodynia vary among different neuropathic pain conditions. For example, allodynia is a prominent feature of postherpetic neuralgia and traumatic neuropathy due to what is thought to be loss and damage of C fiber innervation in the epidermis.[34] However, although diabetic peripheral neuropathy is considered painful, allodynia is unusual.[38]

Mechanisms of neuropathic pain

Current understandings of neuropathic pain mechanisms suggest that a nerve lesion can lead to dramatic changes in the nervous system.[32] Nicvkel and colleagues suggest that changes in peripheral, central, and autonomic systems lead to the activation and overlap of several sensitization process:[39]

Chapter 9

- peripheral sensitization of nociceptors

- abnormal ectopic excitability of affected neurons

- increased nociceptive facilitation at the spinal cord

- disinhibition of spinal inhibitory neurons

- sympathetically maintained pain

- central nervous system reorganization.

Peripheral mechanisms

As reviewed in previous chapters, pain sensations are normally initiated by activity of high-threshold unmyelinated C and thinly myelinated Aδ primary afferent neurons. However, after peripheral nerve lesion, neurons become atypically sensitive and prone to pathological spontaneous activity. As with nociception, peripheral sensitization is an important mechanism of neuropathic pain, contributing to conditions such as herpes zoster, postherpetic neuralgia, and CRPS.[39] Directly after a nerve injury, the site becomes heavily populated by macrophages, mast cells, and T lymphocytes from peripheral blood flow, which congregate around the injured nerve fiber.[40] At the same time, Schwann cells begin to proliferate and release proteases (key components of the inflammatory response), which attack endoneurial blood vessels, leading to a disruption in the blood–nerve barrier. This further causes the release of inflammatory mediators such as substance P, bradykinin, nitric oxide, and calcitonin gene-related peptide from injured axons, which, in turn, activate adjacent nociceptors (Figure 9.3).[41] Peripheral signaling pathways between primary afferent neurons, Schwann cells, and the immune system are complex, with chemokines attracting and guiding monocytes to a damaged neuron. Once differentiated, macrophages and mast cells release a series of inflammatory mediators that in turn cause Schwann cells to release signal molecules, including nerve growth factor (NGF) (Chapter 1), which not only promote local axonal growth and remyelination but also significantly contribute to the sensitization of peripheral nociceptors. Thus, it is not surprising that

Scholtz and Woolf suggest that neuropathic pain conditions and neuroimmune disorders share similar features.[40]

Abnormal ectopic excitability after nerve injury

Inflammatory and immune mediators induce ectopic spontaneous activity after a nerve injury at both injured and adjacent non-injured primary afferent nociceptors. This spontaneous activity is most likely due to molecular and cellular changes such as damaged VGSCs that accumulate on an injured nerve causing a shift forwards in threshold potential.[37] Additionally, nerve injury also causes increases in expression of messenger RNA for VGSCs, thus increasing their concentration at both injured sites and more proximally within the dorsal root ganglion. Such ongoing ectopic discharges may initiate or maintain both peripheral and central sensitization, which then amplifies nociceptive AΔ and C fiber inputs from adjacent intact afferent nerves.[42] Damage to peripheral nerves also causes upregulation of receptor proteins such as TRPV1 receptors (Chapter 1). Studies provide evidence for the upregulation of TRPV1 receptors on both injured and non-injured nociceptive afferent fibers[43] due mostly to increased expression of second messengers such as protein kinases.[44] More recently, lipid metabolites such as lysophosphatidic acid (LPA) released after nerve damage have also been shown to play a significant role in neuropathic pain. Here, animal studies show that LPA receptor-deficient mice do not develop neuropathic pain, whereas mice receiving intrathecal LPA injections develop signs of neuropathic pain commonly seen after peripheral nerve injury.[45]

Damage to peripheral nerves is also associated with Wallerian degeneration. This term refers to the vigorous reaction of non-neuronal cellular responses, especially at the distal stump of a damaged nerve, which lead to clearing of debris in the peripheral nerve to sustain an environment that supports axonal regrowth.[46] Here, the axon and myelin sheath of the damaged nerve are degraded

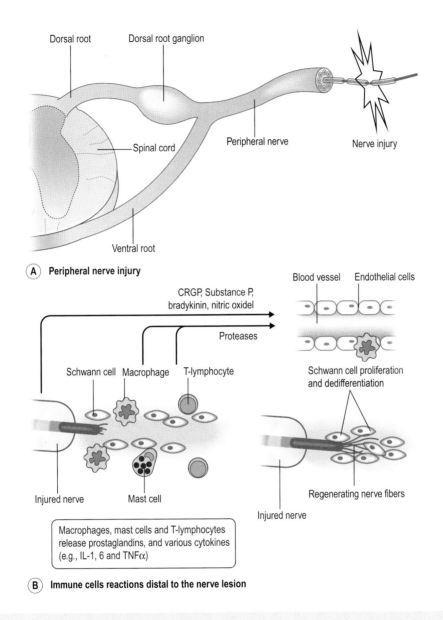

Figure 9.3

Peripheral nerve injury provokes local invasion of macrophages, mast cells and T-lymphocytes causing Schwann cells to both proliferate and dedifferentiate (lose their specialist function) and to release a multitude of signaling molecules that facilitate Wallerian degeneration in injured peripheral nerves

by the action of inflammatory infiltrates such as TNFα, NGF, macrophages, and other immune cells described above,[40] thus encouraging symptoms such as hyperalgesia and allodynia. Animal studies show that hyperalgesic symptoms after partial nerve injury are relieved by anti-NGF antibodies.[47]

Chapter 9

Dorsal root ganglion mechanisms

Although proximal to a peripheral nerve damage site, immune cells in the dorsal root ganglion (DRG) react to nerve injury, their response being influenced by incoming macrophages.[40] Indeed, significant spontaneous discharge has been shown in large myelinated fibers at the DRG after cutting spinal nerves distal to the DRG.[48] Thus, nociceptive activity in large fiber neurons that are not normally nociceptive may induce central sensitization and clinical allodynia.[49] Like neuropathic pain mechanisms in the periphery, both neuro and immune pro-inflammatory mediators are released at the DRG. Schwann cells and glial cells release a cascade of inflammatory mediators, in particular TNFα, which in turn sensitize and lower thresholds in the glial cells at the DRG. This activity thus directly modulates ectopic action potential discharges.[40,49]

Spinal cord mechanisms

Despite evidence suggesting the importance of peripheral sensitization, there is a considerable degree of reorganization in the spinal cord in response to peripheral nerve injuries.[50] Thus, many researchers now consider central pain mechanisms as the main pathophysiological mechanism underlying neuropathic pain.[32,40] For example, although large myelinated fibers normally terminate at laminae III–V, after peripheral nerve damage they also sprout to lamina II of the superficial dorsal horn (Figure 9.4). Ongoing spontaneous activity due to peripheral nerve injury leads to an increase in excitability in spinal cord nociceptive neurons, multireceptive wide dynamic range neurons, and inputs from incoming non-nociceptive Aβ neurons.[3] General dorsal horn hyperexcitability causes expansion in neuronal receptive fields as well as a spread of this increased excitability to adjacent segments.[3] So, while the spread of pain beyond the boundaries of affected peripheral nerves was once considered to indicate hysteria, Woolf and Mannion sensibly suggest it to be more a result of central sensitization.[35]

As described in Chapter 2, the release of glutamate from incoming nociceptive and non-nociceptive neurons acts on postsynaptic N-methyl-D-aspartate

Figure 9.4

A schematic diagram showing the reorganization of large myelinated fibers that normally signal non-noxious sensory input, sprout to the more superficial laminae receiving nociceptive peripheral input

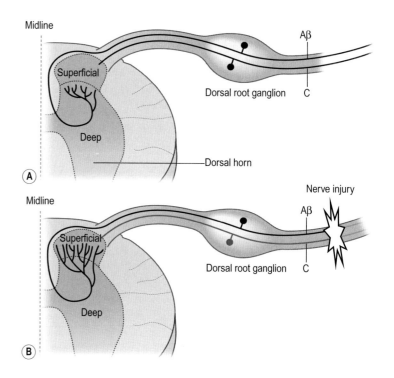

(NMDA) receptors. Activation of these ion channels in turn stimulates a multitude of intracellular cascades that ultimately contribute to central sensitization, principally that of the protein kinase system. Importantly, evidence now suggests that NMDA receptor antagonists may have a role in the relief of neuropathic pain.[50] Peripheral nerve injury leads to the upregulation and overexpression of sodium channels in dorsal horn neurons. Animal studies show that upregulation of these sodium channels is strongly associated with hyperexcitability in second order projection neurons. These gene knockdown (gene silencing) studies show that animals lacking Nav1.3 ion channels (Chapter 1) reduce hyperexcitability in these neurons, thus reducing pain-related behavior in spinal cord-injured rats.[51,52]

Neuroimmune activation in the spinal cord

As reviewed in Chapter 2, microglia and astrocytes play key roles in the response to injuries both peripherally and centrally,[40,53] and their negative effect in chronic pain states has been substantially validated. Microglia act as resident macrophages and are inactive in normal conditions. They become active in response to a number of insults, those being injury, infection, ischemia, tumors, and neurodegenerative disorders such as multiple sclerosis.[53] Once activated, microglia both proliferate towards cell bodies of injured nerves as well as around central terminals of injured afferent sensory nerves.[54,55] Activated microglia also show changes in functional activities such as phagocytosis, increases in expression of nociceptor-specific receptors, and the release of pro-inflammatory mediators. Unlike microglia, astrocytes respond relatively slowly to nerve injury, but are sustained for longer periods.[40] However, although it is not known what triggers astrocyte activation and proliferation, it is suggested that direct pathways of communication exist between these glial cells that coordinate patterns of activation.[40]

Evaluating neuropathic pain

Aims of evaluation

When assessing people with possible neuropathic pain it is important to assess what type(s) of pain they have: nociceptive, neuropathic, or a mixture of both.[56]

Although there are many available tools that help in the assessment of neuropathic pain, the practitioner's ability to let the patient tell their story, careful observation, and thorough examination remain the most reliable sources of information.

Case history and observation

In the absence of obvious trauma, pain of neurological origin can develop slowly over time. Thus, care must be taken in allowing the patient to fully describe their pain history as they understand it.[56] The history should include questions regarding the location, intensity, and character of the pain, temporal factors, and any exacerbating or relieving factors. Additionally, enquiry relating to previous medical and surgical history is important as this may point to factors relating to the onset and maintenance of neuropathic pain. Patients should also be observed from the first moment of an initial appointment. It is important to note not only their movements and gait, but also how they understand and express their symptoms. If neuropathic pain is suspected, there are several well-validated screening tools available. Neuropathic pain, like other forms of pain, has a significant impact on general activity, fitness, independence, mood, sleep, occupation, and social functioning. If not addressed, these factors not only affect patients and their families, but also become obstacles in the treatment of neuropathic pain.

Screening tools

Several self-reporting and classification tools have been developed to validate neuropathic pain. In this section, four of the most widely validated general screening tools are reviewed.

The Leeds Assessment of Neuropathic Symptoms and Signs (LANSS)

The LANSS contains five symptom items and two clinical examination items and is based on analysis of sensory description and examination of sensory dysfunction.[57] The symptom items relate to altered sensations such as pricking and tingling as well as increased sensitivity and skin changes. The two clinical items test for symptoms of allodynia using light touch and pinprick thresholds. A score of 12 or more out of a possible 24 is suggestive of neuropathic pain. A self-reporting version, the S-LANSS, was later developed and like the LANSS, this 11-point Likert-scale questionnaire has been validated in many settings, showing good to excellent sensitivity and specificity when compared to clinical diagnosis.[58]

The Douleur Neuropathique en 4 (DN4)

The DN4 is a practitioner-administered questionnaire consisting of 10 items, seven of which are related to pain quality (i.e., sensory and pain descriptors), while three items are based on clinical examination and are related to the presence or absence of touch or pinprick hypoesthesia and tactile allodynia.[59] Scoring is simple since each question has a yes/no answer. People scoring four or more out of 10 are likely to have neuropathic pain. Although originally developed in France, the DN4 has been translated into 15 languages, including Spanish and Thai.[58]

The Neuropathic Pain Questionnaire (NPQ)

The NPQ contains 12 items and is aimed at differentiating neuropathic pain patients from non-neuropathic pain patients.[60] The NPQ has 10 items related to sensation (e.g., numbness, tingling) and sensory responses (e.g., increased pain response to touch) and two items relating to the effects of symptoms on patients. The NPQ has been shown to be reliable for (1) initial screening and (2) monitoring neuropathic pain treatments as an outcome measure.[61]

painDETECT

The painDETECT, designed in Germany, is a nine-item self-reporting questionnaire, seven items of which relate to sensory descriptors, while the other two relate to spatial and temporal features of patients' pain patterns.[62] The painDETECT was originally developed for people with neuropathic pain related to the low back; however, validity studies also show it to be applicable to other types of neuropathic pain.

Recommendations from the International Association for the Study of Pain (IASP) suggest that due to a lack of a gold standard diagnostic approach to neuropathic pain, the above screening tools provide a simple and easy option for practitioners and patients alike since they can be completed in clinical, online, or telephone settings, as appropriate.[63]

Clinical examination

Mechanisms of neuropathic pain lead to substantial changes in the nervous system that are significantly different to CP occurring in an intact nociceptive system.[32] Clinical examination of a pain patient with a possible neuropathic pain condition therefore aims to confirm or reject the possibility of a lesion or disease within the nervous system.[58] Patients with neuropathic pain will have areas of altered sensation or hypersensitivity in the affected area.[32] In order to diagnose neuropathic pain, it is important to evaluate the precise quality of abnormal somatosensory function by identifying the location, quality, severity, and pattern of pain. Thus, a neurological examination must assess the presence or absence of specific stimulus-evoked signs[6] in addition to asking the patient to report the particular quality of sensation (e.g., burning). Neuropathic pain is typically confined to part or the total innervation of an affected nerve. However, it is important to understand that pain in the region of an affected nerve may not be neuropathic in origin. For example, surrounding altered muscle tone and associated nociceptive pain may also arise due to a nerve injury.[1]

A standard examination of a person presenting with neuropathic pain must include the components of touch, pressure, vibration, cold, heat, and temporal summation.[32,64] Responses to these stimuli should be recorded as 'normal,' 'decreased,' or 'increased.' Additionally, positive pain responses to these stimuli should be reported as 'hyperalgesic' or 'allodynic' and classified as either dynamic or static in character of the stimulus (e.g., dynamic light touch). There are various bedside assessments available; for example, light touch can be assessed with the application of cotton wool to the skin, pinprick with a single pin or stick,

Table 9.3: Clinical evaluation of hyperalgesia and allodynia (adapted from references 32 and 63)

Stimuli type	Clinical assessment	Expected response
Mechanical		Focal
Dynamic mechanical	Cotton bud/artist's brush	Sharp burning pain in affected zone and possibly in adjacent skin areas
Punctate	Prick with stick or pin	Sharp burning pain in affected zone and possibly in adjacent skin areas
Static (superficial tissue)	Light finger pressure to skin	Dull pain at reduced thresholds in affected area of skin
Static (deep tissue)	Finger pressure applied to tissue underlying skin	Dull pain at reduced thresholds in underlying muscles
Thermal		
Cold	Cold water/metal filled tubes at 20°C	Burning temperature sensation in affected area
Heat	Warm metal/water filled tubes at 40°C	Burning temperature sensation in affected area
Temporal summation	Pricking skin with safety pin at intervals of >3/ second for 30 seconds with equal intensity	Sharp superficial pain that increases in intensity

and heat and cold with a metal object (e.g., water filled tubes) at either 20° C or 40°C.[32] Additionally, temporal summation is the clinical equivalent of increasing nociceptive activity during repetitive noxious C fiber activation. This 'wind-up' of pain can be reproduced easily using a mechanical stimulus, usually pinprick. Table 9.3 summarizes methods used to examine people with neuropathic pain.

Additional investigation

In order to confirm initial diagnosis, CT and MRI scans also help to identify causes of nerve damage that require further treatment. Furthermore, neurophysiological tests such as quantitative sensory testing are reliable in detecting small fiber neuropathies by measuring sensory responses to mechanical, thermal, and electrical stimuli. However, this equipment is expensive and mostly available to those working in research and tertiary care settings. Although clinical findings may fit well with distinct neuropathic pain syndromes such as diabetic peripheral neuropathy, painful

neuropathy may also be caused by other less obvious, but treatable conditions such as vitamin B_{12} and copper deficiencies.[65] Thus, further investigation may be required to find evidence of nerve dysfunction.

Treatment

Although there are consensus-based guidelines for the treatment of neuropathic pain based on high evidence level trials, significant gaps in the literature exist.[66] This is mostly due to a lack of studies that (1) compare different treatment approaches; (2) use the same study design; and (3) compare the use of different outcome measures. Thus, many patients receiving treatment for neuropathic pain do not experience sufficient pain relief, with at least a 30% reduction being generally accepted as meaningful.[32] This is most likely due to the heterogeneity of mechanisms associated with neuropathic pain as well as the influence of comorbid psychological factors such as anxiety and depression. Thus, a first step is a thorough diagnosis that is able to unravel the cause, such as diabetes or local nerve compression, with treatment of the underlying conditions addressed first.[32] If these first-line interventions do not alleviate the pain, then management of pain symptoms is then addressed. Here, patient education is important, as patients should understand the reasons for the continuation of their pain and their treatment plan, and be aware that there may be side-effects of medication. Additionally, given the effect of psychological factors on the treatment of pain symptoms, assessment of emotional, cognitive, and social function is also important.[67]

Generally, pharmacological and interventional approaches are recommended for the first-line treatment of neuropathic pain. However, cognitive behavioral therapy,[68] graded motor imagery,[69] and virtual reality tasks[70] have also been shown to reduce pain in certain neuropathic pain conditions, such as phantom limb and complex regional pain syndrome. The remainder of this section will briefly review pharmacological treatments and other interventional types of treatment shown to benefit people with neuropathic pain.

Pharmacological approaches

The International Association for the Study of Pain (IASP) guidelines recommend medications in the treatment of neuropathic pain that show consistent effectiveness in neuropathic pain.[66] First-line treatments showing the greatest efficacy are antidepressants that involve both norepinephrine/noradrenaline and serotonin reuptake inhibition.[71] Additional first-line medication also includes: antiepilepsy drugs acting on sodium channels (e.g., carbamazepine, lamotrigine), medications acting as calcium channel blockers (e.g., pregabalin, gabapentin), and topical lidocaine.[72] Opioids and tramadol (opioid-SNRI combinations) are also useful in the treatment of neuropathic pain, but are considered as second-line, mainly due to concerns over their side-effects and long-term safety compared to the above mentioned first-line drugs.[66] However, in situations such as the treatment of acute neuropathic pain and cancer-related neuropathic pain, these drugs are used as first-line treatments. Due to inconsistent findings in different RCTs, several other

antidepressants, such as citalopram, paroxetine (both SSRIs), and topical capsaicin, are considered as third-line.[73]

First-line medications

A significant number of RCTs have found tricyclic antidepressants (TCAs) (e.g., nortriptyline, amitriptyline) to be effective in the treatment of several types of peripheral neuropathic pain conditions, including diabetic neuropathy, postherpetic neuropathy, and neuropathies invoked by spinal cord injury.[16] Not surprisingly, TCAs are also effective in the treatment of depression, a common comorbidity in patients with neuropathic pain. However, TCAs have several side-effects, in particular because of their additional anticholinergic action on the parasympathetic nervous system (e.g., dry mouth, constipation, difficulty in urination, and hypotension).

Although antidepressants have several modes of action, they mainly inhibit the reuptake of both serotonin and norepinephrine in descending pain pathways. Selective norepinephrine and serotonin reuptake inhibitors, such as duloxetine and venlafaxine, have been found to be effective for several painful neuropathies, especially diabetic peripheral neuropathy, but not for postherpetic neuropathy.[16,72] However, neither drug has been studied in the treatment of other peripheral neuropathies.[32] Although nausea is a common side-effect of both medications, venlafaxine has been shown to cause cardiac conduction and blood pressure abnormalities, and thus is prescribed with caution in patients with cardiac disease.[74]

Pregabalin and gabapentin are anticonvulsive drugs that bind to calcium channels on the central terminals of primary afferent nociceptors and thus decrease the release of glutamate and substance P.[32] Like antidepressants, these drugs have been found to be effective in the treatment of peripheral and centrally mediated neuropathic pain while pregabalin has also been found to improve sleep disturbance and anxiety. However, both pregabalin and gabapentin produce dose-related dizziness and drowsiness.[66]

Topical lidocaine, a local anesthetic that blocks VGSCs in nociceptor cell membranes, shows both efficacy and excellent tolerability in people with neuropathic pain, especially those with allodynia.[73] Given the lack of systemic absorption and thus reduced likelihood of side-effects and drug interactions, lidocaine is particularly useful in older people with neuropathic pain. However, given its topical application, it does not benefit those with centrally mediated pain.[75]

Second-line medications

Opioid medications are agonists at both presynaptic and postsynaptic opioid receptors and provide pain-relief at least as great as that found with all first-line medications.[9] However, due to long-term safety issues concerning side-effects, immunosuppressive effects, and the potential for misuse, opioids are mostly used in patients who do not respond to first-line medication. Additionally, as patients on long-term opioid therapies develop dependence, it is especially important to consider this line of medication in people with a current or previous history of substance abuse (including abuse of alcohol and prescription medication), as they are more likely to misuse opioids.[66]

Another common second-line drug is tramadol. This medication has a dual effect in that it (1) inhibits the reuptake of serotonin and (2) acts as a weak opioid mu-receptor agonist. Although the risk of dependence is relatively low, it can interact with other serotonin reuptake inhibitor medication, and thus increase the potential for the potentially fatal condition serotonin syndrome.[16]

Interventional therapies

As pharmacological relief of neuropathic pain is often inadequate, forms of neurostimulation have been shown to be effective in people with chronic neuropathic pain. Systematic reviews of RCTs show spinal cord stimulation to be effective in patients with neuropathic pain from failed low back surgery and CRPS, while neural blockade is recommended for people with postherpetic peripheral neuropathy.[76] The aim of spinal cord stimulation is to apply adequate electrical current over the dorsal columns that cause paresthesias which overlap the painful areas while minimizing paresthesias externally.[77] Guidelines based on meta-analysis also show that although not of high evidence levels, transcutaneous electrical stimulation (TENS) and electro-acupuncture are more effective than placebo in both central and peripheral neuropathic pain conditions.[78] Here, it is suggested that TENS activates central mechanisms to provide analgesia by acting on various opioid receptors, depending on the frequency.[79] Laser therapy, although not rigorously researched, shows promise as a treatment approach. Human studies have found very low laser therapy to result in perceived decreases in pain and disability, while animal studies show laser therapy decreases levels of hypoxia-induced factor 1a, an important modulator in neurogenic inflammation.[80]

Psychological therapies

There are a number of treatment approaches that fall under the umbrella term 'psychological' and which are specifically designed to change psychological processes involved in the modulation of pain, distress, and disability.[81] Overall, there is a clear lack of evidence both for and against the effectiveness of psychological interventions for neuropathic pain in altering the experience of pain, disability, and altered mood.[81] However, cognitive and behavioral therapies aimed at social and emotional functioning have shown promise in conditions such as diabetic peripheral neuropathy, postherpetic neuralgia, and CRPS. However, more rigorous trials, using larger samples that include placebo comparison groups, are required.[81] For example, in a small non-blinded pilot study, Otis and colleagues showed that participants receiving CBT showed significant decreases in pain severity and pain-related interference at four-month follow-up compared to those receiving 'treatment as usual.'[68] Additionally, psychological therapy is also shown to be a useful adjunct to ongoing pharmacological treatment for neuropathic pain.[67]

Motor imagery and virtual reality therapies

Virtual reality (VR) and motor imagery therapies are showing increasing evidence in the effective treatment of a range of chronic pain conditions. The following sections review and briefly discuss current evidence for these therapies.

Graded motor imagery

Graded motor imagery (GMI) is a modified approach using both visual and imagery techniques. It is made up of three sequential treatment techniques that include left/right limb discrimination training, motor imagery exercises, and mirror therapy.[82] Resources include flash cards, phone/tablet applications, handbooks, mirror boxes, and web-accessible software. Developed by Moseley and colleagues, GMI has been shown to be effective in producing short-term reductions in pain intensity with chronic regional pain syndrome and in phantom limb pain patients.[83] While these techniques have only been used as a collective by Moseley's group, other researchers have used components of GMI to show alterations in brain activity.[84] However, the focus of studies investigating the effect of GMI on levels of pain intensity is narrow, with only a few studies investigating its effects on phantom limb pain, CRPS, and post-stroke pain. Further studies are required on other neuropathic pain disorders such as spinal cord and peripheral nerve injury and diabetes as well as chronic somatic pain syndromes such as fibromyalgia and irritable bowel syndrome. It should

also be noted that none of the above studies incorporated baseline anxiety or depression scores (potential latent variables).[85,86] These limitations make simple interpretation of the results difficult.

Virtual reality applications

Research shows that virtual reality (VR)/imagery application technology is in its infancy. VR technology is currently used as a method of pain distraction for patients who have difficulty diverting attention away from their ongoing pain.[87] VR technology is also being developed to provide ways of subjecting patients to movement that they may avoid due to fear of pain, such as walking[88] (Figure 9.5). VR technology has also been used to simulate movement of specific body parts that patients are unable to control (phantom limb pain) or avoid using (CRPS).[89,90] Currently, VR applications are being developed for both expensive high-resolution head-mounted units and relatively inexpensive desktop computers that also require the use of polarized or shutter glasses in combination with large 3-D monitors.[87]

Physical therapy

Although physical modalities such as hot and cold packs, ultrasound, and short-wave diathermy show

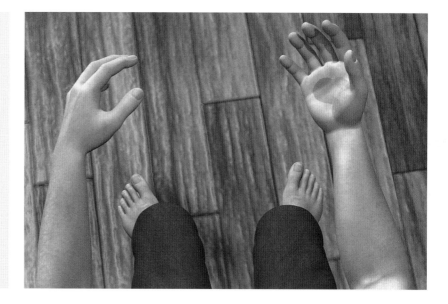

Figure 9.5

An image of a typical virtual reality walking computer application for people with spinal cord injury or people with phantom limb pain

anecdotal efficacy in people with chronic pain, these modalities are not recommended for people with neuropathic pain.[79] However, there is evidence showing these and other physical therapeutic techniques are beneficial in mobilizing associated joint contracture and mobilization of connective tissue and improving movement function in people with neuropathic pain. Here, only small studies show promise using soft-tissue techniques such as Thai massage and reflexology for changes in foot mobility and function in people with diabetic peripheral neuropathy.[91,92] Concerning the effect of manual therapy on neuropathic pain, evidence comes from isolated pilot and case studies. Here for example, massage therapy is shown to be effective in decreasing symptoms and increasing quality of life in a patient suffering severe chemotherapy-induced peripheral neuropathy.[93] Similarly, spinal cord injury patients report partial decreases in levels of neuropathic pain at two-month follow up following a six-week course of either acupuncture or massage.[94]

Exercise therapy

The use of therapeutic exercise is increasing rapidly as a treatment for many diseases. Exercise has been shown to activate afferent sensory nerves from active muscles to the spinal cord; for example, the exercise-pressor reflex changes during activity that alters blood pressure and heart rate via sympathetic pathway activation.[95] More pertinently, research also shows improvements in regeneration of nerve injuries after exercise, due probably to increased production of neurotransmitters associated with the stimulation of axonal growth.[96] Given this effect on spinal cord neurons, it is not surprising that therapeutic exercise may also affect central pain modulatory pathways.[97] However, although partly evident, the effects of exercise on the central nervous system are not well studied.

Most studies have investigated the effect of exercise on diabetic painful neuropathies. Findings suggest that long-term exercise does not so much reduce levels of pain as delay the onset of diabetes-associated neuropathy.[98] However, importantly, animal studies currently suggest that physical exercise can improve mechanical allodynia and thermal hyperalgesia.[99,100] These reductions in neuropathic pain symptoms have also recently been shown to be due to increased anti-inflammatory and decreased proinflammatory cytokines.[101]

Summary

Neuropathic pain is a complex chronic pain state that is accompanied by nerve tissue injury which not only alters neurophysiological function but also neuroanatomical wiring. Although not all patients with nerve lesions develop neuropathic pain, many people receiving treatment for neuropathic pain symptoms do not gain any pain relief. Thus, effective treatment for neuropathic pain continues to be a challenge and current therapeutic options are confined to pharmacological treatments normally approved for other conditions which include antidepressants and anticonvulsants. However, as stated by Baron and colleagues, increased knowledge concerning the mechanisms of neuropathic pain and their translation into more accurate evaluation of symptoms and signs should allow observations of potentially differing mechanisms between patients. While this systematic approach allows more accurate prescription of medication that acts on particular mechanisms, studies are now showing that other forms of non-pharmacological treatments may also be effective. However, given the complex nature of neuropathic pain, individualized care is recommended, employing multiple therapies to address not only pain, but also pain-related disability and psychological dysfunction, and paying attention to patient education.

Chapter 9

References

1. Treede RD, Jensen TS, Campbell JN, Cruccu G, Dostrovsky JO, Griffin JW, et al. Neuropathic pain: redefinition and a grading system for clinical and research purposes. Neurology. 2008;70(18):1630–5.

2. Campbell JN, Meyer RA. Mechanisms of neuropathic pain. Neuron. 2006;52(1):77–92.

3. Baron R. Mechanisms of disease: neuropathic pain – a clinical perspective. Nature Clinical Practice Neurology. 2006;2(2):95–106.

4. Naleschinski D, Baron R. Complex regional pain syndrome type I: neuropathic or not? Current Pain and Headache Reports. 2010;14(3):196–202.

5. Finnerup NB, Jensen TS. Mechanisms of disease: mechanism-based classification of neuropathic pain – a critical analysis. Nature Clinical Practice Neurology. 2006;2(2):107–15.

6. Harden RN. Chronic neuropathic pain. Mechanisms, diagnosis, and treatment. Neurologist. 2005;11(2):111–22.

7. International Association for the Study of Pain. Epidemiology of neuropathic pain: how common is neuropathic pain, and what is its impact? Seattle: IASP Press; 2015.

8. Davies M, Brophy S, Williams R, Taylor A. The prevalence, severity, and impact of painful diabetic peripheral neuropathy in type 2 diabetes. Diabetes Care. 2006;29(7):1518–22.

9. Smith BH, Torrance N. Epidemiology of neuropathic pain and its impact on quality of life. Current Pain and Headache Reports. 2012;16(3):191–8.

10. Sampathkumar P, Drage LA, Martin DP. Herpes zoster (shingles) and postherpetic neuralgia. Mayo Clinic Proceedings. 2009;84(3):274–80.

11. Verma S, Estanislao L, Simpson D. HIV-associated neuropathic pain: epidemiology, pathophysiology and management. CNS Drugs. 2005;19(4):325–34.

12. Fishbain DA, Cole B, Lewis JE, Gao J. What is the evidence that neuropathic pain is present in chronic low back pain and soft tissue syndromes? An evidence-based structured review. Pain Medicine (Malden, Mass). 2014;15(1):4–15.

13. Bennett MI, Rayment C, Hjermstad M, Aass N, Caraceni A, Kaasa S. Prevalence and aetiology of neuropathic pain in cancer patients: a systematic review. Pain. 2012;153(2):359–65.

14. Bennett MI, Smith BH, Torrance N, Potter J. The S-LANSS score for identifying pain of predominantly neuropathic origin: validation for use in clinical and postal research. Journal of Pain. 2005;6(3):149–58.

15. Bouhassira D, Attal N, Alchaar H, Boureau F, Brochet B, Bruxelle J, et al. Comparison of pain syndromes associated with nervous or somatic lesions and development of a new neuropathic pain diagnostic questionnaire (DN4). Pain. 2005;114(1–2):29–36.

16. Dworkin RH, Panarites CJ, Armstrong EP, Malone DC, Pham SV. Healthcare utilization in people with postherpetic neuralgia and painful diabetic peripheral neuropathy. Journal of the American Geriatric Society. 2011;59(5):827–36.

17. Torrance N, Smith BH, Bennett MI, Lee AJ. The epidemiology of chronic pain of predominantly neuropathic origin. Results from a general population survey. Journal of Pain. 2006;7(4):281–9.

18. Tesfaye S, Vileikyte L, Rayman G, Sindrup SH, Perkins BA, Baconja M, et al. Painful diabetic peripheral neuropathy: consensus recommendations on diagnosis, assessment and management. Diabetes/Metabolism Research and Reviews. 2011;27(7):629–38.

19. Jung BF, Johnson RW, Griffin DR, Dworkin RH. Risk factors for postherpetic neuralgia in patients with herpes zoster. Neurology. 2004;62(9):1545–51.

20. Shipton E. Post-surgical neuropathic pain. ANZ Journal of Surgery. 2008;78(7):548–55.

21. Haythornthwaite JA, Benrud-Larson LM. Psychological assessment and treatment of patients with neuropathic pain. Current Pain and Headache Reports. 2001;5(2):124–9.

22. Gault D, Morel-Fatio M, Albert T, Fattal C. Chronic neuropathic pain of spinal cord injury: what is the effectiveness of psychocomportemental management? Annals of Physical Rehabilitation Medicine. 2009;52(2):167–72.

23. Jensen TS, Backonja MM, Hernandez Jimenez S, Tesfaye S, Valensi P, Ziegler D. New perspectives on the management of diabetic peripheral neuropathic pain. Diabetes and Vascular Disease Research. 2006;3(2):108–19.

24. Cole BE. Diabetic peripheral neuropathic pain: recognition and management. Pain Medicine (Malden, Mass). 2007;8(Suppl 2):S27–32.

25. Evans SR, Ellis RJ, Chen H, Yeh T–m, Lee AJ, Schifitto G, et al. Peripheral neuropathy in HIV: prevalence and risk factors. AIDS (London, England). 2011;25(7):919–28.

26. Schifitto G, McDermott MP, McArthur JC, Marder K, Sacktor N, Epstein L, et al. Incidence of and risk factors for HIV-associated distal sensory polyneuropathy. Neurology. 2002;58(12):1764–8.

27. Beerthuizen A, Stronks DL, Van't Spijker A, Yaksh A, Hanraets BM, Klein J, et al. Demographic and medical parameters in the development of complex regional pain syndrome type 1 (CRPS1): prospective study on 596 patients with a fracture. Pain. 2012;153(6):1187–92.

28. Terkelsen AJ, Bach FW, Jensen TS. Experimental forearm immobilization in humans induces cold and mechanical hyperalgesia. Anesthesiology. 2008;109(2):297–307.

29. Naleschinski D, Baron R. Complex regional pain syndrome type I: neuropathic or not? Current Pain and Headache Reports. 2010;14(3):196–202.

30. O'Connell NE, Wand BM, Gibson W, Carr DB, Birklein F, Stanton TR. Local

anaesthetic sympathetic blockade for complex regional pain syndrome. Cochrane Database of Systematic Reviews. 2016;7:Cd004598.

31. Ali Z, Raja SN, Wesselmann U, Fuchs PN, Meyer RA, Campbell JN. Intradermal injection of norepinephrine evokes pain in patients with sympathetically maintained pain. Pain. 2000;88(2):161–8.

32. Baron R, Binder A, Wasner G. Neuropathic pain: diagnosis, pathophysiological mechanisms, and treatment. Lancet Neurology. 2010;9(8):807–19.

33. Treede RD, Meyer RA, Raja SN, Campbell JN. Peripheral and central mechanisms of cutaneous hyperalgesia. Progress in Neurobiol. 1992;38(4):397–421.

34. Meyer RA, Rinkamp M, Campbell JN, Srinivasa NR. Neural mechanisms of hyperalgesia after tissue injury. John Hopkins APL Technical Digest. 2005;26(1).

35. Woolf CJ, Mannion RJ. Neuropathic pain: aetiology, symptoms, mechanisms, and management. Lancet. 1999;353(9168):1959–64.

36. Ochoa J, Torebjork HE, Culp WJ, Schady W. Abnormal spontaneous activity in single sensory nerve fibers in humans. Muscle and Nerve. 1982;5(9s):S74–7.

37. Woolf CJ, Mannion RJ. Neuropathic pain: aetiology, symptoms, mechanisms, and management. Lancet. 1999;353(9168):1959–64.

38. Khan GM, Chen SR, Pan HL. Role of primary afferent nerves in allodynia caused by diabetic neuropathy in rats. Neuroscience. 2002;114(2):291–9.

39. Nickel FT, Seifert F, Lanz S, Maihofner C. Mechanisms of neuropathic pain. European Neuropsychopharmacology. 2012;22(2):81–91.

40. Scholz J, Woolf CJ. The neuropathic pain triad: neurons, immune cells and glia. Nature Neuroscience. 2007;10(11):1361–8.

41. Julius D, Basbaum AI. Molecular mechanisms of nociception. Nature. 2001;413(6852):203–10.

42. Sun Q, Tu H, Xing G–G, Han J–S, Wan Y. Ectopic discharges from injured nerve fibers are highly correlated with tactile allodynia only in early, but not late, stage in rats with spinal nerve ligation. Experimental Neurology. 2005;191(1):128–36.

43. Zakir HM, Mostafeezur RM, Suzuki A, Hitomi S, Suzuki I, Maeda T, et al. Expression of TRPV1 channels after nerve injury provides an essential delivery tool for neuropathic pain attenuation. PLoS One. 2012;7(9):e44023.

44. Malek N, Pajak A, Kolosowska N, Kucharczyk M, Starowicz K. The importance of TRPV1-sensitisation factors for the development of neuropathic pain. Molecular and Cellular Neurosciences. 2015;65:1–10.

45. Inoue M, Rashid MH, Fujita R, Contos JJ, Chun J, Ueda H. Initiation of neuropathic pain requires lysophosphatidic acid receptor signaling. Nature Medicine. 2004;10(7):712–8.

46. Vargas ME, Barres BA. Why is Wallerian degeneration in the CNS so slow? Annual Review of Neuroscience. 2007;30:153–79.

47. Pezet S, McMahon SB. Neurotrophins: mediators and modulators of pain. Annual Review of Neuroscience. 2006;29:507–38.

48. Sukhotinsky I, Ben–Dor E, Raber P, Devor M. Key role of the dorsal root ganglion in neuropathic tactile hypersensibility. European Journal of Pain. 2004;8(2):135–43.

49. Krames ES. The Dorsal root ganglion in chronic pain and as a target for neuromodulation: a review. Neuromodulation: Technology at the Neural Interface. 2015;18(1):24–32.

50. Bridges D, Thompson SWN, Rice ASC. Mechanisms of neuropathic pain. British Journal of Anaesthesia. 2001;87(1):12–26.

51. Leone C, Biasiotta A, La Cesa S, Di Stefano G, Cruccu G, Truini A. Pathophysiological mechanisms of neuropathic pain. Future Neurology. 2011;6(4):497–509.

52. Hains BC, Klein JP, Saab CY, Craner MJ, Black JA, Waxman SG. Upregulation of sodium channel Nav1.3 and functional involvement in neuronal hyperexcitability associated with central neuropathic pain after spinal cord injury. Journal of Neuroscience. 2003;23(26):8881–92.

53. Zhang J. Peripheral and central immune mechanisms in neuropathic pain. Neuroinflammation. John Wiley & Sons, Inc; 2015. p. 107–21.

54. Marchand F, Perretti M, McMahon SB. Role of the immune system in chronic pain. Nature Reviews Neuroscience. 2005;6(7):521–32.

55. Gosselin R-D, Suter MR, Ji R-R, Decosterd I. Glial cells and chronic pain. The Neuroscientist. 2010;16(5):519–31.

56. Haanpää M, Attal N, Backonja M, Baron R, Bennett M, Bouhassira D, et al. NeuPSIG guidelines on neuropathic pain assessment. Pain. 2011;152.

57. Bennett M. The LANSS Pain Scale: the Leeds assessment of neuropathic symptoms and signs. Pain. 2001;92(1–2):147–57.

58. Haanpää M, Attal N, Backonja M, Baron R, Bennett M, Bouhassira D, et al. NeuPSIG guidelines on neuropathic pain assessment. PAIN®. 2011;152(1):14–27.

59. Pérez C, Gálvez R, Insausti J, Bennett M, Ruiz M, Rejas J. Adaptación lingüística y validación al español de la escala LANSS (Leeds Assessment of Neuropathic Symptoms and Signs) para el diagnóstico diferencial del dolor neuropático. Med Clin (Barc). 2006;127.

60. Krause SJ, Backonja MM. Development of a neuropathic pain questionnaire. Clinical Journal of Pain. 2003;19(5):306–14.

61. Krause SJ, Backonja M. Development of a neuropathic pain questionnaire. Clinical Journal of Pain. 2003;19.

62. Gauffin J, Hankama T, Kautiainen H, Hannonen P, Haanpää M. Neuropathic pain and use of PainDETECT in patients with fibromyalgia: a cohort study. BMC Neurology. 2013;13(1):21.

63. Haanpää M. Diagnosis and classification of neuropathic pain. Pain Clinical Updates. 2010;XVII(7).

64. Jensen TS, Finnerup NB. Allodynia and hyperalgesia in neuropathic pain: clinical manifestations and mechanisms. Lancet Neurology. 2014;13(9):924–35.

65. Hammond N, Wang Y, Dimachkie M, Barohn R. Nutritional Neuropathies. Neurologic Clinics. 2013;31(2):477–89.

66. O'Connor AB, Dworkin RH. Treatment of neuropathic pain: an overview of recent guidelines. American Journal of Medicine. 2009;122(10 Suppl):S22–32.

67. Turk DC, Audette J, Levy RM, Mackey SC, Stanos S. Assessment and treatment of psychosocial comorbidities in patients with neuropathic pain. Mayo Clinic Proceedings. 2010;85(3 Suppl):S42–S50.

68. Otis JD, Sanderson K, Hardway C, Pincus M, Tun C, Soumekh S. A randomized controlled pilot study of a cognitive–behavioral therapy approach for painful diabetic peripheral neuropathy. Journal of Pain. 2013;14(5):475–82.

69. Moseley GL. Using visual illusion to reduce at-level neuropathic pain in paraplegia. Pain. 2007;130(3):294–8.

70. Li A, Montaño Z, Chen VJ, Gold JI. Virtual reality and pain management: current trends and future directions. Pain management. 2011;1(2):147–57.

71. Magrinelli F, Zanette G, Tamburin S. Neuropathic pain: diagnosis and treatment. Practical Neurology. 2013;13(5):292–307.

72. Attal N, Cruccu G, Baron R, Haanpää M, Hansson P, Jensen TS, et al. EFNS guidelines on the pharmacological treatment of neuropathic pain: 2009 revision. Eur J Neurol. 2010;17.

73. Finnerup NB, Attal N, Haroutounian S, McNicol E, Baron R, Dworkin RH, et al. Pharmacotherapy for neuropathic pain in adults: a systematic review and meta-analysis. Lancet Neurology. 2015;14(2):162–73.

74. Johnson EM, Whyte E, Mulsant BH, Pollock BG, Weber E, Begley AE, et al.

Cardiovascular changes associated with venlafaxine in the treatment of late-life depression. American Journal of Geriatric Psychiatry. 2006;14(9):796–802.

75. Delorme C, Navez ML, Legout V, Deleens R, Moyse D. Treatment of neuropathic pain with 5% lidocaine-medicated plaster: five years of clinical experience. Pain Research and Management. 2011;16(4):259–63.

76. Cruccu G, Anand P, Attal N, García-Larrea L, Haanpää M, Jørum E, et al. EFNS guidelines on neuropathic pain assessment. European Journal of Neurology. 2004;11.

77. Wallace M. Interventional and nonpharmacological therapies for neuropathic pain. In: Raja S, Somner C, editors. World Congress of Pain; Buenos Aires IASP Press; 2014.

78. Cruccu G. Treatment of painful neuropathy. Current Opinion in Neurology. 2007;20(5):531–5.

79. Akyuz G, Kenis O. Physical therapy modalities and rehabilitation techniques in the management of neuropathic pain. American Journal of Physical Medicine and Rehabilitation. 2014;93(3):253–9.

80. Hsieh YL, Chou LW, Chang PL, Yang CC, Kao MJ, Hong CZ. Low-level laser therapy alleviates neuropathic pain and promotes function recovery in rats with chronic constriction injury: possible involvements in hypoxia-inducible factor 1alpha (HIF-1alpha). Journal of Comparative Neurology. 2012;520(13):2903–16.

81. Eccleston C, Hearn L, C. WAd. Psychological treatments for chronic pain involving damage or disease to nerves responsible for pain. Cochrane Database of Systematic Reviews. 2015(10).

82. Moseley G, Butler D, Beames T, GIles T. The graded motor imagery handbook. Adelaide: Neuro Orthopaedic Institute; 2012. 143 p.

83. Bowering KJ, O'Connell NE, Tabor A, Catley MJ, Leake HB, Moseley GL, et al. The effects of graded motor imagery and its components on chronic pain: a systematic review and meta-analysis. Journal of Pain. 2013;14(1):3–13.

84. Diers M, Christmann C, Koeppe C, Ruf M, Flor H. Mirrored, imagined and executed movements differentially activate sensorimotor cortex in amputees with and without phantom limb pain. PAIN®. 2010;149(2):296–304.

85. Moseley GL. Is successful rehabilitation of complex regional pain syndrome due to sustained attention to the affected limb? A randomised clinical trial. Pain. 2005;114(1–2):54–61.

86. Moseley GL. Graded motor imagery for pathologic pain: a randomized controlled trial. Neurology. 2006;67(12):2129–34.

87. Keefe FJ, Huling DA, Coggins MJ, Keefe DF, Zachary Rosenthal M, Herr NR, et al. Virtual reality for persistent pain: a new direction for behavioral pain management. Pain. 2012;153(11):2163–6.

88. Gromala D, Song M, Yim J–D, Fox T, Barnes SJ, Nazemi M, et al. Immersive VR: a non–pharmacological analgesic for chronic pain? CHI '11 Extended Abstracts on Human Factors in Computing Systems; Vancouver, BC, Canada. 1979704: ACM; 2011. p. 1171–6.

89. Murray D, Patchick E, Pettifer S, Howard T, Caillette F, Kulkarni J, et al. Investigating the efficacy of a virtual mirror box in treating phantom limb pain in a sample of chronic sufferers. International Journal on Disability and Human Development 2006. p. 227.

90. Sato K, Obata D, Morita K, Fukumori S, Miyake K, Gofuku A. A novel application of virtual reality for pain control: virtual reality-mirror visual feedback therapy. 2012 2012–10–24.

91. Chatchawan U, Eungpinichpong W, Plandee P, Yamauchi J. Effects of Thai foot massage on balance performance in diabetic patients with peripheral neuropathy: a randomized parallel-controlled trial. Medical Science Monitor Basic Research. 2015;21:68–75.

92. Dalal K, Maran VB, Pandey RM, Tripathi M. Determination of efficacy of reflexology in managing patients with diabetic neuropathy: a randomized controlled clinical trial. Evidence-Based

Complementary and Alternative Medicine. 2014;2014:11.

93. Cunningham JE, Kelechi T, Sterba K, Barthelemy N, Falkowski P, Chin SH. Case report of a patient with chemotherapy-induced peripheral neuropathy treated with manual therapy (massage). Supportive Care in Cancer. 2011;19(9):1473–6.

94. Norrbrink C, Lundeberg T. Acupuncture and massage therapy for neuropathic pain following spinal cord injury: an exploratory study. Acupuncture in Medicine. 2011;29(2):108–15.

95. Cooper MA, Kluding PM, Wright DE. Emerging relationships between exercise, sensory nerves, and neuropathic pain. Frontiers in Neuroscience. 2016;10:372.

96. Molteni R, Zheng JQ, Ying Z, Gomez–Pinilla F, Twiss JL. Voluntary exercise increases axonal regeneration from sensory neurons. Proceedings of the National Academy of Sciences of the United States of America. 2004;101(22):8473–8.

97. Denk F, McMahon SB, Tracey I. Pain vulnerability: a neurobiological perspective. Nature Neuroscience. 2014;17(2):192–200.

98. Dobson JL, McMillan J, Li L. Benefits of exercise intervention in reducing neuropathic pain. Frontiers in Cellular Neuroscience. 2014;8:102.

99. Kami K, Taguchi MSS, Tajima F, Senba E. Improvements in impaired GABA and GAD65/67 production in the spinal dorsal horn contribute to exercise-induced hypoalgesia in a mouse model of neuropathic pain. Molecular Pain. 2016;12:1744806916629059.

100. Shen J, Fox LE, Cheng J. Swim therapy reduces mechanical allodynia and thermal hyperalgesia induced by chronic constriction nerve injury in rats. Pain Medicine (Malden, Mass). 2013;14(4):516–25.

101. Chen YW, Tzeng JI, Lin MF, Hung CH, Wang JJ. Forced treadmill running suppresses postincisional pain and inhibits upregulation of substance P and cytokines in rat dorsal root ganglion. Journal of Pain. 2014;15(8):827–34.

Introduction

Pain perceived within the abdomen may arise via a range of different mechanisms, many of which remain poorly understood. Visceral pain is one of the most frequent causes of morbidity in the general population, with unexplained abdominal symptoms accounting for between 15% and 40% of cases.[1-3] Typically, patients undergo many diagnostic tests and examinations though no specific cause of pain can be found. While substantial progress has been made in the assessment and treatment of chronic somatic pain, there has been little success in the management of visceral pain.[4] Visceral pain is unique in that pain is not evoked from all visceral structures; it is infrequently linked to visceral pathology, refers to other body regions, is poorly localized, and is often accompanied by motor and autonomic signs.[5] Despite significant increases in our understanding of visceral pain, mechanisms are less clearly understood than in somatic pain and this is most likely due to greater difficulties in accessing visceral structures with visceral stimuli in experimental settings.[6]

Functional gastrointestinal disorders (FGIDs) are the most prevalent form of visceral pain. However, it is also important to recognize that while pain is the most apparent and intolerable of abdominal symptoms, it is not the only one. Thus, other complaints such as bloating, constipation, and satiety must also be considered. Irritable bowel syndrome (IBS) and functional dyspepsia are two common FGIDs, with IBS being characterized by abdominal pain and altered bowel habit, while functional dyspepsia is characterized by epigastric pain, discomfort, and gastroesophageal reflux. This chapter reviews the epidemiology, mechanisms, and clinical manifestations of chronic visceral pain.

Epidemiology

Prevalence

Chronic visceral pain (CVP) makes up a major component of the clinical spectrum in both primary and secondary care settings. Epidemiological data show a wide prevalence of visceral pain with rates in adults of 25% for intermittent abdominal pain, 20% for chest pain, and 16–25% for pelvic pain in women.[5] Nonspecific abdominal pain is now the tenth most common cause of hospital admission in men and the sixth for women where it accounts for up to 67% of consecutive hospital admissions.[7] While abdominal pain can be an indication of underlying disease, in most cases diagnostic tests are either normal or negative. Importantly, it has been shown that nonspecific abdominal pain costs the UK over £100 million each year.[7] For example, population-based studies show IBS, a symptom-based condition, having a prevalence of between 7% and 15%.[8] Like most other chronic pain conditions, clinicians consider IBS to be a diagnosis of exclusion, given after organic and other functional causes of visceral pain have been ruled out.

Chronic pelvic pain is also a debilitating condition, especially among women, with a major impact on health-related quality of life.[9] However, there is a lack of research into its prevalence.[10] The prevalence rate in the general population ranges between 6% and 27%. However, Halder and colleagues suggest that nonspecific pelvic pain is estimated at about 16% in population studies in the USA and UK.[7] The authors further state that one-third of women with pelvic pain will have no obvious gynecological pathology, while one-third will have persistent pain despite hysterectomy. It is further suggested that persistent pelvic pain accounts for health care costs of £158 million and £24 million in indirect costs such as loss of earnings.[5]

Gender

Extensive evidence shows that females and males differ greatly in their nociceptive processing.[11] The menstrual cycle, dysmenorrhea, and pregnancy all have unique effects on pain thresholds and an individual's affective reaction to the painful stimuli. While the reason for female predominance for abdominal pain is not clear, studies show differences in basic GI function such as gallbladder emptying, colon transit timing, visceral sensitivity, central pain processing, and effects of estrogen and progesterone on gut function.[12,13] For example, estrogen-dependent hyper-responsiveness to stress can promote immune activation resulting in altered gut barrier permeability and function.[14] Thus, clinical studies stress the importance of early treatment concerning gynecological viscera in women, as it is often underestimated and undertreated as it regarded as 'physiological or normal' in relation to natural events such as giving birth.[15]

Mechanisms of visceral pain

Visceral pain is, to an extent, dependent on the nature of the provoking stimulus. While some non-painful sensations arise from the gastrointestinal (GI) tract (e.g., the feeling of satiety, gas, urge to defecate), the only conscious sensation from most viscera is pain.[16] During daily activities, these sensations can increase to mild discomfort, but when viscera become diseased or inflamed, the same stimuli can produce overwhelming sensations that can stop activity and demand complete attention.[17] Nausea and other autonomic responses such as sweating, piloerection, and dyspnea also occur commonly with visceral pain. Additionally, visceral pains generate strong emotional responses and, in many cases, appear out of proportion to the perceived intensity of the pain. Visceral pain also presents with distinctive features different to that of somatic pain (Table 10.1). These features are described further in the sections that follow.

There is often no obvious link between reported visceral pain intensity and pathology. For example, chronic pancreatitis typically has a known pathology, but alterations in pain do not consistently correlate

Table 10.1: Distinctive features of visceral pain

1	Initially, poorly localized and diffuse, most often perceived along the midline of the trunk
2	Increased intensity and duration of a stimulus is distinctly referred to superficial tissue
3	Stimulation at referred pain sites may be perceived as hyperalgesic
4	Intense visceral stimuli evoke nonspecific or whole body motor responses, strong autonomic responses and strong affective responses

with the degree of change shown by radiographic and laboratory findings.[17] Other disorders such as IBS, noncardiac chest pain, and post-cholecystectomy syndrome appear to have no histopathological changes and are termed 'functional.' Functional visceral pain is associated with changes in luminal pressure due to altered motility, production of gas, and the ingestion of food; the term 'visceral hypersensitivity' was created to describe this collection of symptoms in the absence of pathology.[17]

An unusual feature of visceral pain is that tissue damaging stimuli may not produce pain such as cutting, crushing, and burning of the GI tract, whereas stimuli that induce visceral pain are luminal distension, stretching, shearing forces, inflammation, and ischemia.[18,19] Inflating a balloon inside hollow organs evokes transient pain in the absence of tissue damage.[20–22] Moreover, severe abdominal pain is associated with mild occurrences such as gas or cramping from irritable bowel syndrome, while relatively mild pain (or no pain) can be associated with severe life-threatening conditions such as cancer of the colon. Solid organs are the least pain sensitive, with the serosal membranes of hollow organs (Figure 10.1) being the most sensitive.[23,24]

Neuroanatomy of visceral pain

Unlike somatic tissue, the viscera are dually innervated by primary afferents that project to separate regions of the neuroaxis and contribute to different

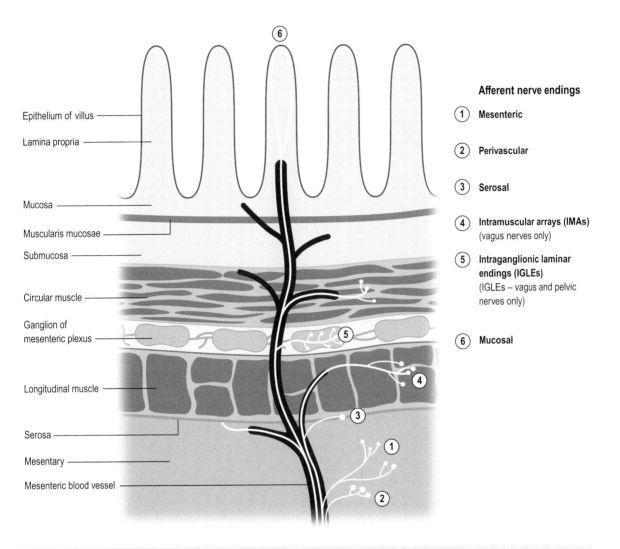

Afferent nerve endings

(1) **Mesenteric**

(2) **Perivascular**

(3) **Serosal**

(4) **Intramuscular arrays (IMAs)**
(vagus nerves only)

(5) **Intraganglionic laminar
endings (IGLEs)**
(IGLEs – vagus and pelvic
nerves only)

(6) **Mucosal**

Epithelium of villus

Lamina propria

Mucosa

Muscularis mucosae

Submucosa

Circular muscle

Ganglion of
mesenteric plexus

Longitudinal muscle

Serosa

Mesentary

Mesenteric blood vessel

Figure 10.1

A schematic representation of afferent nerve endings both in and around the gut wall. Current evidence suggests that afferent nerves involved in nociception innervate the mesentery,[1] blood vessels,[2] serous membrane,[3] and mucosa.[4] Although vagal nerve endings (IGLEs and IMAs) respond to mechanical stimuli (muscle stretch and contraction), their role in nociception is not known

aspects of visceral pain.[25,26] Most indications are that splanchnic innervation conveys nociception while vagal/pelvic pathways contribute to homeostatic functions. However, recent studies suggest this functional dichotomy is far more complex.[27] Additionally, somatic sensory afferent pathways are precisely organized and pass along defined peripheral nerves, extend into one or two spinal segments, and are organized unilaterally. However, visceral sensory afferents originate from multiple branches of nerves organized in web-like plexuses distributed throughout the abdominal and thoracic cavities and extend into multiple spinal segments (Figure 10.2). Once they have entered the spinal cord, visceral afferent fibers have

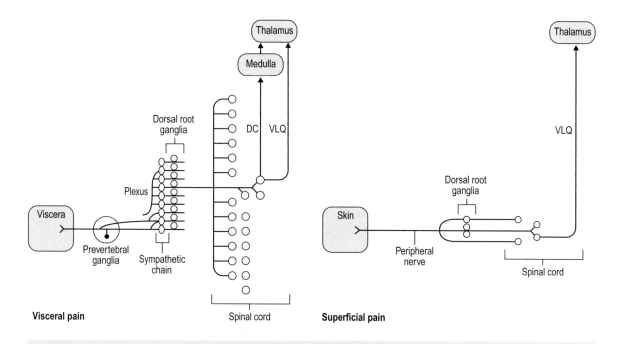

Visceral pain

Superficial pain

Figure 10.2

A schematic representation showing differences between visceral pain somatic pain pathways. Visceral pain pathways are more diffuse with multiple peripheral branches through prevertebral ganglia and sympathetic chain before entering the spinal cord. Somatic pain pathways are more organized, with distinct peripheral nerves entering the spinal cord at only one or two segments

extensive terminal branches in the spinal cord extending rostrocaudally for 5–10 segments, and cover the mediolateral and dorsoventral extent of the dorsal horn (DH) (Figure 10.4). Additionally, these branches project to the contralateral DH. It is this that provides the basis for bilateral distribution of visceral pain and viscerosomatic convergence[28,29] (Figure 10.3).

Visceral sensory processing is also different to somatic sensory processing: peripheral sites of visceral neuronal synaptic contact occurs in the cell bodies of the prevertebral ganglia such as the celiac and superior mesenteric ganglia.[17] Thus, the location of these synapses can lead to alterations in visceral function that are independent of central control. Furthermore, the gut carries the enteric nervous system, also a self-contained 'visceral brain' that regulates the numerous functions of digestion and absorption.

Viscerosomatic convergence

Another unique characteristic is referral of pain to distal somatic sites. This is due to viscerosomatic convergence of afferent fibers that together synapse with wide dynamic range neurons (WDR) in the spinal cord and higher centers of the CNS. Because of viscerosomatic convergence, somatic injury and visceral dysfunction can respectively affect central processing of somatic and visceral inputs.[30] Importantly, the convergence of both visceral and somatic inputs may also account for visceral pain being accompanied by somatic pain conditions and vice versa.[6]

The brain–gut axis

Knowledge of bidirectional communication between the enteric nervous system of the gut and the brain is essential for the understanding of the established influence of psychological factors on GI sensation and

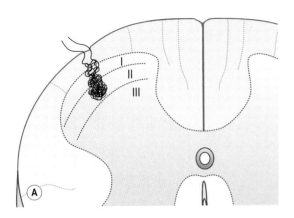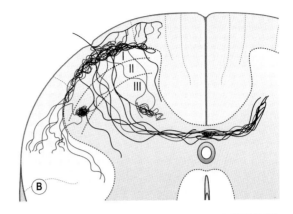

Figure 10.3

A schematic representation showing differences between central projections of visceral and somatic neurons. Visceral afferent fibers have extensive terminal branches that extend between five and 10 segments, multiple laminae, and also extend to the contralateral dorsal horn. In contrast, somatic afferent pathways entering the spinal cord are precisely organized, only extend into one or two segments, and are organized unilaterally

motor function.[1] Brain–gut interactions are essential in the regulation of digestive processes (e.g., appetite, digestion), modulation of the gut-associated immune system (e.g., T-cell and Peyer's patch function), and the organization of the global physical and emotional state of an organism (e.g., sleep and anxiety) with activity of the GI tract.[31] Here, the enteric nervous system (ENS) and the brain communicate through neural (ANS), neuroendocrine (HPA axis), and neuroimmune pathways (Figure 10.5). The ANS with sympathetic and parasympathetic arms modulate afferent signals arising from the gut lumen and are transmitted via enteric, spinal, and vagal pathways to the CNS. Equally, efferent signals from the CNS are communicated to the intestinal wall. Although, reflex circuits within the ENS can regulate GI functions such as motility, secretion, and blood flow, coordination and general homeostasis requires constant communication between the GI tract and the CNS. Here, descending corticolimbic efferent influences can alter and increase responsiveness of ENS sensory and motor activity and thus modulate visceral pain transmission (e.g., altered gut motility, gut distension).[31] For example, extrinsic (e.g., vision, smell) or intrinsic (e.g., emotion, thought) information has, by the nature of its higher center connections, the capability

to affect GI sensation, motility, secretion, and inflammation.[32] Conversely, visceral afferent information to brain reciprocally affects central pain perception. The ANS drives afferent signals from both the lumen and the ENS, via spinal and vagal pathways to the CNS. Visceral afferent signals to the brain also affect mood and behavior. For example, Elsenbruch and colleagues show that altered central processing of visceral stimuli in IBS patients is mediated by symptoms of anxiety and depression.[33]

Psychological modulation of visceral pain

Psychological morbidities are common in patients with visceral pain, and an understanding of this problem is crucial for the management of these conditions. The perception of visceral sensation is mediated by emotional mechanisms such as stress and anxiety. In threatening situations, stress evokes adaptive responses that serve to stabilize the internal environment of an organism to aid survival. This involves the ANS, HPA, and neuroimmune systems that are referred to by Meyer as the emotional motor system.[34] The body is subjected to many stressors that are generally divided into two categories: exteroceptive (e.g., psychological) and interoceptive

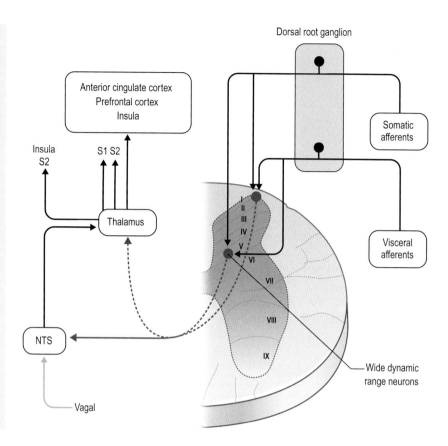

Figure 10.4

A schematic representation of somatic and visceral primary afferent neurons entering laminae I and V of the dorsal horn. Supraspinal and vagal neurons project to cortical sites via the nucleus tractus solitarius (NTS) and the thalamus. Primary somatosensory cortex (S1), secondary somatosensory cortex (S2)

(altered bodily function).[35] Exteroceptive stressors become stressful only after being processed in the context of previous experience and are therefore limbic-sensitive. Interoceptive stressors in contrast are limbic-insensitive and represent threats to homeostasis (i.e., immune stress). Here, cognitive processing is bypassed as brainstem/pontine nuclei, including the nucleus of solitary tract, the ventrolateral medulla and the locus coeruleus, receive afferent visceral input.[35] However, in patients with CVP, conscious perception of interoceptive signals from the GI tract can occur in the form of abdominal discomfort and pain.[31]

Chronic stress and visceral pain

Despite being poorly understood, chronic stress is shown to be strongly associated with visceral hypersensitivity and altered bowel function. Previous studies show that chronic stress prompts changes

in both peripheral and central antinociceptive and pronociceptive pain pathways as well as a function of the HPA axis. Peripherally, alterations in the substance P/neurokinin-1 receptors, disruption in intestinal epithelial barrier function, and changes in types and concentrations of gut microbiota correlate with levels of peripheral nociceptive sensitization.[36] Centrally, altered function has been shown in the HPA axis and sympathetic nervous system function in the form of increased ACTH, cortisol, and catecholamine levels in several functional disorders such as IBS and functional dyspepsia (FD).[37,38] In healthy people, these physiological responses are rapidly turned on and off to coordinate the stress response to the duration of the stressors.[39]

Stress can modulate both pain processing and perception, in particular, sub-regions of the hypothalamus, amygdala, and periaqueductal gray. These structures also receive input from somatic

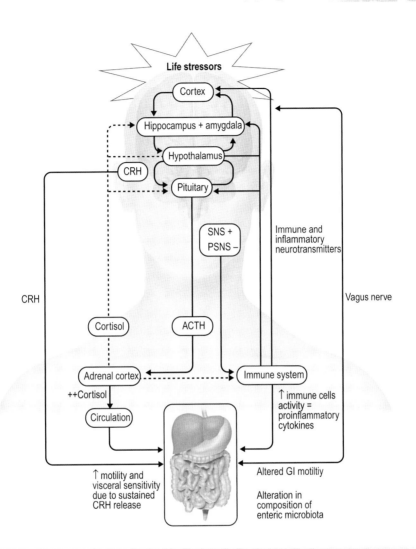

Life stressors

Cortex

Hippocampus + amygdala

Hypothalamus

CRH

Pituitary

SNS +
PSNS –

Immune and
inflammatory
neurotransmitters

CRH

Vagus nerve

Cortisol

ACTH

Adrenal cortex

Immune system

++Cortisol

↑ immune cells
activity =
proinflammatory
cytokines

Circulation

↑ motility and
visceral sensitivity
due to sustained
CRH release

Altered GI motiltiy

Alteration in
composition of
enteric microbiota

Figure 10.5
A diagram showing communication between the CNS and ENS via autonomic pathways that modulate
gastrointestinal function. The HPA axis is key to brain–gut signaling, especially in times of external and internal
stress or increased immune activity. In normal situations, circulating cortisol feeds back to limbic brain regions to
switch off the HPA axis. However, in times of prolonged stress, GI tract activity can be altered by ongoing release of
CRH. Additionally, there are increases in systemic proinflammatory cytokines which act on the pituitary to maintain
activation of the HPA axis

⟶ Positive feedback during normal function

- - - - -➔ Negative feedback during normal function

ACTH – adrenocorticotropic hormone; CRH – corticotropin-releasing hormone; PSNS – parasympathetic nervous
system; SNS – sympathetic nervous system; CNS – central nervous system; ENS – enteric nervous system; HPA axis –
hypothalamic–pituitary–adrenal axis

and visceral afferents as well as higher center regions (prefrontal cortex, anterior cingulate cortex, insular cortex), which in turn project to the locus coeruleus and pituitary gland, which subsequently facilitate HPA axis and ANS output to the body.[40,41] In ongoing stressful situations, increased release of corticotropin-releasing hormone are shown to contribute to increases in sympathetic nervous system (SNS) activity. This increased responsiveness to stressful situations also modulates (1) increases in endogenous pain facilitation and (2) decreases in endogenous pain inhibition. Here, cumulative data suggest that people with unexplained visceral pain show a high incidence of psychological problems and experimental evidence in both humans and animals shows that stress alters GI function. However, although psychological therapy is shown to improve well-being and improved quality of life in people with chronic visceral pain, it does not decrease the severity of visceral symptoms.[42] These findings suggest that psychological issues such as catastrophizing and self-efficacy may be more related to health care seeking behavior rather than underlying disease process.

Stress and the response of gut microbiota

Increasing evidence now supports the concept that organisms within the gut contribute to the early programming and later responsiveness of the stress system.[43] The gut plays host to 10^{13}–10^{14} microorganisms (10 times the number of cells in the body) and contains 150 times the number of genes in our genome.[44] Intestinal microbiota are essential for maintaining health, including normal GI function. Here, their functions are mainly metabolic and protective. Gut microbiota make up an intestinal barrier, help to stimulate epithelial cell regeneration, and produce compounds (short chain fatty acids) that nourish the mucosa while also acting as a barrier to pathogens by adhering to the mucosa generating an immune response.[45] Studies repeatedly show the impact of microbiota on CNS function and stress perception while stress (and HPA axis activity) can influence the composition of gut microbiota.[46] In particular, early-life stressors are shown to have long-term effects on the type and

concentrations of microbiota and thus increases in HPA axis activity.[47] However, chronic stress also increases permeability of the gut allowing bacteria and bacteria antigens to cross the epithelial barrier and activate an immune response, which in turn leads to enhanced HPA activation. Data from patients with IBS and anxiety/depression indicate that alteration in HPA activity may induce increased gut permeability. Furthermore, such changes in types and concentrations of microbiota produce increased amounts of gas by fermenting poorly absorbable carbohydrates, which in turn causes abdominal pain and bloating.[48] Microbiota influence the brain directly by vagal activation via the nucleus tractus solitarius to the insula cortex and more indirectly by spinal pathways via the spinothalamic tracts to the thalamus and primary sensory cortex (Figure 10.6).[49] Hence microbiota in the

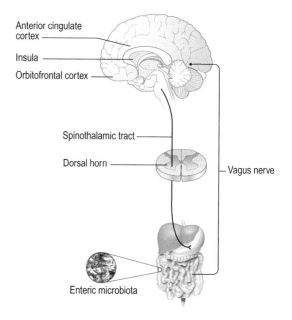

Anterior cingulate cortex

Insula

Orbitofrontal cortex

Spinothalamic tract

Dorsal horn

Vagus nerve

Enteric microbiota

Figure 10.6

Microbiota can influence pain perception in the brain via vagal pathways through the NTS and spinal afferents via the spinothalamic tracts. These pathways project to higher centers such as the insula, cingulate, and orbitofrontal cortices where visceral pain is perceived

gut can be altered by brain function, and microbial alteration can, in turn, influence brain function.

The gastrointestinal tract and serotonin

Serotonin (5-HT) is a well-characterized neurotransmitter in the central nervous system and plays a crucial role in regulating mood, body temperature, sleep, appetite, and metabolism.[50] However, over 90% of the body's 5-HT is synthesized and stored in enterochromaffin cells situated in the gut. Here it plays a critical role in the motility (contraction/relaxation of smooth muscle), sensation (pain and satiety), and secretory reflexes of the GI tract.[51] Recent studies also show that 5-HT receptors are also expressed extraneuronally in immune cells (e.g., monocytes and macrophages) in the GI tract. Once activated, these 5-HT receptors trigger the synthesis and release of proinflammatory cytokines.[52] These findings suggest that 5-HT regulated pathways are associated with immune and inflammatory responses involved in inflammatory intestinal diseases.[53] There is also growing evidence that serotonergic mechanisms are involved in FGID pathophysiology.[54] Findings also show increased postprandial levels of circulating 5-HT in diarrhea-predominate IBS and decreased levels in people with constipation-predominant IBS (IBS-C).[55] However, despite much evidence for the different 5-HT receptor subunits, the actual role of 5-HT in the GI tract remains both perplexing and difficult to identify specifically.

Clinical manifestations of chronic visceral pain

Functional gastrointestinal disorders

Irritable bowel syndrome

IBS is a relapsing GI disorder typified by recurring abdominal pain and cramping associated with altered bowel habit,[56] in the absence of detectable organic disease.[57] Longitudinal population-based studies show that although prevalence of IBS is constant over time, the severities of symptoms do vary. Additionally, IBS symptom severity alone does not explain illness behavior. Instead, psychological symptoms and reduced quality of life are the most important to the experience of GI symptoms and health care seeking patterns.[58] IBS affects around 11% of the global population with rates varying from 5% in France[59] to 32% in Nigeria.[60] In most populations women report more IBS symptoms, with rates two to three times higher than in men.[61] Over 50% of all patients with IBS report depression or anxiety and these patients experience more severe symptoms.[61] Interestingly, evidence also shows that IBS subtypes are more frequent in different genders with diarrhea being found predominantly in men and IBS with constipation being more prevalent in women.[62,63]

Functional dyspepsia

Functional dyspepsia refers to a group of upper GI symptoms that are common in adults. Symptoms include postprandial fullness, recurrent epigastric pain, and epigastric burning in the absence of pathology and other upper GI symptoms such as nausea, vomiting, and belching.[64,65] Population studies report high prevalences of around 25% in the US, China, and Australia,[66] with greater prevalence rates in women.[65] Adults with functional dyspepsia also score highly on anxiety scales, but less on depression scales, with large population studies showing considerably more psychological morbidity in these people than in healthy controls.[67]

Noncardiac chest pain

Due to the high morbidity and prevalence of coronary artery disease, chest pain is treated as cardiac in origin until shown otherwise. However, many patients initially thought to have cardiac disease are later diagnosed with esophageal disease. Studies show that around 33% of chest pain cases are diagnosed as noncardiac chest pain with no other GI (dysphagia, heartburn, and acid reflux) or psychological (anxiety and/or depression) symptoms being significantly associated.[68] Although the prevalence in the community is similar, more women than men are referred to tertiary care clinics and women are more likely to report anxiety-related symptoms.[69,70] Both peripheral and central pain mechanisms have been proposed to be responsible for visceral hypersensitivity in patients with noncardiac chest pain leading to heightened responses to stimulation of the esophageal mucosa.[71] These alterations in pain mechanisms are thought to be due to acute tissue irritation following repeated mechanical stimuli, inflammation, or spasm.[71]

Chronic abdominal wall pain

Chronic pain originating in the abdominal wall is often unrecognized or confused with pain arising from the viscera and is thus subjected to exhaustive diagnostic testing. Prevalence rates for chronic abdominal wall pain are uncertain. Indeed, a few cross-sectional studies have shown prevalence rates ranging from 11% to 74%.[72] Pain in the abdominal wall may arise from three or more sources including referral from abdominal and thoracic viscera, T7–T12 radicular lesions, and peritoneal or abdominal wall lesions originating from the ribcage or the rectus sheath.[73] Entrapment of the anterior cutaneous nerve (Figure 10.7) has been shown to be the most common cause of chronic abdominal wall pain due to intra- or extra-abdominal compression, such as scarring.[74] As with other CVP conditions, comorbid disorders are common, especially overweight and obesity (84%).[75] Other CVP conditions (IBS/gastroesophageal reflux disease (GORD)) are also commonly associated, as is chronic depression, where in one study, around 20% of subjects were treated with antidepressant medication.[75]

Pelvic pain syndromes

There are many different types of chronic pelvic pain conditions with different etiologies and functional effects.[76] Most of these conditions are sex-specific while a few are common in both men and women. This section presents an overview of some of the more common pelvic pain conditions.

Dysmenorrhea

Dysmenorrhea is typified by painful menstrual cramps, associated both with and without heavy menstrual flow.[77] Such pain during menses in the absence of identifiable pathology is referred to as primary dysmenorrhea, and is highly prevalent in adolescence and

shown to be associated with the hypercontractility of uterine tissue.[78] However, secondary dysmenorrhea refers to painful menses where underlying pathology has been identified.[77] Common conditions associated with secondary dysmenorrhea include endometriosis, pelvic inflammatory disease, ovarian cysts, and benign uterine growths such as fibroids and polyps.[76]

Endometriosis

Endometriosis is a disorder characterized by the outgrowth of tissue lining the inside of the uterus onto the surface of adjacent organs in the pelvis. Endometrial tissue can also spread to more distant organs in the abdomen and thoracic cavities where such tissue does not normally exist.[79,80] Pain symptoms of endometriosis include acute and chronic pelvic pain that includes dysmenorrhea, dyspareunia (pain during sexual intercourse), and dyschezia (pain with defecation);[79,80] however, many women are asymptomatic. Studies investigating endometriosis-related pain in animal models show endometrial tissue to be heavily vascularized and innervated with both sensory and autonomic nerve fibers.[81] These fibers are shown to release nociceptive neurotransmitters such as substance P and CGRP,[79] and thus are considered likely candidates for symptoms of pelvic pain.

Dyspareunia

Dyspareunia is reported as pain during and after intercourse, on tampon insertion, urination, and gynecological examination, and pain due to vaginal atrophy (postmenopausal). Dyspareunia is also reported as the most common female dysfunction, affecting between 10% and 15% of the female population.[76] The symptoms of dyspareunia are associated with some underlying conditions such as vulvar vestibulitis, vaginismus (involuntary spasm), endometriosis, and pelvic inflammatory disease. Histopathological studies show that peripheral innervation of the vestibular mucosa is significantly increased in women with vulvar vestibulitis compared to healthy controls.[82] Here, samples taken from vulvar vestibular tissue show increased densities of free

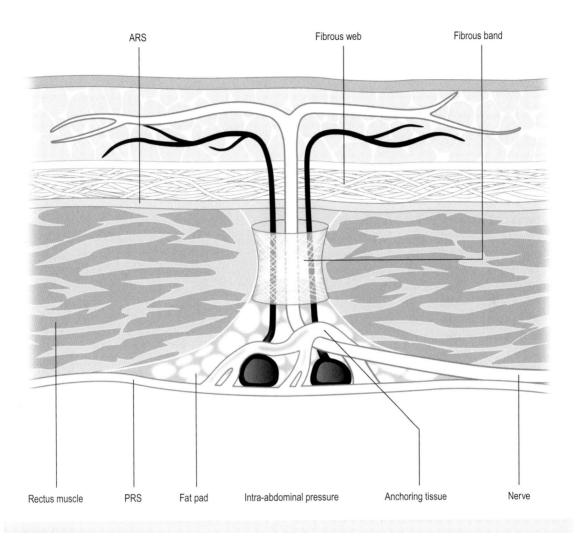

ARS Fibrous web Fibrous band

Rectus muscle PRS Fat pad Intra-abdominal pressure Anchoring tissue Nerve

Figure 10.7
A diagram showing the effect of intra-abdominal pressure and/or scarring of musculoskeletal tissue surrounding branches of the anterior cutaneous nerve

nociceptive nerve endings between epithelial cells.[83] However, there is no evidence yet showing sprouting of sympathetic nerve fibers.

Vulvodynia

Vulvodynia is characterized by pain and discomfort due to burning and itching of female genitalia in the absence of skin disease or infection for more than three months.[76] Pain may be spontaneous or provoked by touch or pressure. Vulvodynia has been exclusively diagnosed in Caucasian women and often coexists with dyspareunia.[84] Mechanisms underlying vulvodynia are not entirely understood; however, factors associated with neuropathic pain are likely to be involved (e.g., pelvic levator ani, pudendal nerves). Additionally, the mammalian vagina has an extensive supply of sympathetic, parasympathetic, and nociceptive nerve fibers.[85] Thus, not surprisingly, repetitive stimulation of these pain receptors, as in contact dermatitis and yeast infections, leads to chronic inflammation and, as described previously, increased excitability in the dorsal horn.[86]

Pelvic pain in men

The terms prostatodynia and chronic pelvic pain are used to describe unexplained chronic pelvic pain in men. Common symptoms include pain in the groin, genitalia, and perineum, and discomfort during urination in the absence of pathology.[87] Thus, prostatitis/chronic pelvic pain is subdivided into categories of convenience in which male patients meet three criteria: inflammatory and noninflammatory chronic pelvic pain syndrome and asymptomatic inflammatory prostatitis.[76] Additionally, recent experimental evidence further indicates the involvement of autoimmune processes with recent findings, suggesting lower numbers or defects in androgen receptors.[88]

Chronic testicular pain (orchialgia) is a diffuse type of pelvic pain which refers to the back and groin and as such is often misdiagnosed.[76] Such pain can be caused by direct sources including infection, torsion, tumor, and obstruction.[89] However, while over 50% of patients present with pain for which no etiology can be found, some present with post-vasectomy pain syndrome, which, while not common, is distressing.[89] Furthermore, psychiatric issues, as with other chronic pain disorders must also be considered. The lack of understanding of testicular pain is partly due to the organ's mixed innervation. The contents of the scrotum (epididymis) are innervated by the spermatic nerves while the scrotum is innervated by the genitofemoral and pudendal nerves. However, pain originating in pelvic areas can also refer to the testes, thus adding to diagnostic confusion.

Coccydynia (men and women)

Coccydynia is a condition in which pain presents in the coccyx, sacrum, and surrounding soft tissue; it is five times more common in females than in males. Most cases occur due to either a subluxation or a hypermobile coccyx. Most patients report a traumatic event they associate with their symptoms, in particular

posterior subluxation.[90] Body mass has also been shown to be an influence, with obesity being three times more common in coccydynia patients.[90] Additionally, despite its small size, the coccyx has several important functions. Together with being the insertion site for many ligaments and tendons, it serves as one leg of a tripod, along with the ischial tuberosities, that provides weight-bearing support when a person is seated. Maigne and colleagues suggest that due to the lack of sagittal rotation in the pelvis when sitting, where the BMI increases, the degree of pelvic rotation decreases. Thus, the coccyx in obese patients is exposed to an increased risk of posterior subluxation.

Chronic pain related to previous organic visceral disease and surgery

The pathogenesis of pain in organic visceral disease is both inadequately researched and poorly understood. Nevertheless, chronic pain is a common complication after surgery, whether it be due to the surgery itself or tissue damage.[91] Evidence currently shows that pain in chronic pancreatitis is initially caused by increased intrapancreatic pressure, inflammation, and pancreatic and extrapancreatic complications.[92] Subsequent studies have shown that ongoing pain is maintained by altered nociceptive transmission, both peripherally, due to increased excitability of nerves innervating the pancreas, and centrally, due to altered descending pain modulation commonly associated with centrally mediated pain.[93] Drewes and colleagues also suggest that spontaneous and postprandial pain in chronic pancreatitis reflect characteristic pain features of those patients with neuropathic pain.[94] Other researchers propose that neuropathic pain mechanisms also apply to chronic cholecystitis and post-cholecystectomy syndrome due to the hypersensitivity of biliary nociceptive nerve fibers, especially in the sphincter of Oddi.[95,96]

Abdominal and pelvic adhesions are shown to be the largest cause of lower abdominal and pelvic pain related to previous surgery and disease.[97,98] Surgery is the most common cause of adhesions, with mechanical injury of the peritoneum and peritoneal ischemia due to manipulation of abdominal tissue predisposing tissue to the formation of adhesions.[99] Peritoneal adhesions can also develop in the absence of surgery cased by inflammatory disease affecting the gut, peritoneum, and ovarian tubes.[97] In addition to the potential emergency of intestinal bowel obstruction commonly found in those undergoing abdominal surgery, chronic pain is an important sequela of adhesions.[97] In such cases, persistent pain is thought to occur when adhesions retract the viscera without obstructing them.[100] Sulaiman and colleagues assessed the distribution and type of nerve fibers present in peritoneal adhesions. They found that both C and A-δ neurons expressing the sensory neuronal markers CGRP and substance P were present in all adhesions irrespective of reports of chronic abdominopelvic pain.

The assessment and management of chronic visceral pain

Current diagnostic criteria

There are currently no known gold standard tests for the diagnosis of CVP disorders. Consequently, clinicians base their diagnosis on specific clusters of abdominal symptoms including non-painful symptoms such as constipation, nausea, and vomiting rather than an understanding of underlying mechanisms.[101] Presently, the Rome Foundation (Rome IV criteria) offers symptom-based criteria for adult and pediatric functional GI disorders (FGIDs) associated with chronic pain developed through expert consensus from 18 countries worldwide.[102] These disorders are now classified by GI symptoms related to a combination of:[103]

- motility disturbance

- visceral hypersensitivity

- altered mucosal and immune function

- altered microbiota

- altered CNS processing.

Although abnormal findings such as altered gut motility and increases in colonic mast cells feature in many FGIDs, these findings are not sufficient for

the definition of a disorder.[103] Additionally, the Rome process is taking steps to eliminate the term 'functional' by acknowledging the interaction of multifactorial pathophysiological factors involved in the onset and maintenance of FGIDs. Thus, the most recent definition is: 'disorders of gut-brain interaction' due to combinations of the above listed processes.

Current therapeutic models

Although there are a number of pharmacological and non-pharmacological therapies available for people with CVP, these treatments fail for most patients. Below, therapeutic options and more novel approaches being currently investigated are briefly reviewed.

Pharmacological approaches affecting the peripheral nervous system

Although NSAIDs are the most widely used analgesic drug, their association with several GI side effects (i.e., gastric ulceration, dyspepsia, and hepatic toxicity) exclude their long-term use.[104] Additionally, as NSAIDs inhibit inflammatory mediators and prostaglandins, their influence is not effective due to CVP not being associated with injury or inflammation. Thus, novel drugs targeting different physiological mechanisms are discussed.

Alterations in 5-HT receptor function in the gut are shown to be associated with abdominal pain.[105] Although the 5-HT receptor agonist tegaserod has been shown to be effective in the treatment of IBS-C and related abdominal pain, it was withdrawn from the market after post-marketing analysis reported increased incidents of cerebrovascular and cardiac events.[106,107] Similarly, the 5-HT antagonist alosetron has also been shown in many studies to be an effective agent for the treatment of IBS-D, with improvements in abdominal pain and reduced fecal urgency.[108] However, as with tegaserod, there are serious adverse events including severe constipation and ischemic colitis, and therefore the drug has very limited approval for patients presenting with severe IBS-D.[109]

Emerging pharmaceuticals currently under investigation for CVP target voltage-gated ion channels such as the TRPV1 and Na$_v$1.1 channels, thought to underlie the onset and maintenance of visceral hypersensitivity.[107,110] Additionally, antagonists for neurotransmitters shown to have a role in the maintenance of CVP, especially the tachykinins (e.g., substance P, NKA, and B), have also proven effective in decreasing abdominal pain.[111]

Pharmacological approaches affecting the central nervous system

Tricyclic antidepressants (e.g., amitriptyline and nortriptyline) have been extensively used in somatic pain conditions, but less extensively investigated for their use in relieving CVP. Besides its antidepressant effects in a patient group showing associations with psychological factors, these drugs also have independent analgesic effects. The mechanism of analgesic action has not been confirmed but is thought to be related to its action as 5-HT and norepinephrine/noradrenaline reuptake inhibitors in addition to the possible increase of endogenous opioids.[112] While other classes of antidepressants, such as SSRIs (e.g., citalopram and paroxetine) and SNRIs (e.g., duloxetine and venlafaxine), show limited evidence concerning analgesic effects in CVP, they do have superior tolerability compared to tricyclic antidepressants.[113]

Anticonvulsants (e.g., pregabalin and gabapentin) have been evaluated in chronic somatic pain syndromes such as neuropathic pain; however, they have not been evaluated specifically for most abdominal and pelvic pain disorders. While some animal studies have investigated such anticonvulsant effects for visceral pain, only the role of pregabalin has been examined in human studies. Here, pregabalin has been demonstrated to have inhibitory effects on pain hypersensitivity in chronic pancreatitis patients.[114]

Opioids are one of the most overprescribed drugs for people with chronic pain. There are opioid receptors in many areas of the GI tract, the spinal cord, and many nuclei in the higher centers. Thus, opioids have a widespread action and therefore can have significant adverse effects such as respiratory depression, somnolence, and, importantly regarding the GI tract, decreased bowel motility.[104] Thus, they are not recommended for people with visceral pain complaints.

Psychological interventions

Psychological factors have strong associations with the onset, maintenance, and treatment of chronic pain. While much of the literature focuses on specific somatic pain disorders such as low back pain and headaches, recent research has investigated psychological variables in abdominal and pelvic pain.[115,116] Studies of such psychological variables in people with CVP have also shown associations between treatment-seeking behaviors, excessive use of health care, and pain sensitivity.[117] Thus, if endogenous and pharmaceutical modulation of the CNS can relieve chronic pain, then it can be argued that other forms of CNS modulation may also relieve visceral pain. For example, cognitive behavioral therapy (CBT) has been found to reduce levels of visceral pain and improve health-related quality of life.[104,118] Compared to medical treatment alone, CBT combined with medical treatment is more effective in improving abdominal and psychological symptoms in IBS patients.[118] However, what is not clear is which patients are more likely to respond to psychological treatments. Further studies are therefore required to (1) identify baseline pain and psychological scores and (2) from these scores to accurately predict likely treatment responses. Other psychological treatments such as hypnotherapy have been shown to be consistently effective in both short- and long-term symptom scores in both IBS and FD.[119,120]

Manual therapy

There are many popular manual therapy approaches for chronic musculoskeletal pain conditions such as fibromyalgia, back pain, and post-injury pain. However, much less is known about manual therapeutic effects for abdominal and pelvic pain. Although a few controlled trials and systematic reviews exist, these focus predominantly on the use of manual therapy to treat IBS and chronic pelvic pain.[121–124] While results from studies investigating the treatment of IBS using osteopathic manipulative techniques show promise, sample sizes in all studies are low. Furthermore, very few studies acquired psychometric baseline scores. Lack of such data reduces the ability of investigations to (1) accurately predict the efficacy of any treatment and (2) predict those individuals likely to benefit (or not benefit) from a given treatment. Thus, future studies using larger sample sizes that obtain baseline psychological data will help to predict more accurately the effect of manual intervention on CVP patients.

Although other manual therapies such as physiotherapy, chiropractic, and massage are used for musculoskeletal pain, there is scant literature and virtually no evidence of their efficacy or use for the treatment of CVP. Each therapy offers forms of manipulation to soft and deep tissue, spinal segments and their impact on the spinal ganglia, as well as neural stimulation via peripheral afferents as potentially beneficial for internal problems such as visceral pain. However, there are, at present no studies showing either sufficient methodological rigor or sufficient explanation for potential mechanisms of manual therapy for the treatment of CVP.

Future therapeutic roles for manual therapy

In the absence of observable pathology, CVP appears to be driven by altered receptor and neurotransmitter function in both the peripheral and the central nervous system due to stress-related inputs. To date, only a few studies have explored the effect of manipulative and body-based therapies for the treatment of CVP, with all investigations focusing on the treatment of IBS. While results show improvements in symptom severity and improvement in quality of life, there remains no demonstrable scientific basis for these positive findings. Thus, at present there are no valid methods showing or describing either the physiological effects of manual therapeutic techniques on visceral tissue or how these techniques affect or inhibit visceral pain or other IBS symptoms.

However, manual therapy techniques may be relevant to some conditions within the CVP spectrum.

For example, visceral manipulation textbooks describe manual techniques that treat postoperative scar tissue and adhesions.[125,126] More interestingly, recent animal studies show that post mortem rats given visceral mobilization techniques for postoperative adhesions showed significantly reduced adhesion severity and lower numbers of adhesions compared to control groups.[127] Given that abdominal surgery can cause temporary ileus,[128] which is implicated in the formation of adhesions,[129] the authors, in later research, show that mobilization of viscera in animals also reduces experimental postoperative ileus.[130] Additionally, Rice and colleagues describe two case reports that show the benefit of soft tissue physical therapy in patients presenting with small bowel obstruction secondary to abdominal and pelvic surgery[131] and a motor vehicle accident.[132]

While these results are encouraging, further investigations are necessary to determine the efficacy of such treatments in larger multicenter randomized blinded human trials. Moreover, it has been suggested that mechanical stimulation to the abdomen could disrupt intestinal surgical repairs or increase the severity of adhesions, with the risk of tissue damage or internal bleeding. While valid, these arguments also have no clinical or experimental support. Interestingly, Bove and Chapelle state that their investigations show that even vigorous massages in rat models do not disrupt even very delicate sutures. However, these findings need to be further examined in both hospital and community settings using protocols that specify clear communications between manual therapists and physicians regarding manual procedures, types of surgical procedures, and time between surgery and manual intervention.

Summary

Major challenges still exist in all areas of therapy for visceral pain disorders, largely due to the lack of understanding of the etiology and mechanisms of CVP. Visceral nociceptive pathways are being identified and pharmacological treatments being discovered that have been shown to modulate both peripheral and central pathways. However, clinicians in all areas of health care need to accept a biopsychosocial understanding of these conditions, as singular or disease-based approaches are ineffective.[133] The role of manual therapy for the treatment of CVP is controversial. This is due to largely to claims that manual therapy is beneficial as a form of treatment, while there is virtually no evidence of its efficacy.

Moreover, most CVP conditions are likely generated by peripheral and central driven neuroimmune processes. However, if manual therapy can be shown to be reliable in the treatment of CVP, it should be recognized as an adjunct therapy in a multidisciplinary management strategy that includes one or more centrally acting agents in addition to ongoing psychological and behavioral interventions.

References

1. Anand P, Aziz Q, Willert R, van Oudenhove L. Peripheral and central mechanisms of visceral sensitization in man. Neurogastroenterology and Motility. 2007;19(1 Suppl):29–46.

2. Endo Y, Shoji T, Fukudo S. Epidemiology of irritable bowel syndrome. Annals of Gastroenterology. 2015;28(2):158–9.

3. Chang FY, Chen PH, Wu TC, Pan WH, Chang HY, Wu SJ, et al. Prevalence of functional gastrointestinal disorders in Taiwan: questionnaire-based survey for adults based on the Rome III criteria. Asia Pacific Journal of Clinical Nutrition. 2012;21(4):594–600.

4. Austin PD, Henderson SE. Biopsychosocial assessment criteria for functional chronic visceral pain: a pilot review of concept and practice. Pain Medicine. 2011;12(4):552–64.

5. Collett B. Visceral pain: the importance of pain management services. British Journal of Pain. 2013;7(1):6–7.

6. Sikandar S, Dickenson AH. Visceral pain: the ins and outs, the ups and downs. Current Opinion in Supportive and Palliative Care. 2012;6(1):17–26.

7. Halder S, Locke GI. Epidemiology and social impact of visceral pain. In: Giamberardino MA, editor. Visceral pain: clinical, pathophysiological and therapeutic aspects. Oxford: Oxford University Press; 2009. p. 1–7.

8. Hungin AP, Chang L, Locke GR, Dennis EH, Barghout V. Irritable bowel syndrome in the United States: prevalence, symptom patterns and impact. Alimentary Pharmacology and Therapeutics. 2005;21(11):1365–75.

9. Latthe P, Mignini L, Gray R, Hills R, Khan K. Factors predisposing women to chronic pelvic pain: systematic review. BMJ (Clinical Research edition). 2006;332(7544):749–55.

10. Ahangari A. Prevalence of chronic pelvic pain among women: an updated review. Pain Physician. 2014;17(2):E141–7.

11. Chang L, Toner BB, Fukudo S, Guthrie E, Locke GR, Norton NJ, et al. Gender, age, society, culture, and the patient's perspective in the functional gastrointestinal disorders. Gastroenterology. 2006;130(5):1435–46.

12. Arendt-Nielsen L, Bajaj P, Drewes AM. Visceral pain: gender differences in response to experimental and clinical pain. European Journal of Pain. 2004;8(5):465–72.

13. Meleine M, Matricon J. Gender-related differences in irritable bowel syndrome: potential mechanisms of sex hormones. World Journal of Gastroenterology. 2014;20(22):6725–43.

14. Wada-Hiraike O, Warner M, Gustafsson JA. New developments in oestrogen signalling in colonic epithelium. Biochemical Society Transactions. 2006;34(Pt 6):1114–6.

15. Giamberardino MA. Women and visceral pain: are the reproductive organs the main protagonists? Mini-review at the occasion of the 'European Week Against Pain in Women 2007'. European Journal of Pain. 2008;12(3):257–60.

16. Traub RJ. Sensitization in visceral pain and hyperalgesia. Seminars in Pain Medicine. 2003;1(3):150–8.

17. Ness T. Distinctive clinical and biological characteristics of visceral pain. Pasricha P,

Willis W, Gebhart G, editors. New York, London: Informa Healthcare; 2007.

18. Robinson DR, Gebhart GF. Inside information: the unique features of visceral sensation. Molecular Interventions. 2008;8(5):242–53.

19. Drewes AM, Gregersen H. Multimodal pain stimulation of the gastrointestinal tract. World Journal of Gastroenterology. 2006;12(16):2477–86.

20. Gregersen H, Drewes AM, McMahon BP, Liao D. Balloon-distension studies in the gastrointestinal tract: current role. Digestive Diseases. 2006;24(3–4):286–96.

21. Petersen P, Gao C, Arendt-Nielsen L, Gregersen H, Drewes AM. Pain intensity and biomechanical responses during ramp-controlled distension of the human rectum. Digestive Diseases and Sciences. 2003;48(7):1310–6.

22. Drewes AM, Pedersen J, Liu W, Arendt-Nielsen L, Gregersen H. Controlled mechanical distension of the human oesophagus: sensory and biomechanical findings. Scandinavian Journal of Gastroenterology. 2003;38(1):27–35.

23. Mertz H. Review article: visceral hypersensitivity. Alimentary Pharmacology and Therapeutics. 2003;17(5):623–33.

24. Giamberardino MA, Vecchiet J, Affaitati G, Vecchiet L. Visceral pain mechanisms. In: Tiengo MA, editor. Neuroscience: focus on acute and chronic pain. Topics in Anaesthesia and Critical Care. Milan: Springer; 2001. p. 59–70.

25. Traub R. Spinal mechanisms of visceral pain and sensitisation. In: Pasricha P, Willis W, Gebhart G, editors. Chronic abdominal

and visceral pain. 1. New York, London: Informa Healthcare; 2007. p. 85–98.

26. Meller ST, Gebhart GF. A critical review of the afferent pathways and the potential chemical mediators involved in cardiac pain. Neuroscience. 1992;48(3):501–24.

27. Meen M, Coudore-Civiale MA, Eschalier A, Boucher M. Involvement of hypogastric and pelvic nerves for conveying cystitis induced nociception in conscious rats. Journal of Urology. 2001;166(1):318–22.

28. Cervero F, Laird JM. Visceral pain. Lancet. 1999;353(9170):2145–8.

29. Sugiura Y, Terui N, Hosoya Y. Difference in distribution of central terminals between visceral and somatic unmyelinated (C) primary afferent fibers. Journal of Neurophysiology. 1989;62(4):834–40.

30. Cameron DM, Brennan TJ, Gebhart GF. Hind paw incision in the rat produces long-lasting colon hypersensitivity. Journal of Pain. 2008;9(3):246–53.

31. Mayer EA, Tillisch K. The brain-gut axis in abdominal pain syndromes. Annual Review of Medicine. 2011;62:10.1146/annurev-med-012309–103958.

32. Mayer EA, Tillisch K. The brain-gut axis in abdominal pain syndromes. Annual Review of Medicine. 2011;62:381–96.

33. Elsenbruch S, Rosenberger C, Enck P, Forsting M, Schedlowski M, Gizewski ER. Affective disturbances modulate the neural processing of visceral pain stimuli in irritable bowel syndrome: an fMRI study. Gut. 2010;59(4):489–95.

34. Mayer EA. The neurobiology of stress and gastrointestinal disease. Gut. 2000;47(6):861–9.

35. Herman JP, Cullinan WE. Neurocircuitry of stress: central control of the hypothalamo-pituitary-adrenocortical axis. Trends in Neurosciences. 1997;20(2):78–84.

36. Larauche M, Mulak A, Taché Y. Stress and visceral pain: from animal models to clinical therapies. Experimental Neurology. 2012;233(1):49–67.

37. Dinan TG, Quigley EMM, Ahmed SMM, Scully P, O'Brien S, O'Mahony L, et al. Hypothalamic-pituitary-gut axis dysregulation in irritable bowel syndrome: plasma cytokines as a potential biomarker? Gastroenterology. 130(2):304–11.

38. Kim SE, Chang L. Overlap between functional GI disorders and other functional syndromes: what are the underlying mechanisms? Neurogastroenterology and Motility. 2012;24(10):895–913.

39. Sharma A, Aziz Q. Mechanisms of visceral sensitisation in humans. In: Pasricha P, Willis W, Gebhart G, editors. Chronic abdominal and visceral pain: theory and practice. 1. New York, London: Informa Healthcare; 2007. p. 141–55.

40. Sawchenko PE, Li HY, Ericsson A. Circuits and mechanisms governing hypothalamic responses to stress: a tale of two paradigms. Progress in Brain Research. 2000;122:61–78.

41. Buller KM. Neuroimmune stress responses: reciprocal connections between the hypothalamus and the brainstem. Stress. 2003;6(1):11–7.

42. Creed F, Guthrie E, Ratcliffe J, Fernandes L, Rigby C, Tomenson B, et al. Does psychological treatment help only those patients with severe irritable bowel syndrome who also have a concurrent psychiatric disorder? Australian and New Zealand Journal of Psychiatry. 2005;39(9):807–15.

43. Dinan TG, Cryan JF. Regulation of the stress response by the gut microbiota: implications for psychoneuroendocrinology. Psychoneuroendocrinology. 2012;37(9):1369–78.

44. Lozupone CA, Stombaugh JI, Gordon JI, Jansson JK, Knight R. Diversity, stability and resilience of the human gut microbiota. Nature. 2012;489(7415):220–30.

45. Lee W-J, Hase K. Gut microbiota-generated metabolites in animal health and disease. Nature Chemical Biology. 2014;10(6):416–24.

46. Dinan TG, Cryan JF. Regulation of the stress response by the gut microbiota: implications for psychoneuroendocrinology. Psychoneuroendocrinology. 37(9):1369–78.

47. Cryan JF, Dinan TG. Mind-altering microorganisms: the impact of the gut microbiota on brain and behaviour. Nature Reviews. Neuroscience. 2012;13(10):701–12.

48. Lee KN, Lee OY. Intestinal microbiota in pathophysiology and management of irritable bowel syndrome. World Journal of Gastroenterology : WJG. 2014;20(27):8886–97.

49. Wang H-X, Wang Y-P. Gut microbiota-brain axis. Chinese Medical Journal. 2016;129(19):2373–80.

50. Kato S. Role of serotonin 5-HT(3) receptors in intestinal inflammation. Biological and Pharmaceutical Bulletin. 2013;36(9):1406–9.

51. Camilleri M. Serotonin in the gastrointestinal tract. Current Opinion in Endocrinology, Diabetes and Obesity. 2009;16(1):53–9.

52. Ghia JE, Li N, Wang H, Collins M, Deng Y, El-Sharkawy RT, et al. Serotonin has a key role in pathogenesis of experimental colitis. Gastroenterology. 137(5):1649–60.

53. Seidel MF, Fiebich BL, Ulrich-Merzenich G, Candelario-Jalil E, Koch FW, Vetter H. Serotonin mediates PGE2 overexpression through 5-HT2A and 5-HT3 receptor subtypes in serum-free tissue culture of macrophage-like synovial cells. Rheumatology International. 2008;28(10):1017–22.

54. Stasi C, Bellini M, Bassotti G, Blandizzi C, Milani S. Serotonin receptors and their role in the pathophysiology and therapy of irritable bowel syndrome. Techniques in Coloproctology. 2014;18(7):613–21.

55. Crowell MD. Role of serotonin in the pathophysiology of the irritable bowel syndrome. British Journal of Pharmacology. 2004;141(8):1285–93.

56. Halder SLS, Locke GR. Epidemiology and socioeconomic impact of visceral and abdominal paion syndromes. In: Pasricha PJ WW, Gebhart GF, editor. Chronic abdominal and visceral pain: theory and practice. New York, London: Inroma Healthcare; 2007.

57. Talley NJ, Spiller R. Irritable bowel syndrome: a little understood organic bowel disease? Lancet. 2002;360:165–77.

58. Ringstrom G, Abrahamsson H, Strid H, Simren M. Why do subjects with irritable bowel syndrome seek health care for their symptoms? Scandinavian Journal of Gastroenterology. 2007;42(10):1194–203.

59. Dapoigny M, Bellanger J, Bonaz B, Bruley des Varannes S, Bueno L, Coffin B, et al. Irritable bowel syndrome in France: a common, debilitating and costly disorder. European Journal of Gastroenterology and Hepatology. 2004;16(10):995–1001.

60. Okeke EN, Ladep NG, Adah S, Bupwatda PW, Agaba EI, Malu AO. Prevalence of irritable bowel syndrome: a community survey in an African population. Annals of African Medicine. 2009;8(3):177–80.

61. Canavan C, West J, Card T. The epidemiology of irritable bowel syndrome. Clinical Epidemiology. 2014;6:71–80.

62. Herman J, Pokkunuri V, Braham L, Pimentel M. Gender distribution in irritable bowel syndrome is proportional to the severity of constipation relative to diarrhea. Gender Medicine. 2010;7(3):240–6.

63. Quigley EMM, Fried M, Gwee K, Olano C, Guarner F, Khalif I et al. Irritable bowel syndrome: a global perspective. World Gastroenterological Global Guideline 2009.

64. Talley NJ, Stanghellini V, Heading RC, Koch KL, Malagelada JR, Tytgat GN. Functional gastroduodenal disorders. Gut. 1999;45(Suppl 2):Ii37–42.

65. Mahadeva S, Goh K. Epidemiology of functional dyspepsia: a global perspective. World Journal of Gastroenterology. 2006;12(17):2661–6.

66. Westbrook JI, Talley NJ. Empiric clustering of dyspepsia into symptom subgroups: a population-based study. Scandinavian Journal of Gastroenterology. 2002;37(8):917–23.

67. Van Oudenhove L, Aziz Q. The role of psychosocial factors and psychiatric disorders in functional dyspepsia. Nature Reviews Gastroenterology and Hepatology. 2013;10(3):158–67.

68. Eslick GD, Jones MP, Talley NJ. Non-cardiac chest pain: prevalence, risk factors, impact and consulting – a population-based study. Alimentary Pharmacology and Therapeutics. 2003;17(9):1115–24.

69. Carmin CN, Ownby RL, Wiegartz PS, Kondos GT. Women and non-cardiac chest pain: gender differences in symptom presentation. Archives of Womens Mental Health. 2008;11(4):287–93.

70. Taylor AL, Bellumkonda L. Minority women and cardiovascular disease. Cardiovascular disease in racial and ethnic minorities. Contemporary Cardiology. New York: Humana Press Inc; 2009. p. 297–320.

71. Hollerbach S, Bulat R, May A, Kamath MV, Upton AR, Fallen EL, et al. Abnormal cerebral processing of oesophageal stimuli in patients with noncardiac chest pain (NCCP). Neurogastroenterology and Motility. 2000;12(6):555–65.

72. Srinivasan R, Greenbaum DS. Chronic abdominal wall pain: a frequently overlooked problem. Practical approach to diagnosis and management. American Journal of Gastroenterology. 2002;97(4):824–30.

73. Greenbaum D. Abdominal Wall Pain. In: Pasricha P, Willis W, Gebhart G, editors. Chronic abdominal and visceral pain. 1. New York, London: Informa Healthcare; 2007. p. 427–35.

74. Applegate WV, Buckwalter NR. Microanatomy of the structures contributing to abdominal cutaneous nerve entrapment syndrome. Journal of the American Board of Family Practice. 1997;10(5):329–32.

75. Costanza CD, Longstreth GF, Liu AL. Chronic abdominal wall pain: clinical features, health care costs, and long-term outcome. Clinical Gastroenterology and Hepatology. 2(5):395–9.

76. Hubscher C, Harpreet K, Kaddumi E. Pelivc pain syndromes: pathophysiology. In: Pasricha P, Willis W, Gebhart G, editors. Chronic abdominal and visceral pain. 1. New York, London: Informa Healthcare; 2007.

77. French L. Dysmenorrhea. American Family Physician. 2005;71(2):285–91.

78. Dawood MY. Primary dysmenorrhea: advances in pathogenesis and management. Obstetrics and Gynecology. 2006;108(2):428–41.

79. Berkley KJ, Rapkin AJ, Papka RE. The pains of endometriosis. Science. 2005;308(5728):1587–9.

80. Bloski T, Pierson R. Endometriosis and chronic pelvic pain: unraveling the mystery behind this complex condition. Nursing for Womens Health. 2008;12(5):382–95.

81. Berkley KJ, Dmitrieva N, Curtis KS, Papka RE. Innervation of ectopic endometrium in a rat model of endometriosis. Proceedings of the National Academy of Sciences of the United States of America. 2004;101(30):11094–8.

82. Granot M, Friedman M, Yarnitsky D, Zimmer EZ. Enhancement of the perception of systemic pain in women with vulvar vestibulitis. BJOG: An International Journal of Obstetrics and Gynaecology. 2002;109(8):863–6.

83. Bohm-Starke N, Hilliges M, Falconer C, Rylander E. Neurochemical characterization of the vestibular nerves in women with vulvar vestibulitis syndrome. Gynecologic and Obstetric Investigation. 1999;48(4):270–5.

84. Reed BD, Harlow SD, Sen A, Legocki LJ, Edwards RM, Arato N, et al. Prevalence and demographic characteristics of vulvodynia in a population-based sample. American Journal of Obstetrics and Gynecology. 2012;206(2):170.e1–9.

85. Ventolini G. Vulvar pain: anatomic and recent pathophysiologic considerations. Clinical Anatomy. 2013;26(1):130–3.

86. Sadownik LA. Etiology, diagnosis, and clinical management of vulvodynia. International Journal of Women's Health. 2014;6:437–49.

87. Watson R. Chronic pelvic pain in men. California, USA: Medscape; 2015

88. Pontari MA, Ruggieri MR. Mechanisms in prostatitis/chronic pelvic pain syndrome. Journal of Urology. 2008;179(5 Suppl):S61–7.

89. Levine L. Chronic orchialgia: evaluation and discussion of treatment options. Therapeutic Advances in Urology. 2010;2(5–06):209–14.

90. Maigne JY, Doursounian L, Chatellier G. Causes and mechanisms of common coccydynia: role of body mass index and coccygeal trauma. Spine. 2000;25(23):3072–9.

91. Kehlet H, Jensen TS, Woolf CJ. Persistent postsurgical pain: risk factors and prevention. Lancet. 2006;367(9522):1618–25.

92. Steer ML, Waxman I, Freedman S. Chronic pancreatitis. New England Journal of Medicine. 1995;332(22):1482–90.

93. Bouwense SA, Ahmed Ali U, ten Broek RP, Issa Y, van Eijck CH, Wilder-Smith OH, et al. Altered central pain processing after pancreatic surgery for chronic pancreatitis. British Journal of Surgery. 2013;100(13):1797–804.

94. Drewes AM, Krarup AL, Detlefsen S, Malmstrom ML, Dimcevski G, Funch-Jensen P. Pain in chronic pancreatitis: the role of neuropathic pain mechanisms. Gut. 2008;57(11):1616–27.

95. Stawowy M, Bluhme C, Arendt-Nielsen L, Drewes AM, Funch-Jensen P. Somatosensory changes in the referred pain area in patients with acute cholecystitis before and after treatment with laparoscopic or open cholecystectomy. Scandinavian Journal of Gastroenterology. 2004;39(10):988–93.

96. Kurucsai G, Joo I, Fejes R, Szekely A, Szekely I, Tihanyi Z, et al. Somatosensory hypersensitivity in the referred pain area in patients with chronic biliary pain and a sphincter of Oddi dysfunction: new aspects of an almost forgotten pathogenetic mechanism. American Journal of Gastroenterology. 2008;103(11):2717–25.

97. Vrijland WW, Jeekel J, van Geldorp HJ, Swank DJ, Bonjer HJ. Abdominal adhesions: intestinal obstruction, pain, and infertility. Surgical Endoscopy. 2003;17(7):1017–22.

98. Hammoud A, Gago LA, Diamond MP. Adhesions in patients with chronic pelvic pain: a role for adhesiolysis? Fertility and Sterility. 2004;82(6):1483–91.

99. Menzies D. Postoperative adhesions: their treatment and relevance in clinical practice. Annals of the Royal College of Surgeons of England. 1993;75(3):147–53.

100. Sulaiman H, Gabella G, Davis MC, Mutsaers SE, Boulos P, Laurent GJ, et al. Presence and distribution of sensory nerve fibers in human peritoneal adhesions. Annals of Surgery. 2001;234(2):256–61.

101. Austin P, Henderson S, Power I, Jirwe M, Alander T. An international Delphi study to assess the need for multiaxial criteria in diagnosis and management of functional gastrointestinal disorders. Journal of Psychosomatic Research. 2013;75(2):128–34.

102. Rome Foundation. Rome III diagnostic questionnaire for the adult functional GI disorders (including alarm questions) and scoring algorithm. Raleigh: Rome Foundation Inc; 2006.

103. Schmulson MJ, Drossman DA. What is new in Rome IV. Journal of Neurogastroenterology and Motility. 2017;23(2):151–63.

104. Patrizi F, Freedman SD, Pascual-Leone A, Fregni F. Novel therapeutic approaches to the treatment of chronic abdominal visceral pain. ScientificWorld Journal. 2006;6:472–90.

105. Camilleri M. Serotonin in the Gastrointestinal Tract. Current Opinion in Endocrinology, Diabetes, and Obesity. 2009;16(1):53–9.

106. Ashburn TT, Gupta MS. The IBS market. Nature Reviews. Drug Discovery. 2006;5(2):99–100.

107. Osteen JD, Herzig V, Gilchrist J, Emrick JJ, Zhang C, Wang X, et al. Selective spider toxins reveal a role for the Nav1.1 channel in mechanical pain. Nature. 2016;534(7608):494–9.

108. Sanger GJ, Chang L, Bountra C, Houghton LA. Challenges and prospects for pharmacotherapy in functional gastrointestinal disorders. Therapeutic Advances in Gastroenterology. 2010.

109. Vanuytsel T, Tack JF, Boeckxstaens GE. Treatment of abdominal pain in irritable bowel syndrome. Journal of Gastroenterology. 2014;49(8):1193–205.

110. Lapointe TK, Basso L, Iftinca MC, Flynn R, Chapman K, Dietrich G, et al. TRPV1 sensitization mediates post-inflammatory visceral pain following acute colitis. American Journal of Physiology. Gastrointestinal and Liver Physiology. 2015:ajpgi.00421.2014.

111. Lecci A, Capriati A, Altamura M, Maggi CA. Tachykinins and tachykinin receptors in the gut, with special reference to NK2 receptors in human. Autonomic Neuroscience. 2006;126–127:232–49.

112. Dharmshaktu P, Tayal V, Kalra BS. Efficacy of antidepressants as analgesics: a review. Journal of Clinical Pharmacology. 2012;52(1):6–17.

113. Mika J, Zychowska M, Makuch W, Rojewska E, Przewlocka B. Neuronal and immunological basis of action of antidepressants in chronic pain – clinical and experimental studies. Pharmacological Reports. 2013;65(6):1611–21.

114. Olesen SS, Graversen C, Olesen AE, Frokjaer JB, Wilder-Smith O, van Goor H, et al. Randomised clinical trial: pregabalin attenuates experimental visceral pain through sub-cortical mechanisms in patients with painful chronic pancreatitis. Alimentary Pharmacology and Therapeutics. 2011;34(8):878–87.

115. Farmer AD, Coen SJ, Kano M, Naqvi H, Paine PA, Scott SM, et al. Psychophysiological responses to visceral and somatic pain in functional chest pain identify clinically relevant pain clusters. Neurogastroenterology and Motility. 2014;26(1):139–48.

116. Alappattu MJ, Bishop MD. Psychological factors in chronic pelvic pain in women: relevance and application of the fear-avoidance model of pain. Physical Therapy. 2011;91(10):1542–50.

117. Buenaver L, Edwards R, Haythornthwaite J. Psychological interventions for patients with chronic abdominal and pelvic pain. In: Pasricha P, Willis W, Gebhart G, editors. Chronic abdominal and visceral pain. London, New York: Informa Healthcare; 2007.

118. Mahvi-Shirazi M, Fathi-Ashtiani A, Rasoolzade-Tabatabaei SK, Amini M. Irritable bowel syndrome treatment: cognitive behavioral therapy versus medical treatment. Archives of Medical Science. 2012;8(1):123–9.

119. Wilson S, Maddison T, Roberts L, Greenfield S, Singh S. Systematic review: the effectiveness of hypnotherapy in the management of irritable bowel syndrome. Alimentary Pharmacology and Therapeutics. 2006;24(5):769–80.

120. Calvert EL, Houghton LA, Cooper P, Morris J, Whorwell PJ. Long-term improvement in functional dyspepsia using hypnotherapy. Gastroenterology. 2002;123(6):1778–85.

121. Muller A, Franke H, Resch KL, Fryer G. Effectiveness of osteopathic manipulative therapy for managing symptoms of irritable bowel syndrome: a systematic review. Journal of the American Osteopathic Association. 2014;114(6):470–9.

122. Piche T, Pishvaie D, Tirouvaziam D, Filippi J, Dainese R, Tonohouhan M, et al. Osteopathy decreases the severity of IBS-like symptoms associated with Crohn's disease in patients in remission. European Journal of Gastroenterology and Hepatology. 2014;26(12):1392–8.

123. Ferraz BB, Martins MRI, Foss MHDA. Impacto da terapia manual visceral na melhora da qualidade de vida de pacientes com dor abdominal crônica. Revista Dor. 2013;14:124–8.

124. Manley J. The effectiveness of manual therapy on chronic pelvic pain: an evidence-based review. San Francisco: University of California; 2012.

125. Barral J. Visceral manipulation II. Seattle, WA: Eastland Press; 2007.

126. Finet G. Treating Visceral dysfunction: an osteopathic approach to understanding and treating the abdominal organs. Portland, OR: Stillness Press; 2000.

127. Bove GM, Chapelle SL. Visceral mobilization can lyse and prevent peritoneal adhesions in a rat model. Journal of Bodywork and Movement Therapies. 2012;16(1):76–82.

128. Mattei P, Rombeau JL. Review of the pathophysiology and management of postoperative ileus. World Journal of Surgery. 2006;30(8):1382–91.

129. Springall RG, Spitz L. The prevention of post-operative adhesions using a gastrointestinal prokinetic agent. Journal of Pediatric Surgery. 1989;24(6):530–3.

130. Chapelle SL, Bove GM. Visceral massage reduces postoperative ileus in a rat model. Journal of Bodywork and Movement Therapies. 2013;17(1):83–8.

131. Rice A, King R, Reed E, Patterson K, Wurn BF, Wurn LJ. Manual physical therapy for non-surgical treatment of adhesion-related small bowel obstructions: two case reports. Journal of Clinical Medicine. 2013;2(1):1–12.

132. Rice AD, Wakefield LB, Patterson K, Reed ED, Wurn BF, King CR, 3rd, et al. Decreasing adhesions and avoiding further surgery in a pediatric patient involved in a severe pedestrian versus motor vehicle accident. Pediatric Reports. 2014;6(1):5126.

133. Drossman DA. Severe and refractory chronic abdominal pain: treatment strategies. Clinical Gastroenterology and Hepatology. 2008;6(9):978–82.

Introduction

Headaches and facial pain are among the most common complaints and affect almost all people at some point in their lives. Although headaches may be physiological in acute settings, they can also become pathological and persistent conditions in which people report the presence of headache symptoms every day for several months or even years.[1] The vast majority of headache presentations are primary headaches: a set of benign conditions where the headache condition itself is not due to an underlying cause, good examples being tension headaches and migraine headaches. Here, a diagnosis is made based solely on information gained from the case history, in which there are no abnormal signs. Alternatively, there may be secondary headaches caused by an underlying pathology or disorder that includes infection, intracranial hemorrhage, and space-occupying lesions.[2] As the brain contains no primary afferent nociceptors, headache symptoms arise from surrounding meningeal structures such as the dura, vascular structures, and musculoskeletal tissues such as the scalp, skull, and associated musculature. Primary afferents here transmit nociceptive signals from cranial structures via the trigeminal, first, and second cervical dorsal root ganglia to the brainstem.[3] This chapter will follow the latest headache classification of the International Headache Society;[4] however, it is beyond the scope of this chapter to present and review the classification in full. This chapter will therefore first outline the epidemiology and mechanisms of chronic headaches and orofacial pain. Second, it will review the evaluation and modes of treatment shown to be effective for chronic primary headaches and facial pain disorders, with particular attention paid to those used in manual therapy settings.

Epidemiology

Primary headaches are a group of heterogeneous disorders that cause persistent or episodic head pain where there is no underlying pathology. The diagnosis of primary headache is made using information taken from the case history, self-reporting questionnaires, and recognized taxonomies. For ease of reference, this section reviews the epidemiology of individual disorders separately.

Tension-type headaches

Chronic tension-type headaches (CTTH) are the most prevalent of primary headache disorders in all age groups across the general population and is the cause of significant disability.[5,6] Although data on recent prevalence and incidence rates are scarce, the past-year prevalence rate in the general population is approximately 20%.[7] In Europe, the latest prevalence rates differ greatly, ranging from 5.1% in southern Europe[8] to 74% in western Europe.[9] The prevalence of CTTH also varies with age. A large American study showed a one-year prevalence rate peaking at the fourth decade for both men (42%) and women (47%).[10] These data, showing a slightly higher prevalence in women, are echoed by other observations; for example, in New Zealand the prevalence of CTTH in women has been reported to be twice that of men. The prevalence of CTTH also increases with education level. In a large telephone survey of over 10,000 community subjects, prevalence rates increased with increasing education levels, reaching a peak at graduate school education of over 48% in both men and women equally.[10] Not surprisingly, people with CTTH where the headache is more constant also show more lost work days compared to those reporting episodic tension headaches (27.4 versus 8.9 days/year).[10]

Chapter 11

Migraine headaches

Although migraine headaches are less common than CTTHs, these headaches affect over 5% of the general population, causing significantly more individual incapacity, which also creates a substantial socioeconomic burden for both the person and their family and occupational status.[11] Prevalence rates of migraine are significantly higher in females (18%) compared to men (7%) and like CTTH, prevalence rates increase with age, peaking similarly in the fourth decade.[12] Prevalence rates are also higher among Caucasians (15%) than among African Americans (12%) and Asian Americans (7%); evidence suggests that these race-related differences are most likely due to genetic vulnerability.[13] Additionally, people with chronic migraine have significantly lower levels of household income, are less likely to have full time employment, and are more likely to be occupationally disabled.[11]

Chronic migraine sufferers are twice as likely to report depression, anxiety, and other functional pain disorders such as fibromyalgia.[14] In addition to these functional comorbidities, migraine is also associated with medical conditions such as cardiovascular disease, asthma, Raynaud's phenomenon, and systemic lupus erythematosus.[15] Although there are few studies investigating the incidence of migraine headaches, data from the American Migraine Prevalence and Prevention Study showed that, on average, incidence rates peak in females in their early twenties and in mid to late teens in men. Unlike CTTH sufferers, people with chronic migraine also report significantly reduced health-related quality of life, similar to those with chronic diseases such as chronic heart failure and diabetes.[16]

Trigeminal autonomic cephalalgias

Trigeminal autonomic cephalalgias (TAC) are a group of primary headache conditions that are characterized by unilateral head pain, facial pain, or both that present with accompanying autonomic signs and symptoms.[17] The most prevalent and most studied TAC is the cluster headache. Although little data exist on the epidemiology of this set of conditions, several studies show prevalence rates of cluster headaches in the general population as being below 1% with an overall sex ratio of 4:3 (male to female).[18] Interestingly, however, this ratio may be changing with increasing prevalence rates in women, due possibly to higher levels of education and employment rates.[1] The incidence of cluster headaches is difficult to determine as only three studies showing incidence rates ranging from 2–10 per 100,000 per year.[18] Again, while not substantiated, meta-analysis on regional differences suggest that prevalence rates in the northern countries are higher than in countries near the equator.

Temporomandibular disorders

Temporomandibular pain relates to a group of disorders involving the temporomandibular joint (TMJ), masticatory muscles, and surrounding bony and soft tissues. These disorders are often accompanied by headaches, reductions in TMJ motion, and high levels of pain-related disability.[19] Pain in the temporomandibular region is relatively common, with Lipton and co-workers reporting its occurrence in between 6% and 12% of the general population.[20] Temporomandibular disorders (TMDs) are most common in young and middle-aged adults, rather than children or the elderly, and more than twice as common in females compared to males.[21] Temporomandibular symptoms are also more prevalent in women than men. Here, although it is not entirely clear why, findings from animal and preliminary human studies suggest that sex hormones, specifically estrogen and progesterone, may predispose to TMD and subsequent cartilage breakdown.[18] About one third of TMD patients also have psychiatric diagnoses, with several studies showing that post-traumatic stress disorder symptoms are strongly linked to both poorer TMJ function and greater incidence of temporomandibular pain.[22,23] Additionally, TMDs are also related to lifestyle and occupational characteristics, in particular computer users and instrumentalists.[24] In this population, TMD signs and symptoms are caused by heavy use of the mouth and constant tension of the head and neck muscles, for example during recitals.[25] Table 11.1 summarizes the main features of primary headaches.

Table 11.1: General features of primary headaches

Headache type	Frequency	Site	Clinical features
Tension headache	~20%	Bilateral, frontal, temporal, occipital, neck	Dull, band-like, scalp tenderness, episodic
Migraine headache	7–15%	Unilateral, frontal, vertex, occipital	Throbbing, moderate–severe episodic nausea/vomiting, photophobia, familial
Cluster headaches	<1%	Unilateral, retro-orbital	Excruciating, excessive tearing, redness, Horner's syndrome
Temporomandibular disorders	6–12%	Bilateral/unilateral jaw, ear, facial	Dull, ache, limited range of temporomandibular joint motion, noisy temporomandibular joint motion

Mechanisms and clinical features

Chronic tension-type headaches

Peripheral mechanisms

Due to the uncertainty of pathophysiological mechanisms, the term 'tension-type headache' is used to describe a heterogeneous group of headaches previously labeled as 'psychogenic', 'stress', 'muscle contraction', and 'essential' headaches. Previous studies suggest that people with CTTH show increased pain severity in pericranial myofascial tissues compared to healthy controls. Although this type of pain is still considered to be due to prolonged contraction, ischemia, and inflammation to the head and neck muscles, electromyographic (EMG) studies show no significant levels of ischemia or local inflammation.[26,27] These findings suggest that muscle pain is not due to increased or prolonged muscle contraction. However, increased muscle tone without observed EMG activity may cause microtrauma of muscle fibers where tendon insertions may sensitize peripheral nociceptors.[28] Although not substantiated, these concepts also support the argument for the role of trigger points in muscles showing normal EMG activity at rest. Additionally, several assessor-blinded studies show an increase in the number of trigger points in head and neck muscles (Figure 11.1) in both adults and children with CTTH compared to controls.[29] These findings showed not only referred pain patterns provoked by trigger point activation, but also an association between more active trigger points and increased headache severity.

Current understanding also suggests that other peripheral factors such as the increased excitability of peripheral nociceptors due to local tissue edema and metabolic alterations or hyperexcitability of muscle fibers may also play a significant role in the onset and maintenance of CTTH.[30] However, given the current lack of evidence for obvious underlying peripheral abnormalities, further studies are needed to identify possible mechanisms for the activation of peripheral myofascial nociceptors.

Central mechanisms

Although central mechanisms have been sparsely investigated, it is becoming increasingly evident that central factors are involved in the onset and maintenance of CTTH.[31] This is due to (1) sensitization of dorsal horn and second order neurons as a result of increased inputs from primary nociceptive afferent fibers and (2) the effect of descending supraspinal activity due to psychological dysfunction. Here, population studies find that people with episodic TTH show normal levels of stress and anxiety, whereas those with CTTH report significantly higher levels of anxiety and depression.[32,33] Thus, as with other chronic pain disorders, psychological dysfunction is likely comorbid with CTTH.

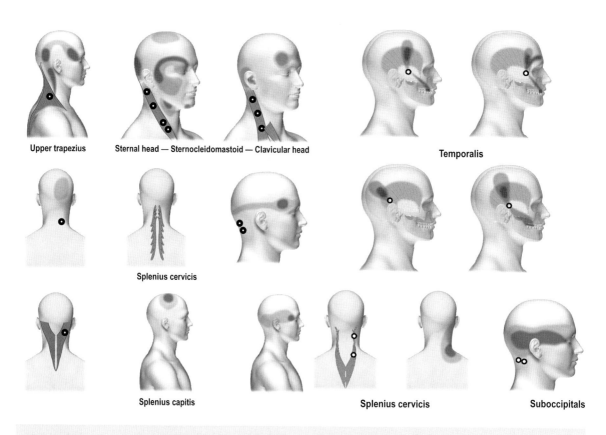

Upper trapezius **Sternal head — Sternocleidomastoid — Clavicular head** **Temporalis**

Splenius cervicis

Splenius capitis **Splenius cervicis** **Suboccipitals**

Figure 11.1

Referred pain from active trigger point in the upper trapezius, sternocleidomastoid, levitator scapulae, suboccipital, and temporalis muscles in people with CTTH (Travell and Simon 1999)

Although pain thresholds are shown to be within normal parameters in people with intermittent TTH, they are reduced in people with CTTH.[34,35] Here, findings from several studies show pain hypersensitivity in many cases where patients report not only cephalic, but additionally extracephalic hyperalgesia, namely in neck and shoulder muscles.[36,37] This expansion of hypersensitivity is suggestive of the involvement of spinal and supraspinal neurons. Such patients also show increased temporal summation (Chapter 2) to both pressure and electrical pain compared to controls.[38] Other factors suggestive of central sensitization (CS), such as involuntary muscle contraction of cephalic muscles and reduced descending pain-inhibitory activity, are also shown in CTTH patients.[39,40] Using conditioned pain modulation protocols (Chapter 3), Sandrini and colleagues found significant impairment of endogenous supraspinal pain modulation not only in CTTH patients but also in migraineurs compared to controls.

Interestingly, nitric oxide (NO), an important molecule in CS pathophysiology, plays an important role in the pathophysiology of CTTH. In the dorsal horn, NO diffuses from the postsynaptic membrane to presynaptic glutaminergic fibers, increasing glutamate release which subsequently acts on NMDA receptors (Chapter 2). Several studies report significant increases in NO synthase production and thus an increase in glutamate levels in dorsal horn neurons.[31,41] Interestingly, Ashina and colleagues show that a NO synthase inhibitor reduces not only the severity of headaches but also hardness in head and neck muscles.[42] Furthermore, the administration of a NO agonist (glyceryl trinitrate) is shown to cause headaches in healthy controls.[43]

Clinical features

People with CTTH usually present with headaches described as dull, pressure-like, or as tightness or a sense of fullness in the head; they are usually experienced as a band extending bilaterally (90% of patients) across the pericranium from the occiput across the side of the head to the frontal region or vice versa.[44] A TTH can last from 30 minutes to several days and is often continuous in severe cases. Patients also report pain in neck and shoulder muscles and this is often described as 'cape-like,' radiating along the medial and lateral trapezius muscles to the scapular and interscapular regions.[45] Overall, physical activity does not influence the intensity of the TTH, unlike migraines, where pain intensity increases with physical activity.[46] Rarely, photophobia or phonophobia may be present, while neurological examination is usually normal.

The most common aggravating factors include stress, lack of sleep, snoring, eating at inappropriate times of the day, alcohol intake, and menstruation.[47] Additionally, factors that aggravate CTTH also aggravate symptoms of migraine headaches, thus, a detailed case history is important to differentiate these conditions. Table 11.2 shows the IHSC diagnostic criteria for CTTH.

Several conditions are associated with CTTH. Probably the most common are psychiatric conditions, especially depression and generalized anxiety disorders;[48,49] however, stress intensity also shows positive correlations with TTH frequency. Sleep disorders are also commonly associated with CTTH, and it is the most common type of headache associated with sleep apnea and other sleep-related breathing disorders.[50,51] Furthermore, CTTH also have a high comorbidity rate with fibromyalgia.[52]

Physical examination

The diagnosis of CTTH involves the exclusion of other causes of headaches. Thus, a thorough physical and neurological examination is required. Manual palpation of the pericranial and neck muscles should elicit general tenderness and the presence of trigger points, but no other physical findings should be noted. Manual pressure to these areas may induce both deep localized tenderness and referred pain to other neck and pericranial tissues.[44] When differentiating from secondary headaches, pain should not be provoked over temporal arteries (more associated with temporal arteritis) and where pain is associated with neck flexion and stretching of paracervical muscles, this

Table 11.2: Diagnostic criteria of a chronic tension-type headache according to the International Headache Society classification

	Description
A	A headache occurring on ≥15 days per month on average for >3 months (≥180 days per year)
B	A headache that last for hours, or may be continuous
C	A headache with at least two of the following characteristics: bilateral location; of a pressing or tightening (non-pulsating) quality; of mild or moderate pain intensity; and not aggravated by routine physical activity, such as walking or climbing stairs
D	Both of the following: no more than one episode of photophobia, phonophobia, or mild nausea; and, either moderate or severe nausea and vomiting

must be distinguished from nuchal rigidity associated with meningeal irritation.[53]

Migraine headaches

Migraine headache is a complex disorder that is incapacitating, reduces health-related quality of life, and is economically costly.[54] Although migraines affect many people, the exact pathogenesis remains undetermined, with concepts having swung between vascular and neuronal mechanisms. However, with the increased availability of imaging techniques such as positron emission tomography (PET) and functional magnetic resonance imaging (fMRI), these theories have been superseded by the neurovascular concept that is now thought to trigger migraine headaches.[55] Current evidence also shows central neuronal hyperexcitability to be a key process in migraine headaches. This section reviews mechanisms of migraine-related auras and mechanisms of migraine pain.

Mechanism of aura

Auras are present in about 30% of migraine patients and are defined as focal neurobiological disturbances that present as visual, sensory, and motor symptoms.[56] Visual auras are the most common, and patients describe it as affecting visual fields, suggesting dysfunction of the visual cortex. These characteristics are related to cortical spreading depression (CSD), described as a slowly spreading wave of altered brain activity that involves alterations in glial cell and vascular function.[57] This spread of cortical depression has a significant effect on neuronal ion homeostasis, with excitatory neurotransmitters such as glutamate leaking into the interstitial fluid.[58] Interestingly, CSD is blocked by NMDA receptor antagonists. By blocking NMDA receptor function, the synthesis of NO (an important vasodilator) is prevented, and thus the extravasation of inflammatory mediators from surrounding blood vessels is inhibited. In human studies, several fMRI studies show this spreading phenomenon to be triggered by visual stimulation (e.g., red-green checkerboard). For example, fMRI methods based on imaging real time blood oxygen levels show headaches are preceded by suppression of brain activity that slowly spreads into the occipital cortex at rates between 3 and 6 mm per minute[59] (Figure 11.2). CSD is also associated with changes in vascular function, with studies showing that focal hyperemia (vasodilatation) is followed by a reactive and often profound oligemia (vasoconstriction) in front of the CSD wave.[57] However, although these vascular changes occur, findings suggest they do so only in the occipital cortex and in no other brain regions.[60]

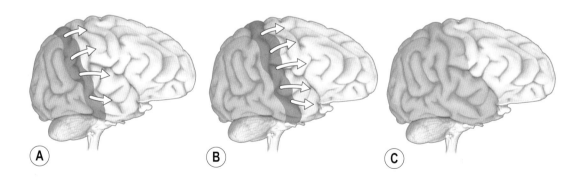

Ⓐ   Ⓑ   Ⓒ

Figure 11.2

Schematic image of CSD. CSD causes migraine auras and involves a wave of depolarization of all cortical elements, spreading at rates between 3 and 6 mm/min (red). Not long after, repolarisation occurs together with a decrease in cerebral blood flow (blue) (from Olesen et al. 2009)

Mechanisms of migraine pain

Experimental and clinical data now show that migraine pain is driven by neurogenic inflammation of the dura mater.[56] The action of CSD is adequate stimulus to initiate a sterile inflammatory response with the release of neuropeptides that activate neurons in the trigeminal ganglion.[60] Neurons innervating cerebral vessels arising from the trigeminal ganglion contain neuropeptides such as substance P and neurokinin A. Thus, stimulation of both dural C and Aδ fibers causes not only plasma extravasation and leakage of plasma, but also increased nociception in dural blood vessels.[61] However, although these inflammatory mechanisms occur, it is not certain if they are sufficient to reduce migraine headache, as blockade of neuropeptide receptors (e.g., substance P antagonists) associated with extravasation does not predict reductions in symptoms.[56]

Given this uncertainty, additional mechanisms have also been proposed. Recent imaging studies in migraine patients show an increase in metabolism in the brainstem (increased trigeminal activity) and decreased cerebral metabolism (CSD), especially in the medial, frontal, and parietal cortices, compared to global flow.[62] Aurora and colleagues suggest that a reduction of inhibitory tone in cortical centers increases activity in the brainstem, namely the trigeminal ganglion. However, although functional imaging techniques lack sufficient resolution during brainstem scans, many animal studies show increased activity of other brainstem nuclei such as the locus coeruleus, substantia nigra, and periaqueductal gray (PAG).[63] The trigeminal complex has direct ascending connections with these nuclei en route towards cortical regions (Figure 11.3).[64] The PAG has a significant influence on nociceptive pathways and has been shown to be hyperactive in people with migraines.[65] Furthermore, the trigeminal complex also has reflex connections with the parasympathetic system via the sphenopalatine ganglion and superior salivatory nucleus that are related to cranial autonomic features such as sweating, nasal congestion, and lacrimation also observed in people with cluster headaches.[66]

Clinical features

Although clinicians and patients believe that migraine is always preceded by an aura this is incorrect. Many migraine patients do not have a visual aura and only 55–65% experience other prodromal symptoms such as mood disturbances, restlessness, gastrointestinal symptoms, and fatigue.[67] For example, patients often describe excessive yawning for several hours prior to the onset of a migraine headache. In such cases, their recognition by patients allows an opportunity to use medications early, so that they are more likely to reduce or halt the headache process.[68] Most auras last less than one hour[4] with the headache following within an hour after the aura dissipates.[67] Migraineurs showing a visual aura describe a combination of visual, sensory (parasthesias in tongue and/or extremities), and aphasic auras.[69] The classic visual aura typically begins as a small defect and gradually enlarges to form flashing lights and 'fortification lines,' a term used to define zig-zag lines, often at right angles to each other, and an accompanying blind spot. From a diagnostic perspective migraine auras differ from those due to cerebral ischemia in which symptoms spread slowly across the visual field and are followed by a gradual return to normal function. Auras due to cerebral ischemia have a sudden onset and are related to areas of vascular compromise.[70]

Typically, migraine pain is throbbing, pulsatile, most often occurs when the person is awake, and is often accompanied by nausea, thought to be due to gastric stasis (abnormal autonomic function), photophobia, phonophobia, impaired cognitive function, and diarrhea. Although migraine pain is unilateral in the frontal region, pain often spreads over the duration of a migraine attack to parietal, occipital, jaw, and neck regions.[71] If left untreated, migraine symptoms typically last between four and 72 hours and, unlike in CTTH, are exacerbated by physical activity, movement, lifting, and stooping.[72] During an attack, migraineurs attempt to find a quiet, dark space where they can remain immobile in a sitting or semi-supine position, rather than lying flat, which can often exacerbate their head pain.[67] The intensity of migraine pain is usually described as moderate to severe; however,

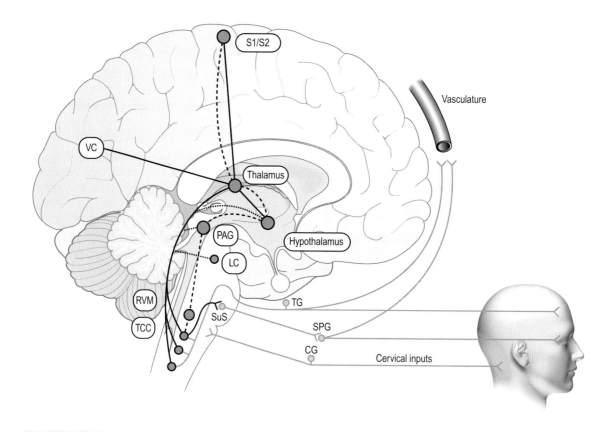

Figure 11.3

A schematic representation of trigeminal complex afferents projecting to (A) cortical sites via the thalamus, (B) via the periaquaductal grey, locus coeruleus (LC) to cortical sites and (C) through reflex connections with the sphenopalatine ganglion (SPG) and superior salivatory nucleus (SuS) that provide parasympathetic outflow to the cranium. Cervical ganglion (CG), rostral ventral medulla (RVM), trigeminocervical complex (TCC), visual cortex (VC)

some people only describe mild discomfort in association with other migraine symptoms. Additionally, patients complain of scalp tenderness in the region of the headache while also describing brief, sharp 'ice-pick headache' pain. Migraine patients further describe postdromal symptoms that can persist for over 24 hours after the headache and that include, fatigue (washed out), irritability, euphoria, muscle weakness, and/or pain, as well as anorexia or food craving.[67]

Diagnostic criteria for migraine without aura are listed in Table 11.3, and criteria for migraine with aura in Table 11.4.

Physical examination

As with CTTH, physical examination of migraine headaches involves the exclusion of other causes of headaches. Although most migraine sufferers show few or no findings, a thorough physical and neurological evaluation of secondary headaches should be performed, including neck flexion for evidence of meningeal irritation.[73] From a manual therapy perspective, it is worth noting that myofascial examination may determine the extent of involvement of neck, shoulder, and pericranial soft tissue. Here, reducing myofascial trigger points at the site of a migraine headaches origin and often reduce

Table 11.3: Diagnostic criteria for migraine without aura according to the International Headache Society classification (ICHD-3)

	Description
A	At least five attacks fulfilling criteria B–D
B	Attacks lasting 4–72 hours if untreated or unsuccessfully treated
C	Headache has at least two of the following characteristics: • unilateral location • pulsating quality • moderate–severe pain intensity • aggravated by or causing avoidance of physical activity
D	During a migraine headache, at least one of the following: • nausea and/or vomiting • photophobia/phonophobia
E	Headache not attributed to any other disorder

Table 11.4: Diagnostic criteria for migraine with aura according to the International Headache Society classification (ICHD-3)

	Description
A	At least two attacks fulfilling criteria B–D
B	Aura consisting of at least one of the following, but no motor weakness: • fully reversible visual symptoms including positive features (e.g., flickering lights, spots, or lines) and/or negative features (i.e., loss of vision) • fully reversible sensory symptoms including positive features (i.e., pins and needles) and/or negative features (i.e., numbness) • fully reversible dysphasic speech disturbance
C	At least two of the following: • homonymous visual symptoms and/or unilateral sensory symptoms • at least one aura symptom develops gradually over ≥5 minutes and/or different aura symptoms occur in succession over ≥5 minutes • each symptom lasts ≥5 and ≤60 minutes
D	Headache fulfilling criteria B–D for migraine without aura begins during the aura or follows aura within 60 minutes
E	Headache not attributed to any other disorder

associated symptoms such as nausea, light, and sound sensitivity.[74] If all other forms of headache have been ruled out, reproducing sites of a migraine headache during an examination also helps to alleviate patient concerns about more sinister causes of their symptoms. For example, an examination should include palpation of neck, head, and facial muscles comparing both the symptomatic and non-symptomatic areas.

Trigeminal autonomic cephalalgias (cluster headaches)

Vascular mechanisms

Like migraine headaches, trigeminal autonomic cephalalgias (TACs) are associated with neurogenic inflammation. Perivascular neurogenic inflammation of the internal carotid artery in its bony canal or elevated pressure within the orbit are also shown to contribute to the onset of cluster headaches.[75] Although evidence shows that pain can continue when vasodilatation is prevented, increased levels of neuropeptides such as calcitonin gene-related peptide and NO in people with TACs indicate the role of neurogenic inflammation in the activation of trigeminal and autonomic nerves.[76] However, while vascular dilatation is also considered to play a role in cluster headaches, they are considered secondary to primary neuronal discharge (Figure 11.4).

Autonomic mechanisms

Pain distribution observed in cluster headaches is largely due to increased activity of the trigeminal and upper cervical nerves and are mediated predominately by the trigeminal autonomic (parasympathetic) reflex.[77] This pathway is activated by a number of triggers such as tooth extraction, lateral cranial trauma, and spicy foods.[78] Cranial parasympathetic fibers arise from the superior salivatory nucleus in the pons and synapse with the sphenopalatine ganglion.[79] These postganglionic fibers then innervate structures such as the lacrimal and nasal mucosa, salivary glands and importantly, craniofacial vasculature.[75] Thus, increased activity of these parasympathetic pathways induces symptoms of lacrimation and

rhinorrhea (Figure 11.4). Additionally, miosis and ptosis (incomplete Horner's syndrome), often seen in people with cluster headaches, are mediated by sympathetic fibers that surround the internal carotid artery.[78]

Neuroendocrine mechanisms

Cluster headaches are shown to be episodic and are strongly associated with sleep. This circadian rhythmicity suggests the role of the hypothalamus in their underlying pathophysiology.[80] Here, the hypothalamic suprachiasmatic nucleus is considered to be responsible for the control of chronobiological regulation.[81] Thus, the relationship between headache attacks, autonomic symptoms, and sleep support the role of the hypothalamus, especially concerning alterations in hormones such as melatonin, cortisol, follicle stimulating hormone, and prolactin.[82] Moreover, cluster headaches are strongly associated with mutations and alterations in release of hypocretin, a neuropeptide released from the posterior hypothalamus whose functions include pain modulation[83] and regulation of the sleep–wake cycle.[75] Although the precise role of the hypothalamus in cluster headaches is still not fully understood, deep brain stimulation therapy in patients with intractable cluster headaches shows 50% reduction in intensity and frequency compared to baseline.[84]

Clinical features

Cluster headaches are typically excruciating attacks that start without warning and last between 15 minutes and three hours. To highlight the intensity of cluster headache pain, it is described as more severe than long-bone fractures, renal stones, or childbirth.[85] Cluster headaches are named as such because they occur in clusters over periods that commonly last between six and 12 weeks and tend to be consistent from period to period, with pain-free periods that may last as long as a year. As described in the previous section, attacks show a circadian rhythm in which they occur at predictable times of the day, usually at 02.00 and 14.00, and may also cluster at a specific time of the month or seasons every year.[78] Cluster headache pain is most often described as boring in quality and occurs in both retro-orbital and temporal regions. Associated symptoms also include

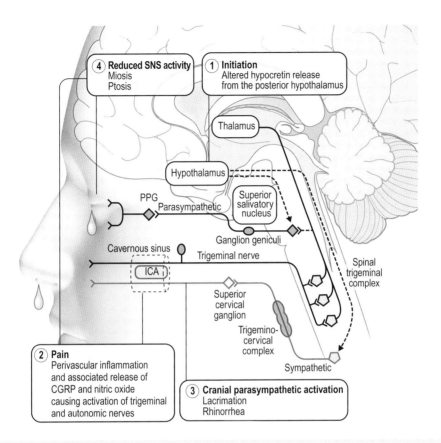

Figure 11.4

A schematic diagram of likely pathophysiological mechanisms of cluster headaches. Here, initiation of an attack is thought to (1) begin in the hypothalamus. This is followed by (2) the onset of pain due to local vasodilatation and the release of inflammatory mediators. These mechanisms are then followed by (3) parasympathetic activation and (4) a partial Horner's syndrome due to reduced sympathetic activity. Internal carotid artery (ICA), calcitonin gene-related peptide (CGRP), pterygopalatine ganglion (PPG)

aural fullness, tearing, and nasal blockage that may occur bilaterally. Table 11.5 shows the International Headache Classification diagnostic criteria for cluster headaches.

Physical examination

As with other primary headaches, examination findings should be normal. The presence of abnormalities other than those signs and symptoms described above suggests another cause of the headache. In addition to the findings in Table 11.5, patients often show distinctive facial characteristics such as multifurrowed and thickened skin with prominent folds as well as vertical forehead creases.[86] Patients are severely distressed, and palpation of pain sites may lead to screaming and/or crying. Other findings include bradycardia, facial flushing, and tenderness.

Temporomandibular pain

Temporomandibular disorders (TMD) are a group of conditions that result in TMJ pain, masticatory muscle pain, or both.[87] For ease of differentiation, Dworkin and LeResche provide diagnostic criteria that divide TMD into three physical categories:[88]

- masticatory muscle pain with or without limited TMJ motion

- TMJ disc displacement (reducing or non-reducing, with or without limited TMJ motion)

- other joint conditions of the TMJ such as arthralgia, arthritis, and arthrosis.

However, as with other chronic pain conditions, underlying mechanisms of pain are not fully understood and there is often poor correlation between the severity of temporomandibular pain and levels of observable tissue damage.[87] Thus, many now believe that such pain may be due more to alterations in central nervous system pain processing.

Peripheral pain mechanisms

The TMJ is commonly affected by degenerative joint disease, disc displacement and disorders are usually caused by excessive or abnormal loading.[89] Excessive loading on the TMJ commonly occurs due to habitual actions such as bruxism (a habit of clenching and/or grinding of teeth), abnormal body postures, trauma and growth abnormalities. Such actions result in activation of C and Aδ fibers and the release proinflammatory mediators such as TNF-α, substance P, and glutamate. This inflammatory response first increases intra-articular pressure due to edema, causing further increasing nociceptive activation, and second, may lead to articular cartilage deterioration, and remodeling of local and adjacent bone, causing both pain and loss of function.[87,90] Additionally, mechanical nociceptors also respond to noxious protrusion, lateral movement, and opening beyond the normal range.[91] These movements, in addition to loading factors, are thought to contribute to disc displacement in which the TMJ may become locked, or in which painful clicking and associated headaches

Table 11.5: Diagnostic criteria for cluster headache according to the International Headache Society classification (ICHD-3)

	Description
A	At least five attacks fulfilling criteria B–D
B	Severe or very severe unilateral orbital, supraorbital, and/or temporal pain lasting 15–180 min (when untreated)[1]
C	Either or both of the following: At least one of the following symptoms or signs, ipsilateral to the headache: a) conjunctival injection and/or lacrimation b) nasal congestion and/or rhinorrhea c) eyelid edema d) forehead and facial sweating e) forehead and facial flushing f) sensation of fullness in the ear g) miosis and/or ptosis A sense of restlessness or agitation
D	Attacks have a frequency between one every other day and eight per day for more than half of the time when the disorder is active
E	Not better accounted for by another ICHD-3 diagnosis

may occur.[92] Not surprisingly, pain originating in the TMJ (especially painful disc displacement) is shown to increase generalized masticatory muscle tone, causing further pain.[93] Additionally, repetitive strain conditions such as clenching and grinding teeth can cause localized ischemia in masticatory muscle, also causing the release of inflammatory mediators that sensitize muscle nociceptors.

Central pain mechanisms

Increased nociceptive input from the TMJ and associated musculature is shown to induce CS, which further lowers TMJ pain thresholds, as well as increase protective masticatory muscle reflexes.[87] Additionally, TMDs are shown to be associated with increases in generalized pain sensitivity during both experimental noxious stimulation and isometric contraction of orofacial muscles.[37] For example, case-control studies show that pressure pain thresholds at multiple sites, including the face, shoulder, and lower limb, are significantly decreased in people with TMD compared to controls.[94] CS has also been confirmed with temporal summation. Here, TMD patients not only reported increases in pain intensity during a series of mildly noxious mechanical stimuli, but also described aftersensations for up to a minute following the last stimulus.[95]

Psychological stress is also shown to play a significant role in TMD pain. Issues such as poor coping skills, occupational stress, and relationship problems are commonly reported by those with TMJ pain. In addition to stress-associated actions such as jaw clenching and teeth grinding, TMD patients also show a high comorbidity with other chronic pain syndromes such as chronic fatigue syndrome and fibromyalgia.[96] It is proposed that there is a clinical overlap between these conditions and that similar underlying mechanisms involving hypothalamic–pituitary–adrenal axis dysregulation directly influence central pain processing.[97] Stress also affects the sympathetic nervous system. Concerning TMDs, increased sympathetic activation affects masticatory muscles due to (1) vasoconstriction (decreased perfusion), (2) reduced contractile force leading to muscle fatigue,

(3) reduced proprioceptive input from muscle spindle afferent fibers causing decreases in the efficiency of complex motor actions such as chewing, and (4) increased nociceptive input.[87]

Clinical features

TMDs represent a broad group of complaints that involve masticatory muscles, the TMJ, and associated orofacial structures.[24] Symptoms of TMD include pain in masticatory muscles, decreased range of movement of the mandible, joint sounds related to TMJ function, and deviation in jaw opening.[19] Other symptoms such as neck pain, headache, periorbital pain, earache, tinnitus, and facial pain are also described by people presenting with TMDs. Patients most often complain of periauricular pain, especially when chewing, with pain radiating to the head. Pain of myofascial origin can be either unilateral or bilateral; however, pain of articular origin is usually unilateral, with the exception of pain in rheumatoid arthritis.[98] Pain is most typically aggravated by wide opening, chewing, and jaw clenching, while 'clicking' and 'popping' usually occur due to the interference of the disc that often results in reflex masticatory muscle spasm. The diagnostic criteria for TMDs are both extensive and controversial, and thus beyond the scope of this overview. The Research Diagnostic Criteria for TMDs is recommended as further reading.[99] However, concerning headaches caused by disorders involving the structure of the temporomandibular region please refer to the ICHD-3 criteria in Table 11.6.

Physical examination

In cases of chronic TMDs, the examination process should include a detailed case history and comprehensive physical examination. TMD pain is generally situated in the masseter muscles, pre-auricular area, and anterior temporalis muscle.[100] Physical examination must include the testing of active mandibular range of movement, TMJ, pain during masticatory and cervical muscle palpation, and inspection of articular joint sounds. Additionally, dental conditions are strongly associated with TMD as are occlusal problems such as overbite[101] and this therefore must be considered during patient reporting and examination. However,

Table 11.6: Headaches attributed to temporomandibular disorders according to the International Headache Society classification (ICHD-3)

	Description
A	Any headache fulfilling criterion C
B	Clinical and/or imaging evidence of a pathological process affecting the temporomandibular joint (TMJ), muscles of mastication and/or or associated structures

C	Evidence of causation demonstrated by at least two of the following:
	
	1. headache has developed in temporal relation to the onset of the temporomandibular disorder
	
	2. either or both of the following
	
	    a headache has significantly worsened in parallel with progression of the temporomandibular disorder
	
	    b headache has significantly improved or resolved in parallel with improvement in or resolution of the temporomandibular disorder
	
	3. the headache is produced or exacerbated by active jaw movements, passive movements through the range of motion of the jaw and/or provocative maneuvers applied to temporomandibular structures such as pressure on the TMJ and surrounding muscles of mastication
	
	4. headache, when unilateral, is ipsilateral to the side of the temporomandibular disorder

D	Not better accounted for by another ICHD-3 diagnosis

like many chronic pain conditions, most clinical findings from a TMD examination come from subjective reporting of pain and altered jaw movement in response to TMJ motion or muscle palpation. Thus, a multiaxial assessment is considered the most appropriate, as detailed in the Research Diagnostic Criteria for TMDs.[88]

Treatment

Chronic tension-type headache

Lifestyle and triggers

On the whole, CTTHs can be managed first by making a detailed analysis of trigger factors, as avoidance of these triggers may have a long-lasting effect on the reduction or elimination of symptoms.[102] For example, CTTHs are triggered by both mental and physical stress, high intake of caffeine products, dehydration, too little or too much sleep, and unsuitable forms of exercise.[103] Given that many patients fail to understand how it is possible to have headaches with

normal findings, patients are encouraged to keep a diary recording frequencies, severity, diet, daily pattern, and medications used. These are helpful for both the clinician and patient in eliciting possible risk factors and the amount of medication used. Additionally, information and reassurance about CTTHs are important; for example, an explanation of how neck and shoulder tension can cause muscle pain leading to alterations in central pain-modulatory systems can be valuable.[31] Furthermore, patients should also be made aware of the fact that if advice is taken, long-term relief is shown to be favorable.[104]

Physical therapy

Physical therapies are the most used non-pharmacological treatments for CTTHs, and they include manual therapy, postural advice, exercise, relaxation, and hot and cold packs.[102] Active treatments are shown to be of most benefit when compared to massage and relaxation techniques.[105] Of these active modalities, the craniocervical training program using low-load endurance exercises to train and regain muscle control of the cervicoscapular and craniocervical regions, in conjunction with other exercises, has been shown to reduce CTTH symptoms.[106] Although other treatments such as spinal manipulation, massage, and relaxation training have short-term benefits,[107] long-term improvements are not shown. However, findings from a recent systematic review show that several randomized controlled trials (RCTs) report manual therapies to be effective in the management of CTTH at six-month follow-up, similar to data from studies investigating treatment using tricyclic antidepressants.[108]

It is important to understand the impact of abnormal sensory features rather than biomechanical factors alone.[109] Thus, clinical management of people with CTTH must extend beyond local tissue dysfunction, with strategies directed towards reducing central and peripheral nervous system sensitivity being implemented. However, studies suggest that people with episodic CTTH, in which peripheral input is dominant, can benefit from manual therapy approaches such as myofascial trigger point work in the upper trapezius,[110] sternocleidomastoid, temporalis, suboccipital and extra-ocular muscles, in conjunction with exercises aimed at improving upper cervical flexor and extensor function.

Different needling therapies are used by manual therapists, the most common being acupuncture and dry needling. However, recent meta-analyses report no statistical difference between acupuncture and sham acupuncture.[111] The authors conclude that findings are affected by factors such as the type of acupuncture stimulation, needle retention, and treatment frequency. Thus, further studies are required to determine treatment parameters in order to ensure effective translation of RCT outcomes. Additionally, to date, there are no data relating to the effects compared to other treatments.

Psychological therapies

There are a large number of psychological approaches available for the treatment of CTTH. First, although methodological rigor is questionable in some studies, cognitive behavioral therapy (CBT) is shown to reduce the physical symptoms of CTTH.[112] EMG biofeedback training has also been investigated as a treatment for CTTH. However, although patients who complete these programs show decreases in frequency and severity of headaches, biofeedback is costly and time-consuming and provides no additional relief when, for example, compared to relaxation techniques.[113] Although evidence is not strong, it is likely, for example, that CBT is of most benefit to people in whom psychological distress plays a major role, whereas relaxation may be a preferred option for people who are anxious.

Pharmacological therapy

In most cases, simple analgesics such as aspirin can be useful. Nonsteroidal anti-inflammatories (NSAIDs) and acetaminophen (paracetamol) are effective as an acute treatment for episodes of CTTH and as such are the mainstay of acute treatment.[102] Indeed, most studies show that NSAIDs are more effective than aspirin or acetaminophen; however, this effectiveness is short-lived, with most patients reporting pain relief for less than two hours post treatment.[114,115] The effect of simple analgesics is enhanced when they are in combination with caffeine;[27] however, as with other combinations, Bendtsen suggests that no recommendations can be made due to the risk of medication overuse headache.[102] Acetaminophen is recommended as the drug of first choice due to the reduced chance of gastric side effects.[116] Preventative treatment must be considered in patients with more constant forms of CTTH. Here, the antidepressant amitriptyline is the only drug shown to be effective.[117] However, although studies investigating analgesic effects of amitriptyline indicate the inhibition of serotonin reuptake, other mechanisms such as norepinephrine reuptake inhibition, NMDA receptor antagonism, and the blockade of muscarinic receptors are also thought to be involved.[118]

Chronic migraine headaches

The treatment of chronic migraines can be divided into three approaches, these being lifestyle triggers, acute management, and preventative management.[119] Alterations in lifestyle and recognition of trigger factors aside, pharmacotherapeutic approaches are shown to be the most studied and the most effective. A detailed review of these approaches is beyond the scope of this chapter and thus the guidelines published by various institutions such as the National Institute for Health and Care Excellence and the American Headache Society are recommended.

Lifestyle, triggers, and education

Trigger factors for people with chronic migraine headaches are similar to those suffering CTTH, the most common being stress, abnormal eating times, fatigue, and lack of sleep.[47] However, trigger factors more particular to migraine include weather, smell, smoke, and depression.[119] As with CTTHs, correct management of these factors are important to not only minimize the frequency and severity of migraine but also to maximize the effect of additional migraine treatments (e.g., caffeine overuse). Here, failure to reduce risk factors will lessen the effectiveness of other preventative treatments;[20] thus, patient education is important in the management of migraine headaches. Several studies show that education has a significant impact, especially in reduction in pain intensity, improvement in levels of depression, and reduced reliance on medical services.[120]

Acute migraine pharmacotherapy

Due to concern about medication overuse, people with chronic migraine find it difficult to know when to take acute treatments.[119] Once risk factors have been identified, acute episodes should be treated early, starting with mild doses of simple analgesics such as aspirin and NSAIDs. If ineffective after maximum tolerated doses, then serotonin receptor agonists should be used.[121] Other pharmacological treatments include dihydroergotamine, a drug thought to be an agonist to several neurotransmitters such as serotonin, dopamine, and epinephrine,[122] and anti-emetic dopamine antagonists such as metoclopramide, which both treats migraine associated nausea and relieves gastric stasis, increasing the absorption of other analgesics.[123]

Preventative pharmacotherapy

Preventative treatment in chronic migraine is used to reduce the frequency, duration, and/or severity of attacks.[124] Most preventative pharmacotherapies are designed to increase antinociception, inhibit cortical spreading depression (antidepressants, calcium channel blockers), decrease or inhibit peripheral and/or CS (anticonvulsants/NSAIDs), modulate autonomic function (beta-blockers) and downregulate serotonin receptors (antidepressants).[124] Although anticonvulsants are shown to be most effective as a first-line preventative, others suggest beta-blockers and antidepressants. Additionally, the renin–angiotensin system has recently been implicated in the pathophysiology of migraine.[125] Here, angiotensin II modulates cerebrovascular blood flow while also having an effect on homeostasis and autonomic function and activating neuroinflammatory transmitters.[126] Thus, recent studies show that ACE inhibitors (lisinopril) and angiotensin II receptor antagonists (candesartan) are effective in reducing the frequency and severity of migraine attacks with minimal side effects.[127]

Physical therapy

Not all patients tolerate acute or preventative medication owing to undesirable side effects, contraindications due to comorbidities such as myocardial dysfunction and asthma, or for other reasons.[108] There are a number of physical therapy approaches such as massage, myofascial release, exercise, and manipulative techniques often used for primary headaches, among them migraines. However, although evidence is encouraging, the overall rigor of RCTs used investigate the effects of these treatments on people with migraine is poor. For example, in an American study using massage therapy, although pain intensity was shown to be reduced by up to 71% compared to controls, data were difficult to interpret as results on migraine frequency and duration were missing.[128] However, in a large single cohort study using physical therapy and relaxation, only 14% of subjects reported reductions in migraine severity using physical therapy alone, compared to 40% with both modalities.[129]

Several chiropractic studies show spinal manipulative techniques to be useful in reducing the frequency of migraine headaches by approximately 50% in follow-up consultations up to 20 months after the first treatment.[130,131] More recently, in a three-armed RCT, osteopathic manipulative treatments (OMT) (and medication), including myofascial release and balanced ligamentous tension techniques, were compared to sham and medication (sham group) and medication only (control group).[132] Results showed that the OMT and medication group demonstrated significant reductions in both pain and disability as well as the use of medication. However, although OMT is shown to be a valid treatment, as with previous studies, practitioners were not blinded from group allocation while comorbidities and related treatments were not verified with their physicians. Additionally, medication treatments were directed by their physicians and thus not described in the methodology, and thus, it cannot be clear if improvements in symptoms are related to OMT or are influenced by changes in doses in drug intake.

A recent Cochrane review investigating the use of acupuncture in preventing migraine attacks located 22 studies with 4985 subjects. Overall results suggest that acupuncture reduces the frequency of headaches compared to sham acupuncture. However, although this mode of treatment should be considered as a treatment option, there are no follow-up studies (> one year) available.[133]

Trigeminal autonomic cephalalgias (cluster headaches)

The management of cluster headaches is divided into acute, intermediate, and preventative treatments that all rely on either pharmacotherapy or neuromodulation.[134] However, because cluster headaches have such a rapid onset, most efficacious acute treatments involve parenteral or pulmonary administration of oxygen and serotonin receptor agonists, somatostatin (octreotide) and lidocaine.[135]

The aim of preventative treatment with cluster headaches is to provoke a fast suppression of attacks and maintain remission with minimal side effects. In the short term, corticosteroids (prednisolone) are highly effective and the most rapidly acting, however, they should be limited to no more than three weeks due side effects.[136] Another drug used in the short term is a serotonin receptor antagonist (methysergide), and this is shown to be ideal for people with short cluster bursts of less than five months in duration.[136]

Concerning long-term treatment of cluster headaches, the calcium channel blocker verapamil is the most effective.[137] However, due to its action, verapamil is contraindicated in people with cardiac conduction problems. Lithium is also used as a long-term preventative; however, related use of NSAIDs and diuretics is contraindicated as they can increase the toxicity of lithium.[138] More radical long-term interventions include radiofrequency blockade of the sphenopalatine ganglion, trigeminal nerve section, occipital nerve stimulation,[139] and deep-brain stimulation of the hypothalamic region.[140] To date, there have been no studies investigating the use of physical therapies on TACs.

Temporomandibular disorders

Like many other chronic pain disorders, there is little high level evidence for physical therapy approaches to TMDs. However, this does not mean manual therapists are without guidance for management of TMDs. Results from several systematic reviews are mixed and all show a high risk of selection bias and low sample numbers. However, while reviews suggest several forms of physical treatment are effective,[141] there are no high-quality evidence data available. The following sections briefly review the above treatment modalities.

Physical therapies

The above reviews generally show that active exercises and manual therapy, alone or in combination, are effective in increasing jaw opening and decreasing pain in people with TMDs due to conditions such as chronic myofascial dysfunction, arthritis, and disk displacement.[142] Manual therapy here includes intra- and extraoral joint mobilization techniques using distraction, anterior glide, and medial-lateral glide forces.[143] Additionally, active and passive stretching of craniomandiubular muscles such as temporalis, in combination with self-care, is also shown to be effective versus waiting list controls and botulinum toxin injection.[144,145] Postural exercises and advice are also recommended to maintain and further optimize jaw opening and correct orientation of the craniomandiubular system. Concerning exercise, stretches addressing cervical and thoracic cage musculature appear to be most beneficial,[146] while postural advice relates to awareness of slouching and sleeping postures.[147]

Acupuncture is increasingly being used to treat TMDs. However, results show that although acupuncture decreases temporomandibular pain compared to no treatment, there are no differences in effect versus sham acupuncture[148] and occlusal splint therapy.[149] Similar findings are shown with electrophysical modalities. However, although radiofrequency energy, TENS, and biofeedback treatments show little benefit in reduction of pain, results are encouraging concerning increased jaw opening and lateral deviation range of motion.[150]

Psychological therapies

Few psychological therapies have been investigated for the treatment of TMDs. Of the ones that have, CBT and relaxation have been most studied. Meta-analysis shows that although psychological interventions showed more long-term improvement in self-reported pain and mood compared to usual treatment (physical therapies), there are greater improvements in psychological outcomes with psychological interventions and increases in physical function with physical treatments.[151] Thus, it is accepted that there is a relationship between levels of psychological dysfunction and the effectiveness of physical treatments. Those with greatest psychological impairment respond best to multimodal therapies while patients without significant psychological impairment respond to interventions such as self-care and manual therapy.[151]

Summary

Recent updates in the classification of primary headaches together with further understanding of pathophysiological mechanisms have contributed to the development of new and improved pharmacological, physical, and psychological treatments. However, due to poor methodology, small sample sizes, and sampling bias, evidence is lacking and provides only modest support for physical therapy modalities for all types of primary headache. Further studies are required to examine the efficacy of these treatments in the reduction of headache severity, frequency, duration, and perceived disability. That being said, methodological design prevents physical therapy studies from competing with the gold standard in pharmacological RCTs. Here, for example, finding placebo treatments that are similar to most physical therapies is challenging and often control or placebo treatments are too similar, or investigators cannot be blinded during the intervention. As with most chronic pain disorders, there is an absence of clear evidence of effect for the treatment of primary headaches, and thus physical treatments are probably more effective when used as part of a multidisciplinary approach.

References

1. Manzoni GC, Torelli P. Epidemiology of typical and atypical craniofacial neuralgias. Neurological Sciences. 2005;26(2):s65–s7.

2. Howlett W. Headache and Facial Pain. In: Howlett W, editor. Neurology in Africa. Bergan: Bergan Open Research; 2012.

3. Shimizu T, Suzuki N. Chapter 3 – Biological sciences related to headache. In: Michael J. Aminoff FB, Dick FS, editors. Handbook of Clinical Neurology. Volume 97: Elsevier; 2010. p. 35–45.

4. International Headache Society. IHS Classification ICHD-3 Beta United Kingdom: Sage Publications Ltd; 2016

5. Waldie K, Buckley J, Bull P, Poulton R. Tension Headache: A Life-Course Review. Journal of Headache and Pain Management. 2015;1(1):1-9.

6. Robbins MS, Lipton RB. The epidemiology of primary headache disorders. Seminars in Neurology. 2010;30(2):107–19.

7. Ferrante T, Manzoni GC, Russo M, Camarda C, Taga A, Veronesi L, et al. Prevalence of tension-type headache in adult general population: the PACE study and review of the literature. Neurological Sciences. 2013;34(1):137–8.

8. Ertas M, Baykan B, Kocasoy Orhan E, Zarifoglu M, Karli N, Saip S, et al. One-year prevalence and the impact of migraine and tension-type headache in Turkey: a nationwide home-based study in adults. The Journal of Headache and Pain. 2012;13(2):147–57.

9. Rasmussen BK, Jensen R, Schroll M, Olesen J. Epidemiology of headache in a general population—A prevalence study. Journal of Clinical Epidemiology. 1991;44(11):1147–57.

10. Schwartz BS, Stewart WF, Simon D, Lipton RB. Epidemiology of tension-type headache. JAMA. 1998;279(5):381–3.

11. Manack A, Buse DC, Serrano D, Turkel CC, Lipton RB. Rates, predictors, and consequences of remission from chronic migraine to episodic migraine. Neurology. 2011;76(8):711–8.

12. Lipton RB, Stewart WF, Diamond S, Diamond ML, Reed M. Prevalence and Burden of Migraine in the United States: Data From the American Migraine Study II. Headache: The Journal of Head and Face Pain. 2001;41(7):646–57.

13. Stewart WF, Lipton RB, Simon D, Liberman J, Von Korff M. Validity of an illness severity measure for headache in a population sample of migraine sufferers. Pain. 1999;79(2–3):291–301.

14. Blumenfeld AM, Varon SF, Wilcox TK, Buse DC, Kawata AK, Manack A, et al. Disability, HRQoL and resource use among chronic and episodic migraineurs: results from the International Burden of Migraine Study (IBMS). Cephalalgia: An International Journal of Headache. 2011;31(3):301–15.

15. Scher AI, Terwindt GM, Picavet HS, Verschuren WM, Ferrari MD, Launer LJ. Cardiovascular risk factors and migraine: the GEM population-based study. Neurology. 2005;64(4):614–20.

16. Turner-Bowker DM, Bayliss MS, Ware JE, Kosinski M. Usefulness of the SF-8™ Health Survey for comparing the impact of migraine and other conditions. Quality of Life Research. 2003;12(8):1003–12.

17. Balasubramaniam R, Klasser GD, Delcanho R. Trigeminal autonomic cephalalgias. The Journal of the American Dental Association. 139(12):1616–24.

18. Fischera M, Marziniak M, Gralow I, Evers S. The incidence and prevalence of cluster headache: a meta-analysis of population-based studies. Cephalalgia: An International Journal of Headache. 2008;28(6):614–8.

19. Wadhwa S, Kapila S. TMJ disorders: future innovations in diagnostics and therapeutics. Journal of Dental Education. 2008;72(8):930–47.

20. Lipton J, Ship J, Larach-Robinson D. Estimated Prevalence and Distribution of Reported Orofacial Pain in the United States. The Journal of the American Dental Association. 1993;124(10):115–21.

21. LeResche L. Epidemiology of temporomandibular disorders: implications for the investigation of etiologic factors. Critical Reviews in Oral Biology and Medicine. 1997;8(3):291–305.

22. Mottaghi A, Zamani E. Temporomandibular joint health status in war veterans with post-traumatic stress disorder. Journal of Education and Health Promotion. 2014;3:60.

23. Afari N, Wen Y, Buchwald D, Goldberg J, Plesh O. Are post-traumatic stress disorder symptoms and temporomandibular pain associated? A twin study. Journal of Orofacial Pain. 2008;22(1):41–9.

24. Jang J-Y, Kwon J-S, Lee DH, Bae J-H, Kim ST. Clinical signs and subjective symptoms of temporomandibular disorders in instrumentalists. Yonsei Medical Journal. 2016;57(6):1500–7.

25. Foxman I, Burgel BJ. Musician health and safety: preventing playing-related musculoskeletal disorders. AAOHN Journal. 2006;54(7):309–16.

26. Ashina S, Bendtsen L, Ashina M. Pathophysiology of tension-type headache. Current Pain and Headache Reports. 2005;9(6):415–22.

27. Ashina S, Ashina M. Current and potential future drug therapies for tension-type headache. Current Pain and Headache Reports. 2003;7(6):466–74.

28. Bendtsen L, Fernández-de-la-Peñas C. The role of muscles in tension-type headache. Current Pain and Headache Reports. 2011;15(6):451–8.

29. Fernández-de-las-Peñas C, Ge H-Y, Alonso-Blanco C, González-Iglesias J, Arendt-Nielsen L. Referred pain areas of active myofascial trigger points in head, neck, and shoulder muscles, in chronic tension type headache. Journal of Bodywork and Movement Therapies. 2011;14(4):391–6.

30. Ashina S, Bendtsen L, Ashina M. Pathophysiology of migraine and tension-type headache. Techniques in Regional Anesthesia & Pain Management. 2012;16(1):14–8.

31. Bendtsen L. Central sensitization in tension-type headache – possible pathophysiological mechanisms. Cephalalgia: An International Journal of Headache. 2000;20(5):486–508.

32. Holroyd KA, Stensland M, Lipchik GL, Hill KR, O'Donnell FS, Cordingley G. Psychosocial correlates and impact of chronic tension-type headaches. Headache. 2000;40(1):3–16.

33. Holroyd KA. Behavioral and psychologic aspects of the pathophysiology and management of tension-type headache. Current Pain and Headache Reports. 2002;6(5):401–7.

34. Gobel H, Weigle L, Kropp P, Soyka D. Pain sensitivity and pain reactivity of pericranial muscles in migraine and tension-type headache. Cephalalgia: An International Journal of Headache. 1992;12(3):142–51.

35. Jensen R. Peripheral and central mechanisms in tension-type headache: an update. Cephalalgia: An International Journal of Headache. 2003;23 Suppl 1:49–52.

36. Fernandez-de-las-Penas C, Schoenen J. Chronic tension-type headache: what is new? Current Opinion in Neurology. 2009;22(3):254–61.

37. Woolf CJ. Central sensitization: Implications for the diagnosis and treatment of pain. Pain. 2011;152(3 Suppl):S2–15.

38. Cathcart S, Winefield AH, Lushington K, Rolan P. Stress and tension-type headache mechanisms. Cephalalgia: An International Journal of Headache. 2010;30(10):1250–67.

39. Sandrini G, Rossi P, Milanov I, Serrao M, Cecchini AP, Nappi G. Abnormal modulatory influence of diffuse noxious inhibitory controls in migraine and chronic tension-type headache patients. Cephalalgia: An International Journal of Headache. 2006;26(7):782–9.

40. Biurrun Manresa JA, Fritsche R, Vuilleumier PH, Oehler C, Mørch CD, Arendt-Nielsen L, et al. Is the conditioned pain modulation paradigm reliable? A test-retest assessment using the nociceptive withdrawal reflex. PLOS ONE. 2014;9(6):e100241.

41. Jensen R. Mechanisms of tension-type headache. Cephalalgia: An International Journal of Headache. 2001;21(7):786–9.

42. Ashina M, Bendtsen L, Jensen R, Lassen LH, Sakai F, Olesen J. Possible mechanisms of action of nitric oxide synthase inhibitors in chronic tension-type headache. Brain: A Journal of Neurology. 1999;122(9):1629.

43. Ashina M, Bendtsen L, Jensen R, Olesen J. Nitric oxide-induced headache in patients with chronic tension-type headache. Brain: A Journal of Neurology. 2000;123(9):1830.

44. Chowdhury D. Tension type headache. Annals of Indian Academy of Neurology. 2012;15(Suppl 1):S83–S8.

45. Millea PJ, Brodie JJ. Tension-type headache. American Family Physician. 2002;66(5):797–804.

46. Ulrich V, Gervil M, Kyvik KO, Olesen J, Russell MB. The inheritance of migraine with aura estimated by means of structural equation modelling. Journal of Medical Genetics. 1999;36(3):225–7.

47. Spierings EL, Ranke AH, Honkoop PC. Precipitating and aggravating factors of migraine versus tension-type headache. Headache. 2001;41(6):554–8.

48. Song T-J, Cho S-J, Kim W-J, Yang KI, Yun C-H, Chu MK. Anxiety and depression in tension-type headache: a population-based study. PLOS ONE. 2016;11(10):e0165316.

49. Bera S, Khandelwal S, Sood M, Goyal V. A comparative study of psychiatric comorbidity, quality of life and disability in patients with migraine and tension type headache. Neurology India. 2014;62:516–20.

50. Rains JC, Davis RE, Smitherman TA. Tension-type headache and sleep. Current Neurology and Neuroscience Reports. 2014;15(2):520.

51. Caspersen N, Hirsvang JR, Kroell L, Jadidi F, Baad-Hansen L, Svensson P, et al. Is there a relation between tension-type headache, temporomandibular disorders and sleep? Pain Research and Treatment. 2013;2013:6.

52. de Tommaso M, Sardaro M, Serpino C, Costantini F, Vecchio E, Prudenzano MP, et al. Fibromyalgia comorbidity in primary headaches. Cephalalgia: An International Journal of Headache. 2009;29(4):453–64.

53. Blanda. M. Tension Headache. In: Pritchard-Taylor J, editor. Medscape neurology. New York: Medscape; 2016.

54. Goadsby PJ, Charbit AR, Andreou AP, Akerman S, Holland PR. Neurobiology of migraine. Neuroscience. 2009;161(2):327–41.

55. Sprenger T, Borsook D. Migraine changes the brain – neuroimaging imaging makes its mark. Current Opinion in Neurology. 2012;25(3):252–62.

56. Goadsby PJ. Pathophysiology of migraine. Annals of Indian Academy of Neurology. 2012;15(Suppl 1):S15–S22.

57. Charles AC, Baca SM. Cortical spreading depression and migraine. Nature Reviews. Neurology. 2013;9(11):637–44.

58. Lauritzen M. Pathophysiology of the migraine aura. The spreading depression theory. Brain: A Journal of Neurology. 1994;117 (Pt 1):199–210.

59. Gardner-Medwin AR, van Bruggen N, Williams SR, Ahier RG. Magnetic resonance imaging of propagating waves of spreading depression in the anaesthetised rat. Journal of Cerebral Blood Flow and Metabolism. 1994;14(1):7–11.

60. Aurora SK, Nagesh V. Pathophysiology of migraine. Handbook of Clinical Neurology. 2010;97:267–73.

61. Markowitz S, Saito K, Moskowitz MA. Neurogenically mediated leakage of plasma protein occurs from blood vessels in dura mater but not brain. The Journal of Neuroscience. 1987;7(12):4129.

62. Aurora SK, Barrodale PM, Tipton RL, Khodavirdi A. Brainstem dysfunction in chronic migraine as evidenced by neurophysiological and positron emission tomography studies*. Headache: The Journal of Head and Face Pain. 2007;47(7):996–1003.

63. Welch KMA, Nagesh V, Aurora SK, Gelman N. Periaqueductal gray matter dysfunction in migraine and chronic daily headache may be due to free radical damage. The Journal of Headache and Pain. 2001;2(Suppl 1):S33–s41.

64. Holland PR, Afridi S. Migraine pathophysiology. Advances in Clinical Neuroscience & Rehabilitation: ACNR 2014;14.

65. Bahra A, Matharu MS, Buchel C, Frackowiak RSJ, Goadsby PJ. Brainstem activation specific to migraine headache. Lancet. 2001;357(9261):1016–7.

66. Ulrich-Lai YM, Herman JP. Neural regulation of endocrine and autonomic stress responses. Nature Reviews. Neuroscience. 2009;10(6):397–409.

67. Kunkel RS. Clinical manifestations of migraine. Clinical Cornerstone. 2001;4(3):18–25.

68. Kelman L. The aura: a tertiary care study of 952 migraine patients. Cephalalgia: An International Journal of Headache. 2004;24(9):728–34.

69. Eriksen MK, Thomsen LL, Olesen J. The visual aura rating scale (VARS) for migraine aura diagnosis. Cephalalgia: An International Journal of Headache. 2005;25(10):801–10.

70. Cutrer FM, Huerter K. Migraine aura. Neurologist. 2007;13(3):118–25.

71. Calhoun AH, Ford S, Millen C, Finkel AG, Truong Y, Nie Y. The prevalence of neck pain in migraine. Headache: The Journal of Head and Face Pain. 2010;50(8):1273–7.

72. Lipton RB, Hamelsky SW, Dayno JM. What do patients with migraine want from acute migraine treatment? Headache. 2002;42 Suppl 1:3–9.

73. Pryse-Phillips W. Evaluating migraine disability: the headache impact test instrument in context. The Canadian Journal of Neurological Science. 2002;29 Suppl 2:S11–5.

74. Goadsby PJ, Lipton RB, Ferrari MD. Migraine – current understanding and treatment. The New England Journal of Medicine. 2002;346(4):257–70.

75. Benoliel R. Trigeminal autonomic cephalgias. British Journal of Pain. 2012;6(3):106–23.

76. Leone M, Bussone G. Pathophysiology of trigeminal autonomic cephalalgias. Lancet Neurology. 8(8):755–64.

77. May A, Goadsby PJ. The trigeminovascular system in humans: pathophysiologic implications for primary headache syndromes of the neural influences on the cerebral circulation. Journal of Cerebral Blood Flow & Metabolism. 1999;19(2):115–27.

78. Eller M, Goadsby PJ. Trigeminal autonomic cephalalgias. Oral Diseases. 2016;22(1):1–8.

79. Knight Y. Brainstem modulation of caudal trigeminal nucleus: a model for understanding migraine biology and future drug targets. Headache Currents. 2005;2(5):108–18.

80. Holle D, Katsarava Z, Obermann M. The hypothalamus: specific or nonspecific role in the pathophysiology of trigeminal autonomic cephalalgias? Current Pain and Headache Reports. 2011;15(2):101–7.

81. Pringsheim T. Cluster headache: evidence for a disorder of circadian rhythm and hypothalamic function. The Canadian Journal of Neurological Sciences. 2002;29(1):33–40.

82. Leone M, Bussone G. A review of hormonal findings in cluster headache. Evidence for hypothalamic involvement. Cephalalgia: An International Journal of Headache. 1993;13(5):309–17.

83. Bartsch T, Levy MJ, Knight YE, Goadsby PJ. Differential modulation of nociceptive dural input to [hypocretin] orexin A and B receptor activation in the posterior hypothalamic area. Pain. 2004;109(3):367–78.

84. Leone M, Franzini A, Cecchini AP, Broggi G, Bussone G. Hypothalamic deep brain stimulation in the treatment of chronic cluster headache. Therapeutic Advances in Neurological Disorders. 2010;3(3):187–95.

85. Bahra A, May A, Goadsby PJ. Cluster headache: A prospective clinical study with diagnostic implications. Neurology. 2002;58(3):354–61.

86. Waldman SD. Targeted headache history. Medical Clinics. 97(2):185–95.

87. Cairns BE. Pathophysiology of TMD pain – basic mechanisms and their implications for pharmacotherapy. Journal of Oral Rehabilitation. 2010;37(6):391–410.

88. Dworkin SF, LeResche L. Research diagnostic criteria for temporomandibular disorders: review, criteria, examinations and specifications, critique. Journal of Craniomandibular Disorders: Facial & Oral Pain. 1992;6(4):301–55.

89. Wang XD, Zhang JN, Gan YH, Zhou YH. Current understanding of pathogenesis and treatment of TMJ osteoarthritis. Journal of Dental Research. 2015;94(5):666–73.

90. Furquim BDA, Flamengui LMSP, Conti PCR. TMD and chronic pain: a current view. Dental Press Journal of Orthodontics. 2015;20(1):127–33.

91. Cairns BE, Sessle BJ, Hu JW. Characteristics of glutamate-evoked temporomandibular joint afferent activity in the rat. Journal of Neurophysiology. 2001;85(6):2446.

92. Costa AL, D'Abreu A, Cendes F. Temporomandibular joint internal derangement: association with headache, joint effusion, bruxism, and joint pain. The Journal of Contemporary Dental Practice. 2008;9(6):9–16.

93. Wang K, Arendt-Nielsen L, Jensen T, Svensson P. Reduction of clinical temporomandibular joint pain is associated with a reduction of the jaw-stretch reflex. Journal of Orofacial Pain. 2004;18(1):33–40.

94. Fernandez-de-las-Penas C, de la Llave-Rincon AI, Fernandez-Carnero J, Cuadrado ML, Arendt-Nielsen L, Pareja JA. Bilateral widespread mechanical

pain sensitivity in carpal tunnel syndrome: evidence of central processing in unilateral neuropathy. Brain: A Journal of Neurology. 2009;132(Pt 6):1472–9.

95. Sarlani E, Grace EG, Reynolds MA, Greenspan JD. Evidence for up-regulated central nociceptive processing in patients with masticatory myofascial pain. Journal of Orofacial Pain. 2004;18(1):41–55.

96. Korszun A, Papadopoulos E, Demitrack M, Engleberg C, Crofford L. The relationship between temporomandibular disorders and stress-associated syndromes. Oral Surgery, Oral Medicine, Oral Pathology, Oral Radiology, and Endodontology. 1998;86(4):416–20.

97. Lambert CA, Sanders A, Wilder RS, Slade GD, Van Uum S, Russell E, et al. Chronic HPA axis response to stress in temporomandibular disorder. Journal of Dental Hygiene: JDH/American Dental Hygienists' Association. 2013;87(2):73–81.

98. Ardic F, Gokharman D, Atsu S, Guner S, Yilmaz M, Yorgancioglu R. The comprehensive evaluation of temporomandibular disorders seen in rheumatoid arthritis. Australian Dental Journal. 2006;51(1):23–8.

99. Schiffman E, Ohrbach R, Truelove E, Look J, Anderson G, Goulet J-P, et al. Diagnostic Criteria for Temporomandibular Disorders (DC/TMD) for clinical and research applications: recommendations of the International RDC/TMD Consortium Network() and Orofacial Pain Special Interest Group(). Journal of Oral & Facial Pain and Headache. 2014;28(1):6–27.

100. Wright EF, North SL. Management and treatment of temporomandibular disorders: a clinical perspective. The Journal of Manual & Manipulative Therapy. 2009;17(4):247–54.

101. Conti ACdCF, Oltramari PVP, Navarro RdL, de Almeida MR. Examination of temporomandibular disorders in the orthodontic patient: a clinical guide. Journal of Applied Oral Science. 2007;15(1):77–82.

102. Bendtsen L, Jensen R. Tension-type headache. Neurologic Clinics. 2009;27(2):525–35.

103. Ulrich V, Russell MB, Jensen R, Olesen J. A comparison of tension-type headache in migraineurs and in non-migraineurs: a population-based study. Pain. 1996;67(2–3):501–6.

104. Lyngberg AC, Rasmussen BK, Jorgensen T, Jensen R. Prognosis of migraine and tension-type headache: a population-based follow-up study. Neurology. 2005;65(4):580–5.

105. Torelli P, Jensen R, Olesen J. Physiotherapy for tension-type headache: a controlled study. Cephalalgia: An International Journal of Headache. 2004;24(1):29–36.

106. van Ettekoven H, Lucas C. Efficacy of physiotherapy including a craniocervical training programme for tension-type headache; a randomized clinical trial. Cephalalgia: An International Journal of Headache. 2006;26(8):983–91.

107. Bronfort G, Assendelft WJ, Evans R, Haas M, Bouter L. Efficacy of spinal manipulation for chronic headache: a systematic review. Journal of Manipulative and Physiological Therapeutics. 2001;24(7):457–66.

108. Chaibi A, Russell MB. Manual therapies for primary chronic headaches: a systematic review of randomized controlled trials. The Journal of Headache and Pain. 2014;15(1):67–.

109. Fernández-de-las-Peñas C, Courtney CA. Clinical reasoning for manual therapy management of tension type and cervicogenic headache. The Journal of Manual & Manipulative Therapy. 2014;22(1):44–50.

110. Fernandez-de-Las-Penas C, Alonso-Blanco C, Cuadrado ML, Miangolarra JC, Barriga FJ, Pareja JA. Are manual therapies effective in reducing pain from tension-type headache?: a systematic review. The Clinical Journal of Pain. 2006;22(3):278–85.

111. Hao XA, Xue CC, Dong L, Zheng Z. Factors associated with conflicting

findings on acupuncture for tension-type headache: qualitative and quantitative analyses. Journal of Alternative and Complementary Medicine (New York, NY). 2013;19(4):285–97.

112. Harris P, Loveman E, Clegg A, Easton S, Berry N. Systematic review of cognitive behavioural therapy for the management of headaches and migraines in adults. British Journal of Pain. 2015;9(4):213–24.

113. Mullally WJ, Hall K, Goldstein R. Efficacy of biofeedback in the treatment of migraine and tension type headaches. Pain Physician. 2009;12(6):1005–11.

114. Prior MJ, Cooper KM, May LG, Bowen DL. Efficacy and safety of acetaminophen and naproxen in the treatment of tension-type headache. A randomized, double-blind, placebo-controlled trial. Cephalalgia: An International Journal of Headache. 2002;22(9):740–8.

115. Stephens G, Derry S, Moore RA. Paracetamol (acetaminophen) for acute treatment of episodic tension-type headache in adults. Cochrane Database of Systematic Reviews. 2016;(6): CD011889.

116. Langman MJS, Weil J, Wainwright P, Lawson DH, Rawlins MD, Logan RFA, et al. Risks of bleeding peptic ulcer associated with individual non-steroidal anti-inflammatory drugs. Lancet. 1994;343(8905):1075–8.

117. Bendtsen L, Mathew N. Prophylactic pharmacotherapy of tension-type headache. In: Olesen J, Goadsby PJ, Ramadan N, Tfelt-Hansen PC, Welsh K, editors. The Headaches. Philadelphia: Lippincot Williams Wilkins; 2005. p. 735–46.

118. Ashina S, Bendtsen L, Jensen R. Analgesic effect of amitriptyline in chronic tension-type headache is not directly related to serotonin reuptake inhibition. Pain. 2004;108(1–2):108–14.

119. Weatherall MW. The diagnosis and treatment of chronic migraine. Therapeutic Advances in Chronic Disease. 2015;6(3):115–23.

120. Andrasik F, Buse DC, Grazzi L. Behavioral medicine for migraine and medication overuse headache. Current Pain and Headache Reports. 2009;13(3):241–8.

121. Ferrari MD, Roon KI, Lipton RB, Goadsby PJ. Oral triptans (serotonin 5-HT(1B/1D) agonists) in acute migraine treatment: a meta-analysis of 53 trials. Lancet (London, England). 2001;358(9294):1668–75.

122. Colman I, Brown MD, Innes GD, Grafstein E, Roberts TE, Rowe BH. Parenteral dihydroergotamine for acute migraine headache: a systematic review of the literature. Annals of Emergency Medicine. 2005;45(4):393–401.

123. Colman I, Brown MD, Innes GD, Grafstein E, Roberts TE, Rowe BH. Parenteral metoclopramide for acute migraine: meta-analysis of randomised controlled trials. BMJ (Clinical research ed). 2004;329(7479):1369–73.

124. Silberstein SD. Preventive migraine treatment. Neurologic Clinics. 2009;27(2):429–43.

125. Tronvik E, Stovner LJ, Schrader H, Bovim G. Involvement of the renin-angiotensin system in migraine. Journal of Hypertension Supplement. 2006;24(1):S139–43.

126. Reuter U, Chiarugi A, Bolay H, Moskowitz MA. Nuclear factor-kappaB as a molecular target for migraine therapy. Annals of Neurology. 2002;51(4):507–16.

127. Nandha R, Singh H. Renin angiotensin system: a novel target for migraine prophylaxis. Indian Journal of Pharmacology. 2012;44(2):157–60.

128. Hernandez-reif M, Dieter J, Field T, Swerdlow B, Diego M. Migraine headaches are reduced by massage therapy. International Journal of Neuroscience. 1998;96(1–2):1–11.

129. Marcus DA, Scharff L, Mercer S, Turk DC. Nonpharmacological treatment for migraine: incremental utility of physical therapy with relaxation and thermal biofeedback. Cephalalgia: An International Journal of Headache. 1998;18(5):266–72; discussion 42.

130. Parker GB, Tupling H, Pryor DS. A controlled trial of cervical manipulation of migraine. Australian and New Zealand Journal of Medicine. 1978;8(6):589–93.

131. Nelson CF, Bronfort G, Evans R, Boline P, Goldsmith C, Anderson AV. The efficacy of spinal manipulation, amitriptyline and the combination of both therapies for the prophylaxis of migraine headache. Journal of Manipulative and Physiological Therapeutics. 1998;21(8):511–9.

132. Cerritelli F, Pizzolorusso G, Renzetti C, Cozzolino V, D'Orazio M, Lupacchini M, et al. A multicenter, randomized, controlled trial of osteopathic manipulative treatment on preterms. PLoS ONE. 2015;10(5):e0127370.

133. Linde K, Allais G, Brinkhaus B, Fei Y, Mehring M, Vertosick EA, et al. Acupuncture for the prevention of episodic migraine. The Cochrane Database of Systematic Reviews. 2016;(6):Cd001218.

134. Tfelt-Hansen PC, Jensen RH. Management of cluster headache. CNS drugs. 2012;26(7):571–80.

135. Cohen AS, Burns B, Goadsby PJ. High-flow oxygen for treatment of cluster headache: a randomized trial. JAMA. 2009;302(22):2451–7.

136. Cohen AS, Goadsby PJ. Prevention and treatment of cluster headache. Progress in Neurology and Psychiatry. 2009;13(3):9–16.

137. Blau JN, Engel HO. Individualizing treatment with verapamil for cluster headache patients. Headache. 2004;44(10):1013–8.

138. Gooriah R, Buture A, Ahmed F. Evidence-based treatments for cluster headache. Therapeutics and Clinical Risk Management. 2015;11:1687–96.

139. Schwedt TJ, Dodick DW, Trentman TL, Zimmerman RS. Occipital nerve stimulation for chronic cluster headache and hemicrania continua: pain relief and persistence of autonomic features. Cephalalgia: An International Journal of Headache. 2006;26(8):1025–7.

140. May A, Leone M, Boecker H, Sprenger T, Juergens T, Bussone G, et al. Hypothalamic deep brain stimulation in positron emission tomography. The Journal of Neuroscience. 2006;26(13):3589–93.

141. Randhawa K, Bohay R, Cote P, van der Velde G, Sutton D, Wong JJ, et al. The effectiveness of noninvasive interventions for temporomandibular disorders: a systematic review by the Ontario Protocol for Traffic Injury Management (OPTIMa) Collaboration. The Clinical Journal of Pain. 2016;32(3):260–78.

142. Medlicott MS, Harris SR. A systematic review of the effectiveness of exercise, manual therapy, electrotherapy, relaxation training, and biofeedback in the management of temporomandibular disorder. Physical Therapy. 2006;86(7):955–73.

143. Shaffer SM, Brismée J-M, Sizer PS, Courtney CA. Temporomandibular disorders. Part 2: conservative management. The Journal of Manual & Manipulative Therapy. 2014;22(1):13–23.

144. Fricton JR. Etiology and management of masticatory myofascial pain. Journal of Musculoskeletal Pain. 1999;7(1–2):143–60.

145. Guarda-Nardini L, Stecco A, Stecco C, Masiero S, Manfredini D. Myofascial pain of the jaw muscles: comparison of short-term effectiveness of botulinum toxin injections and fascial manipulation technique. CRANIO®. 2012;30(2):95–102.

146. Wright EF, Domenech MA, Fischer Jr JR. Usefulness of posture training for patients with temporomandibular disorders. The Journal of the American Dental Association. 2000;131(2):202–10.

147. Komiyama O, Kawara M, Arai M, Asano T, Kobayashi K. Posture correction as part of behavioural therapy in treatment of myofascial pain with limited opening. Journal of Oral Rehabilitation. 1999;26(5):428–35.

148. Goddard G, Karibe H, McNeill C, Villafuerte E. Acupuncture and sham acupuncture reduce muscle pain in myofascial pain patients. Journal of Orofacial Pain. 2002;16(1):71–6.

149. List T, Helkimo M, Karlsson R. Pressure pain thresholds in patients with craniomandibular disorders before and after treatment with acupuncture and occlusal splint therapy: a controlled clinical study. Journal of Orofacial Pain. 1993;7(3):275–82.

150. McNeely ML, Armijo Olivo S, Magee DJ. A systematic review of the effectiveness of physical therapy interventions for temporomandibular disorders. Physical Therapy. 2006;86(5):710–25.

151. Roldan-Barraza C, Janko S, Villanueva J, Araya I, Lauer HC. A systematic review and meta-analysis of usual treatment versus psychosocial interventions in the treatment of myofascial temporomandibular disorder pain. Journal of Oral & Facial Pain and Headache. 2014;28(3):205–22.

Introduction

By 2050, around 25% of the general population will be 65 years of age or older, and this age group is currently considered the fastest growing population.[1] For instance, in the United States, people who had reached the age of 65 previously represented about 5% of the population, but by 2002 this percentage had risen to 13%.[2] Provision for health and social care among this increasing population is therefore moving away from simply prolonging life, towards helping people cope with disability, preventing incapacity, extending quality of life, and encouraging functional independence.[1] Throughout this book, it has been stated that chronic pain (CP) represents one of the most prevalent and costly public health conditions worldwide. Although pain may affect people throughout their lives, older adults are at greater risk of CP and pain-related disability.[3] Despite this significant increase in prevalence of pain in older patients, the relationships between pain and aging are relatively unexplored. Additionally, medical management for older people with pain is often substandard, ranging from failing to prescribe adequate analgesia for patients with intractable pain to exposing potentially life-threatening overdoses and/or drug interactions.[4] Thus, there is a growing requirement to explore pharmacological and non-pharmacological interventions that are effective in reducing pain, suffering, and pain-related disability in older people. After a brief review of the epidemiology of CP in elderly people, this chapter will first examine the effects of aging on a range of physiological mechanisms relating to nociception and pain modulation. Second, the chapter will review psychological factors and dementia and their influence on the course of CP in this population. Finally, the chapter will review both assessment and treatment of chronic pain relevant to the elderly population.

Epidemiology

Age-related distribution of CP conditions varies across different populations, depending on the type of pain symptom being studied.[5] Many epidemiological studies show that pain becomes more bothersome and unremitting as age increases up to the seventh decade of life, after which it plateaus or declines slightly[6] (Figure 12.1). Reports on pain prevalence vary; for example, different studies have suggested that people over 60 years of age experience pain between 45% and 80% of the time.[7,8] However, higher percentages have been reported; for example, Brown and colleagues found that over 90% of elderly people living in the community had experienced pain within the previous month, with over 40% reporting distressing, horrible, or excruciating pain.[9] Reporting of pain is equally, if not more, common among elderly people receiving nursing home care; for example, as many as 80% of inpatients report at least one pain problem.[10] It is also worth noting that more than 50% of those in residential care also suffer from cognitive impairment and dementia[11] and therefore may not be able to report pain symptoms, thus prevalence rates may be falsely reduced.

Older people are most likely to report musculoskeletal pain, especially in the joints, lower extremities, and back.[12] These findings are supported by an extensive Brazilian systematic review including over 116,000 older adults in eight studies where more than half the sample reported lower limb and spine pain.[13] Of these areas of pain, up to 40% of diagnoses were of arthritic conditions. In another systematic review of over 50 accepted articles reporting the prevalence of low back in people over 65, Dionne and colleagues found that although overall back pain prevalence decreases in older age groups, more severe and disabling forms of episodic back pain are reported.[14]

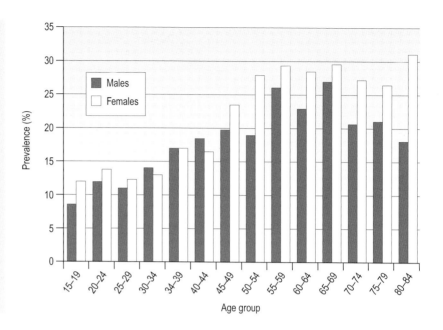

Figure 12.1
Pain prevalence across age-groups based on data from a survey of over 17,000 Australians. Here chronic pain is defined as pain experienced daily for three months in the six months prior to the survey (Blyth et al. 2001)

Comorbidities

Pain in the elderly more often arises because of other coexisting diseases or conditions. Comorbidity is a common problem in older people, in whom chronic diseases increase with age and accumulate over time.[15] For example, a US study of family medicine

Table 12.1
Chronic comorbidities causing pain in elderly patients

Rheumatic disease (e.g., osteoarthritis, rheumatoid arthritis)
Cancer pain
Angina
Postherpetic neuralgia
Temporal arteritis
Atherosclerotic and diabetic peripheral neuropathy
Trigeminal neuralgia
Peripheral vascular disease
Ischemic pain (e.g., cardiac, bowel, brain)

showed the prevalence of comorbidity was 73% in people aged 80 and over.[16] Aside from arthritic conditions mentioned previously, many other age-related conditions are associated with neuropathic pain such as diabetic neuropathy and central post-stroke pain.[3] Conversely, pain arising from visceral organs appears to decline with age; for example, there is a frequent absence of pain in older people with conditions such as myocardial infarction, peptic ulcer, and intestinal blockage.[17] However, decreases in visceral pain in the elderly are not necessarily helpful, as pain from internal organs may indicate potentially life-threatening conditions such as cancer. Table 12.1 shows common conditions causing pain in elderly patients.

Effects of aging on pain sensitivity and modulation

Aging is a multifactorial development that occurs across many different physiological and psychological processes. Important features of aging include an increase in the risk of pathology, a reduced ability to respond to stress, and cumulative homeostatic imbalances that involve nervous, endocrine, and immune systems (Figure 12.2).[3]

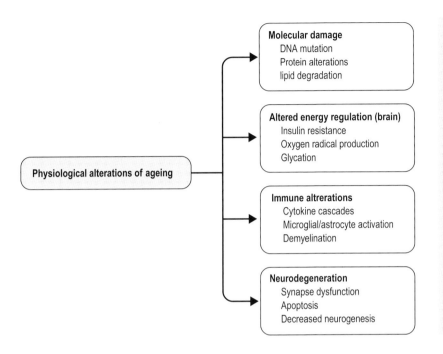

Figure 12.2

Shows different areas of change due to aging that result in damaged molecules, decreased energy metabolism in brain cells, increased activation of microglia and astrocytes resulting in changes in central nervous system plasticity and ultimately neuronal degeneration

Aging and somatosensory function

Like other sensory modalities, age-related anatomical and functional changes occur in the somatosensory system.[18] For instance, it has been long known that peripheral nerves show a reduction of myelinated and non-myelinated fibers, with the proliferative response of Schwann cells decreasing with age.[19,20] Animal studies show that the number and size of dorsal root ganglia also decrease.[21,22] This age-related reduction in the number of peripheral afferents, in combination with coexisting demyelination and increased likelihood of inflammation, shows mechanistic comparisons with neuropathic pain.[18] Age-related changes in pain perception also occur with spinal cord neurotransmitters: immunohistochermical studies show decreases in the expression of neurotransmitters such as calcitonin gene-related-peptide, substance P, and nitric oxide in the spinal cords of old animals and human post-mortem tissue.[23,24] Moreover, potential changes in descending modulation are shown with the age-related loss of serotonergic and noradrenergic terminals in the dorsal horn.[25] There is also a general decline in the opioidergic system, with decreases in the number of opiate receptors in brain regions such as the cortex, striatum, and hypothalamus,[26] as well as the dorsal horns of cervical and thoracic levels of the spinal cord.[27]

Aging and neuroimmune function

Normal aging is associated with neuroimmune changes, something often referred to as 'inflammaging' (a general increase in inflammatory tone).[28] This increase in inflammatory markers with age occurs in various brain regions and in the spinal cord, particularly in the dorsal root ganglion. Results from animal studies show changes in cellular and molecular mechanisms related to aging bear a striking similarity to the development of CP after inflammation and tissue injury in young animals.[25] One common factor lies in the role of free radicals, and it is suggested that due to the production of mitochondrial superoxides in the dorsal horn, free radicals (reactive oxygen species) are involved with the development of increased pain sensitivity through central sensitization. For example, animal studies show that reactive oxygen species are involved in the activation of NMDA receptors.[29] Additionally, microglia, also implicated in the development of CP (as reviewed in Chapter 2), release not only neurotransmitters and various cytokines, but additionally reactive oxygen species[30] that also appear to play a part in the development of central sensitization. Thus, while microglia are involved in the maintenance of CP, they may also represent an important mechanism in the mediation of age-related increases in pain sensitivity.[3]

Aging and autonomic function

Changes in autonomic function are also thought to contribute to increased pain sensitivity in older people. The sympathetic nervous system (SNS) is essential for the maintenance of physiological homeostasis under basal conditions and during the response to stress.[18] In older people, autonomic function is relatively well maintained at rest, but the ability to adapt to environmental and visceral changes becomes diminished.[31] Here, experimental evidence shows that SNS activity increases with age. For example, alterations in central autonomic nerve activity lead to decreased autonomic reactivity (e.g., blood pressure) and reduced autonomic discharge (e.g., bladder function).[31] Interestingly, this increase in SNS tone appears to be specific to regions such as skeletal muscle, the gut, and the heart.[32]

Although the precise relationship between altered autonomic function and CP are not well understood, increased SNS activity is shown to provoke spontaneous pain and reduce thresholds to mechanical and cold stimulation. Like people with chronic regional pain syndrome, the elderly complain of spontaneous burning pain in the affected limb in association with local trophic and motor changes.[33] Here, evidence suggests that psychological stress activates limbic system structures projecting to the hypothalamus, resulting in an increase in SNS tone.[18] Chronic SNS activation is also associated with peripheral vasoconstriction that in turn produces muscular ischemia and thus the potential for myofascial pain.[34]

Aging and pain processing in the brain

Age is also associated with general decreases in gray and white matter volume in brain regions, with some areas being affected more than others.[35,36] Most notable

are the prefrontal cortex and the hippocampus.[37] However, imaging studies show atrophy also occurs in brain regions associated with nociception. For example, compared to younger people, older subjects show significantly reduced gray matter volume in the primary somatosensory and insular cortices;[38] several other studies show inverse associations between reduced gray matter volume and increased pain sensitivity and visceral sensitivity.[3] Similarly, CP in younger age groups is also associated with similar decreases in white and gray matter volume in conditions such as fibromyalgia. Here, most studies show gray matter atrophy at the prefrontal cortex (PFC), the anterior cingulate cortex (ACC), the insula, and the thalamus.[39,40] Although the link between alterations in brain structure and age-related pain processing is not fully understood, Fillingim and colleagues suggest that these morphological changes contribute to pain facilitation and/or reduced pain inhibition observed in younger adults.[41] However, this hypothesis is not clear cut, as loss of brain gray matter due to CP is shown to be reversible even in older adults. For example, Rea and colleagues found that in patients undergoing hip replacement surgery, gray matter in the dorsolateral PFC, ACC, amygdala, and brainstem increased compared to preoperative imaging, especially in the postoperative pain-free patients.[42]

Aging and endogenous pain modulation

Few studies have investigated age-related changes in endogenous pain modulation. It is suggested that increases in pain sensitivity in older people may be due to functional impairment of descending modulatory pathways.[18] Several quantitative sensory methods (Chapter 2) have been used to examine pain modulatory function, the most common being conditioned pain modulation (CPM). CPM refers to a decrease in pain intensity evoked by one (test) stimulus produced by simultaneous application of a second (conditioning) painful stimulus.[43] CPM is based on data from animal studies by LeBars and colleagues, who showed a spinobulbospinal loop through which wide dynamic range neurons in the dorsal horn receive a painful (conditioning) stimulus from one part of the body that then sends an ascending input to the subnucleus dorsalis reticularis in the medulla, which then sends widespread descending inhibition to spinal projection neurons.[44] Cumulative evidence now shows that older adults have reduced levels of CPM and thus reduced pain inhibition. In fact, several studies show that elderly subjects report an increase in pain in response to a conditioning stimulus.[45,46]

Offset analgesia is another experimental model that measures levels of endogenous pain modulation whose neuroanatomical pathways are different from those of CPM.[47] This occurs when a prolonged heat stimulus is given where the stimulus is increased slightly in intensity and then returned to the original temperature. This slight reduction in heat intensity then induces a disproportionate reduction in the subject's perception of pain.[48] Like CPM, recent studies show that offset analgesia is reduced in older people, thus adding to knowledge that endogenous pain inhibition declines in older age.

Psychological factors and pain perception in older adults

Like most areas of CP management, pain in older adults has been dominated by a medical model in which symptoms are a warning sign of tissue damage.[49] However, the influence of psychological and social functioning on the maintenance of pain is now being recognized. As discussed throughout this book, psychological distress disorders such as depression and anxiety and the effects of family, occupational, and social life are all associated with increased pain in older people.

Age-related attitudes and beliefs to chronic pain

Although, people's beliefs and evaluations contribute to the exacerbation and maintenance of CP, older adults show a number of unique attitudes towards health and disability. Many consider that pain and disability are an expected or normal part of aging or that painful arthritic joints are not as debilitating as shortness of breath experienced by people with chronic obstructive pulmonary disease.[37] Additionally, older people are less likely to accept the contribution of psychological factors to pain while also relinquishing control to 'powerful others.'[5] This 'handover' of control is unfortunately associated with increases in depression, pain severity, and pain-related disability.[49] Similarly, older CP patients are more likely to resort to other passive methods of coping such as hoping and praying.[50] Older adults also exchange physical and social activities for more passive ones, sometimes discontinuing many physical activities altogether.[51] Illogically, although these passive strategies are seen as a method of preservation and a way to avoid medical interventions, they serve only to reduce muscle strength, endurance, and flexibility, thus leading to deconditioning and the likelihood of activity-related pain. These issues are highlighted by Larsson and colleagues, who show that kinesiophobia (fear of movement) worsens in elderly people with CP, especially those living in care homes and those with poor self-perceived health.[52] Interestingly, however, studies also show that while older people utilize fewer coping strategies in everyday life than younger adults, they use them more effectively.[53] Similarly, studies report that older people make greater use of emotion-focused coping strategies, thus implying older CP patients would be more open to psychological pain management protocols.[25]

Age-related affective features of chronic pain

Affective consequences of CP are well studied, especially anxiety and/or depression. These comorbidities are of particular importance in older people as they often contribute towards increased health care, accidents, and dependence on others. Although depression and CP are very common in older adults, the prevalence and intensity among CP patients are similar across all age groups.[54] However, compared to younger age groups, pain intensity has a more direct influence on levels of depression, and vice versa in older people.[55] For example, in a large survey of older adults (>90,000) living in the community, results showed that baseline depression increased the likelihood of incapacitating low back pain after two years, regardless of socioeconomic and functional status.[56] This study also showed that older people with disabling low back pain at baseline increased the odds of depression by a similar degree. Similarly, a survey of Danish twins aged 70–100 years found that good physical function at baseline was protective of low back pain and thus the onset of depression.[57]

Although not as well researched, recent evidence shows similar findings regarding anxiety to that of depression and CP in older adults.[5] Like depression, levels of anxiety appear to be related to levels of pain severity and disability so that, in most cases, older people with CP are at risk of becoming frail in relation to higher levels of functional disability in addition to psychological difficulties and social withdrawal.[58] However, in older people, anxiety is also related to the fear of movement and/ or re-injury. Thus, reductions in pain-related anxiety predicts improvements in physical and social functioning and reduced pain-related interference with activity.[3]

Social and family support

Nowhere is the context of family and social support more important than among older adults living with pain and disability. In this population, social isolation and socioeconomic status are the two main factors that have most impact on pain and disability.[49] Generally, the elderly face significant social withdrawal, such as the loss of loved ones, independence, and social and/ or cultural status, all of which combine to exacerbate levels of pain and disability. Interestingly, older people tend to 'downsize' their social networks, not necessarily because of illness or death, but intentionally as it becomes difficult to maintain a large social network. However, small networks are more sensitive to losses and strain so those in the network are less able to provide any meaningful support.[37] Thus, many in elderly communities experience loneliness and loss of connection and find it increasingly difficult to develop new friendships.

Pain and dementia

Clinical pain in dementia

Many studies show that pain in people with cognitive impairment is undertreated and they regularly receive fewer analgesics than people who are cognitively intact.[59] For example, Morrison and colleagues show that dementia patients receive only one-third the dose of opioid analgesics for hip fracture compared to people who are cognitively sound.[60] The authors also found that nearly 80% of the same dementia cohort did not receive any regular postoperative analgesia. These findings are echoed by Pickering and co-workers, who found that CP analgesic consumption of nonsteroidal anti-inflammatories, acetaminophen/paracetamol, and tramadol among dementia patients is also significantly lower.[61] Scherder and colleagues suggest that undertreatment of CP is due mostly to dementia patients not being able to communicate where they are less able to report pain spontaneously and where pain is less intense.[62] Thus, the more severe the dementia, the less able patients become at reporting or expressing pain sensation.

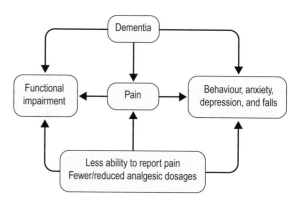

Figure 12.3

A schematic diagram showing the interrelationships between pain, functional impairment and dementia. Impairment and changes in behavior and mood are caused by neuropathological changes in dementia and ongoing painful condtions

Experimental pain and dementia

Neuropathological changes that occur with conditions such as Alzheimer's disease have an impact on the medial pain system compared to the lateral system, suggesting that cognitive and affective factors of pain are more greatly affected than sensory-discriminative factors.[63] Here, people with dementia show unchanged pain thresholds but have higher pain tolerance. This is due to neurodegenerative changes also occurring in central systems involved in pain processing. For example, in patients with early to moderate forms of dementia, there is an increase in nociceptive reactivity observed in facial response to pain and nociceptive motor reflexes.[64] However, in those with more severe forms, nociceptive responses are often blunted. These findings are supported by imaging studies showing alterations in connections between cortical and subcortical regions, those being the dorsolateral prefrontal cortex, the hypothalamus, and the periaqueductal gray.[65] The role of the prefrontal cortex in pain processing is well known (Chapter 3). However, in people with dementia it is hypothesized that Lewy bodies and Lewy neuritis in the prefrontal cortex cause a reduction in suffering from pain.[64] Although evidence from brain imaging and clinical research concerning pain processing and perception is inconsistent, it is generally considered that atrophy of gray matter (processing and cognition) leads to increases in pain tolerance, while white matter (control and coordination of signals) lesions lead to decreases in tolerance.[63]

Assessment of chronic pain in older adults

Barriers to pain assessment

Generally, people believe that pain is an expected and natural consequence of aging. Pain assessment is often hindered by older patients who themselves believe pain is part of the aging process and also do not want to be a bother to health care staff. Additionally, older people often hesitate to report pain for fear of it being a symptom of serious pathology, or indicating the need for hospitalization and/or medications with unpleasant side-effects.[66]

CP assessment often requires patients to complete self-reporting questionnaires or verbally describe sensory-discriminatory and cognitive-affective pain experiences. However, alterations in motor control and cognition in older patients interfere with their ability to communicate or quantify their pain.[67] Additionally, as described above, people with cognitive impairment often struggle to describe pain, as verbal reports decrease and cognitive impairment increases.

Clinical pain assessment

A comprehensive assessment of pain increases the chances of identifying a specific diagnosis; and helps guide pain management.[68] However, clinical assessment of pain in older adults is rarely simple since presentations of persistent pain in this population are often complex and multifactorial due to the presence of coexisting illness, related medication, and difficulties understanding complaints from patients who are cognitively impaired.[69] Pain in the elderly is also more likely to be confounded by poor health and psychosocial issues. Thus, pain assessment requires a multidisciplinary approach that initially involves not only clinicians and psychologists but also physical therapies and occupational therapy to improve functional mobility.

Case history

It is recommended that all older patients presenting with persistent pain should undergo a comprehensive assessment.[68] It is important to gather additional information using a variety of self-reporting measures (if possible) that relate not only to pain characteristics (e.g., intensity, location, quality, and pattern) but also pain-related interference and disability. These latter affects most often cause the biggest problems in older patients, especially those with underlying conditions such as osteoarthritis (Table 12.2). Generally, measures should be simple, brief, and easy to complete. Thus, Carrington-Reid and colleagues suggest the Brief Pain Inventory be used as a routine geriatric pain measure, while measures such as the Abbey Pain Scale is best suited for patients with major cognitive impairment.[68]

Table 12.2
Examples of measures for pain assessment in older adults

Measure	Domain assessed
Multidimensional measures	
Brief Pain Inventory - short form	Pain intensity, location, interference, disability, treatments, degree of relief from treatments
McGill Pain Questionnaire - short-form	Pain descriptors (sensory and affective)
Roland Morris Disability Questionnaire	Pain-related interference or disability
WOMAC*	Pain intensity, interference, and disability related to joint stiffness in osteoarthritis
Checklist of Nonverbal Pain Indicators	Assesses pain behaviors in cognitively impaired older adults
Abbey Pain Scale	Pain measure using nonverbal cues
Unidimensional scales	
Numerical Rating Scale	Pain intensity
Visual Analog Scale	Pain intensity
Wong-Baker Faces Pain Scale	Pain intensity
DN4*	Assesses for possible neuropathic pain

* WOMAC – Western Ontario and McMaster Universities osteoarthritis index; DN4 – Douleur Neuropathique 4 questions

It is also important to identify the impact of pain on daily and social function and sleep. For example, patients should be asked if they are able to bathe or dress, cook, and shop without pain. Furthermore, questions and self-reporting that establish the effect of pain on depressed mood as well as eliciting attitudes and beliefs about pain should also be used. Here, levels of pain catastrophizing, hypervigilance to pain, self-efficacy (one's belief in one's ability to complete tasks when in pain), and wellbeing will help to target appropriate interventions (Table 12.3). It is also important to gain information from family members and/or caregivers about patient behaviors and the impact of pain on their quality of life. This is critical when patients have trouble communicating. Concerning social wellbeing, it is important to identify family, and, if appropriate, faith communities as social support may help to encourage patients to follow treatment plans and alleviate anxiety and/or depression. As discussed above, elderly patients are often unable to describe or assess their pain. Thus, it is important to recognize nonverbal cues and behaviors (Table 12.4).[67]

Physical examination

Physical examination is recommended to focus on musculoskeletal and neuromuscular systems, paying particular attention to weakness, levels of pain sensitivity, and neurological signs.[67,68] In addition to range of motion, gait, and balance testing, it is often helpful to determine physical function by asking about or observing the person's ability to perform activities of daily living. The most common sites for musculoskeletal pain in older people are the back, leg, knee, hip, and other joints.[70] Within the neuromuscular

Table 12.3

Examples of measures for pain-related psychological function and wellbeing

Measure	Domain assessed
Depression, Anxiety and Stress Scale	Depression, anxiety, and stress
Geriatric Depression Scale	Depression in older populations
Pain Catastrophizing Scale	Magnification, rumination of pain, and helplessness to manage pain
Pain Vigilance and Awareness Questionnaire	Attention behaviors to pain
Pain Self-Efficacy Questionnaire	Confidence in ability to perform tasks when in pain
FACIT-Sp*	Spiritual wellbeing (meaning, purpose, faith)

* FACIT-Sp – Functional Assessment of Chronic Illness – Spiritual wellbeing

Table 12.4

Examples of nonverbal indicators of pain (adapted from Herr and Garand 2001)[67]

Behavior	
Nonverbal cues	Agitation, bracing, fidgeting, guarding, rapid eye blinking
Facial expressions	Clenched teeth, wincing, frowning, grimacing, fearful expression
Changes in usual behavior	Aggression, irritability, anxiety, attention-seeking, increased confusion, impaired mobility
Vocalizations	Crying, groaning, sighing

examination, it is important to note neurological impairment such as weakness, hyperalgesia, allodynia, numbness, and paresthesias. Provocation tests such as straight leg raising and joint motion together with palpation for tenderness, deformity, and trigger points will help to determine a more accurate diagnosis. In elderly patients, common pathological conditions such as arthritis, peripheral neuropathies, infections such as pneumonia, and pain at previous fracture sites are important considerations.

Treatment of pain in older adults

There are many treatment approaches to CP in older adults, for example, pharmacological, physical exercise, psychological, educational, and surgical as well as a range of complementary treatments. However, pain management strategies for older adults have not been systematically evaluated and most treatment approaches have been judged by the clinical efficacy of those used in younger patients.[71] Additionally, as stated earlier, between 47% and 80% of community-dwelling older patients do not receive adequate pain treatment and between 16% and 27% of elderly people in care receive no pain treatment at all.[54]

Pharmacological approaches

Analgesic medication, either prescribed or over-the-counter, is the first-line treatment for pain regardless of age.[3] Currently, guidelines for drug interventions in older people provide guidance on both nociceptive and neuropathic pain. The general principles of pharmacology for older people in pain are beyond the scope of this chapter and readers are thus referred to Abdulla et al.'s 'Guidance on the management of pain in older people'.[70] Table 12.5 briefly describes commonly recommended analgesic medication in older adults as adapted from Abdulla and colleagues' guidelines.

Psychological approaches

As with all age groups, psychological factors significantly influence the way people perceive, respond to, and cope with pain. Although medication is helpful in managing pain, older people are particularly vulnerable to adverse effects. Psychological approaches are shown not only to help when drug treatment is ineffective, but more affectively as an adjunct to medication, or as a first-line treatment.[72] Additionally, depression and anxiety are common in older adults, in whom CP impacts most areas of everyday living.

Cognitive behavioral therapy

Cognitive behavioral therapy (CBT) is used to increase patients' control over pain based on the principle that a person's beliefs, attitudes, and behaviors play a key role in the experience of pain.[68] Thus, CBT techniques are used to modify these factors to increase an individual's control over pain and how they manage this. Although meta-analyses and systematic reviews show the benefit of CBT for many pain conditions such as osteoarthritis pain, cancer pain, and low back pain, few studies have focused on older adults. However, studies have examined the effect of CBT in elderly long-term care facilities. First, in a multicentre study, Cook compared the use of CBT and a support control treatment in residents without serious cognitive impairment. Although the author found that residents completing the CBT training reported less pain and related disability, there were no significant treatment effects on depression or clinician medication ratings.[73] A later study examined the effect of CBT on pain, depression, behavioral dysfunction, and functional disability in

long-term care residents. Short-term results showed significant reductions in pain, activity interference, and emotional distress and an increase in daily activities compared to the control group. Still later, in a follow-up study, retrospective chart reviews showed fewer clinician visits and change orders, again compared to the control group.[74] Encouragingly, efforts to train non-psychologists to deliver CBT show much promise, so the reach of such treatments may further help physical therapists in the management of patients with chronic musculoskeletal pain.[75]

Other therapies

Several studies show the benefit of other therapies such as mindfulness, meditation, and biofeedback. For example, Morone and colleagues investigated the effect of an eight-week mindfulness and meditation program on community-dwelling adults over the age of 65 with chronic low back pain. Although they found that the treatment group showed significant improvements in physical function and pain acceptance, no significant reductions in pain intensity were reported. Similar findings are also reported with yoga, where interventions with older adults using chair-based yoga showed improvements in physical function, but again had no effects on pain.[76] Biofeedback has also received attention as a component of multidisciplinary pain management. Here, studies show that older CP patients respond well to biofeedback training and show comparable decreases in pain compared to pain programs as a whole.[77,78]

Exercise therapy

Introducing or maintaining physical activity is an important feature in the management of CP in older adults. However, physical inactivity is more common in older populations and can compromise not only levels of fitness and quality of life, but also increase the risk of falls, especially in those with persistent pain.[70] Exercise is generally acknowledged as a method of reducing pain and improving physical function regardless of age. However, negative sensations associated with exercise in association with self-efficacy expectation often affect motivation in older adults. Although many forms of exercise exist, there is little evidence as to what type is most suitable for older

Table 12.5
Recommended analgesic medication for older adults (adapted from guidelines for pain management in older people, Abdulla et al. 2013)[70]

Analgesic	Recommendations	Side effects
Over-the-counter analgesics		
Acetaminophen/paracetamol	Considered the first-line analgesic in acute and chronic pain	Safest form of analgesia Very rare hepatic effects only with prolonged use of maximum daily dose (4 g/24 h)
Nonsteroidal anti-inflammatory drugs	One of the most widely used primary analgesics More effective for persistent inflammatory pain conditions Recommended when acetaminophen/paracetamol provides insufficient relief	GI toxicity includes bleeding, ulceration that increases in older people especially when combined with low dose aspirin Renal vasoconstriction and increased Na^+ absorption and thus contributes to worsening of chronic renal failure Increased blood pressure with both COX-1 and COX-2, thus risk factors for cardiovascular disease, hypertension, hyperlipidemia, diabetes mellitus
Prescription analgesics		
Weak opioids (e.g., codeine, dihydrocodeine)	Short-term efficacy for moderate pain (osteoarthritis, back pain)	Limited use due to adverse effects of constipation
Strong opioids (e.g., morphine, oxycodone, fentanyl, buprenorphine)	Most studies relating to older adults investigate effect on cancer pain Short-term efficacy for low back pain, osteoarthritis, diabetic peripheral neuropathy Transdermal fentanyl and buprenorphine associated with less constipation in older adults No indication of long-term efficacy	Do not vary with age Sedation, constipation, nausea, vomiting, drowsiness, dizziness Cognitive function not affected in patients taking stable doses
Opioid/SNRI combinations (tramadol)	Recent age-controlled studies show elderly require 20% less dosage than younger adults	Contraindication for patients with seizures To be used with caution in patients taking SSRIs
Antidepressants (SSRIs, SNRIs, tricyclics)	SNRIs (e.g., duloxetine) show most efficacy compared to SSRIs and tricyclics especially for neuropathic pain in older adults	Anticholinergic effects (especially with tricyclics) such as sedation, psychomotor impairment (slowed sensorimotor processes), which may be considered as normal in elderly people
Antiepileptic drugs (e.g., gabapentin, pregabalin)	Newer drugs such as pregabalin, show analgesic efficacy in older people especially in postherpetic and diabetic peripheral neuropathies	Older adults using antiepileptic drugs show fewer central adverse effects such as psychomotor impairment. However, dosage is dependent on renal function

GI – gastrointestinal; SSRI – selective serotonin reuptake inhibitor; SNRI – serotonin norepinephrine/noradrenaline reuptake inhibitor; COX-1/2 – cyclooxygenase-1/2

adults, with studies focusing only on those with OA knee. In general, exercise programs are prescribed depending on the function(s) needed to be improved and the preference of the patient.

There are many types of exercise available for older adults, such as progressive muscle strengthening exercises, aerobic exercise, hydrotherapy, Tai Chi, and yoga. Concerning strength exercise, studies show positive effects in the increases of muscle strength and reduced disability.[79] Ettinger and colleagues, in a randomized controlled trial (RCT) comparing aerobic exercise and resistance exercise, showed both forms to moderately reduce pain severity, decrease pain-related disability, and improve physical performance in older adults disabled by OA knee.[80] Another benefit of exercise in older adults is its effect on the risk of falling. For example, static and dynamic balance exercises such as Tai Chi not only help to reduce the risk of falling but additionally lead to awareness of balance and, equally important, reduce fear of falling.[81] Various groups such as the American College of Cardiology and American College of Sports Medicine recommend several types of exercise, the more relevant of which are reviewed below.

Aerobic exercise

In order to maintain a healthy quality of life, older adults should take part in moderate intensity physical exercise for at least 30 minutes on five days a week, or more vigorous aerobic exercise for 20 minutes on three days a week. To gauge these efforts, moderate intensity aerobic activity equates to 5–6 on a 10-point exertion scale where sitting is 0 and full effort is 10. Using the same scale, vigorous intensity equates to 7–8 and produces large increases in heart rate and breathing. Given the differences in capability among older people, moderate intensity for some may mean a slow walk, while for others it is a brisk walk.[82] Both high and moderate intensity aerobic exercise are shown to produce an analgesic effect both experimentally[83] and clinically, and patients also showed improving function compared to patients attending health education programs.[80]

Muscle strengthening exercise

Muscle strengthening exercise has been repeatedly shown to increase muscle strength, alleviate pain, and improve function.[84] A Cochrane review also provides evidence that progressive resistance training two or three times a week reduces physical disability while also improving balance, gait, speed, and muscle strength in older people.[85] However, although this review shows pain reduction, these data are only reliable concerning older adults with OA. Nevertheless, it is important to note that adverse reactions should be avoided by applying low articular pressures during resisted exercise.[1] Recommendations from the American Geriatrics Society Panel on Exercise and Osteoarthritis suggest that strength training should target all major muscle groups.[86] Their advice also includes a recommendation that intensity of isometric strength exercises should increase from 30% to 75% of maximum voluntary contraction (or using a 10-point scale for effort where 0 is no effort and 10 is maximum effort).[86] It is also recommended that repetitions should be increased from one to 8–10 while also recommending a minimum of two sessions a day, two times per week. However, these recommendations are moderated especially for patients with cardiovascular problems.

Tai Chi

Tai Chi is a traditional Chinese multi-component mind–body exercise that combines aerobic activity, diaphragmatic breathing, relaxation, and mediation through a series of slow, gentle movements and postures that are of low impact and low velocity; they are thus ideal for older people[3]. Tai Chi is also shown to be beneficial for improving physical condition, muscle strength, coordination, flexibility, balance, cardiovascular fitness, and, importantly, decreased risk of falls.[87] Additionally, Tai Chi has been shown to reduce pain and increase health-related quality of life in older people with OA, rheumatoid arthritis, and fibromyalgia.[87,88] For example, it was shown that older adults were able to complete a 12-week program by undertaking Tai Chi exercises while also showing improvement in arthritic symptoms.[89] Longitudinal study data further showed that older patients with OA who continued with Tai Chi three times per week for two years demonstrated significant improvements in both physical and social function as well as decreases in lean body mass.[90]

Physical therapy

Although a few studies show that older patients benefit from physical interventions such as acupuncture, trans/percutaneous electrical stimulation (T/PENS), and massage, there is little research on the use of joint mobilization and manipulation techniques in older adults. In fact, virtually all studies investigate the use of physical therapies and their effects on pain related to osteoarthritis, regardless of age. Although osteoarthritis is associated with aging, very few studies sample subjects solely from older age groups.

Manual therapy

Based on systematic review evidence, several studies report the benefit of mobilization and manipulative techniques to the lumbar region, hips, and pelvis in the treatment of lumbar spine stenosis, especially in conjunction with exercise.[91] Another area of investigation lies with the assessment and treatment of thoracic spine pain, including hyperkyphosis. Here, once red flag risk factors such as vertebral fracture have been ruled out, conservative manual therapy, again in combination with exercise and self-help, such as lying supine on a foam roller, is shown to reduce levels of pain and increase spinal mobility.[92] Concerning hip and knee pain in older adults, there are several studies showing favorable short-term effects in reducing pain intensity and disability.[93,94] However, although results are favorable, current evidence is limited due to the paucity of literature and heterogeneity between study methodologies.[95]

Massage, however, is one area of manual therapy that has been more rigorously studied. For example, results from a prospective RCT show that massage using aromatherapy significantly decreased chronic pain intensity compared to standard nursing visits.[96]

Additionally, slow stroke massage is also shown to reduce shoulder pain and anxiety in elderly post-stroke patients, with effects lasting up to three days.[97] Current literature also suggests that massage helps to influence factors such as sleep and psychosocial health for older people in residential care, while also reducing the need for restraint and pharmacological intervention.[98]

Acupuncture

There are several RCTs showing the positive effects of acupuncture in the treatment of chronic low back pain in the elderly. In an RCT investigating the effectiveness of acupuncture versus usual treatment (medication and exercise prescription), Meng and colleagues found that a five-week course of acupuncture with electrical stimulation was effective in reducing levels of low back pain intensity and pain-related disability in older patients.[99,7] In a further study, Grant and co-workers compared the effectiveness of acupuncture versus TENS. Here, both treatment modalities showed similar significant reductions in back pain intensity directly after the four-week treatment program. At three-month follow-up, only acupuncture showed continued pain reduction; however, this improvement was non-significant.[100] Studies also show that combining acupuncture and TENS appears to have a therapeutic effect.

Summary

Pain in older people is a significant concern and currently presents challenges not only to patients but also to health care providers and caregivers. This is due partly to our poor understanding of age-related changes in pain mechanisms, where older people show increased pain facilitation and decreased pain inhibition. Additionally, older adults are more likely to under-report pain, particularly if it is manageable. This may be due to stoicism (i.e., being brave in the face of pain), fear of serious pathology, or cognitive impairment. Psychosocial factors also influence older people; especially those related to social isolation and likelihood of depression. Given these potential barriers to pain treatment, evaluation must include pain history and previous treatments in addition to the assessment of physical and cognitive function. Concerning treatment, there is a clear need to increase the representation of older adults in clinical trials, especially trials of manual therapy. Although current evidence is encouraging for massage techniques in older people with chronic pain, meta-analysis of studies investigating mobilization and manipulation techniques are impossible

due to there being too few studies and there being a lack of heterogeneity of methods between them. Thus, as described through previous chapters, practitioners and researchers need to progress with well-designed clinical trials and larger prospective observation studies in order to move manual therapy beyond the label of 'encouraging pilot study findings' towards proven forms of treatment for all age groups with CP.

Refererences

1. Edeer AO, Tuna H. Management of chronic musculoskeletal pain in the elderly. Dilemmas and Remedies. 2012;10–24.

2. U.S. Census Bureau. Washington, DC: Global Population Profile;; 2002.

3. Fillingim RB, Turk DC, Yezierski RP. Pain in the elderly. In: Sierra F, Kohanski R, editors. Advances in Geroscience. Cham: Springer International Publishing; 2016. p. 551–92.

4. Arnstein P. Balancing analgesic efficacy with safety concerns in the older patient. Pain Management Nursing. 2010;11(2 Suppl):S11–22.

5. Gagliese L, Katz J, Melzack R. Pain in the elderly. In: Melzack R, Wall P, editors. Handbook of Pain Management. Edinburgh: Churchill Livingstone; 2003.

6. Blyth FM, March LM, Brnabic AJ, Jorm LR, Williamson M, Cousins MJ. Chronic pain in Australia: a prevalence study. Pain. 2001;89(2–3):127–34.

7. Ferrell BA. Pain management in elderly people. Journal of the American Geriatrics Society. 1991;39(1):64–73.

8. Herr K. Pain in the older adult: an imperative across all health care settings. Pain Management Nursing. 2010;11(2 Suppl):S1–10.

9. Brown ST, Kirkpatrick MK, Swanson MS, McKenzie IL. Pain experience of the elderly. Pain Management Nursing. 2011;12(4):190–6.

10. Takai Y, Yamamoto-Mitani N, Okamoto Y, Koyama K, Honda A. Literature review of

pain prevalence among older residents of nursing homes. Pain Management Nursing. 2010;11(4):209–23.

11. Gibson SJ. IASP global year against pain in older persons: highlighting the current status and future perspectives in geriatric pain. Expert Review of Neurotherapeutics. 2007;7(6):627–35.

12. Gibson SJ, Lussier D. Prevalence and relevance of pain in older persons. Pain Medicine. 2012;13(suppl_2):S23–S6.

13. Miranda VS, deCarvalho VB, Machado LA, Dias JMD. Prevalence of chronic musculoskeletal disorders in elderly Brazilians: a systematic review of the literature. BMC Musculoskeletal Disorders. 2012;13(1):82.

14. Dionne CE, Dunn KM, Croft PR. Does back pain prevalence really decrease with increasing age? A systematic review. Age and Ageing. 2006;35(3):229–34.

15. Crimmins EM, Beltrán-Sánchez H. Mortality and morbidity trends: is there compression of morbidity? The Journals of Gerontology Series B: Psychological Sciences and Social Sciences. 2011;66B(1):75–86.

16. Fortin M, Bravo G, Hudon C, Vanasse A, Lapointe L. Prevalence of multimorbidity among adults seen in family practice. Annals of Family Medicine. 2005;3(3):223–8.

17. Moore AR, Clinch D. Underlying mechanisms of impaired visceral pain perception in older people. Journal of the American Geriatrics Society. 2004;52(1):132–6.

18. Yezierski RP. The effects of age on pain sensitivity: pre-clinical studies. Pain Medicine (Malden, Mass). 2012;13(Suppl 2):S27–S36.

19. Komiyama A, Suzuki K. Age-related differences in proliferative responses of Schwann cells during Wallerian degeneration. Brain Research. 1992;573(2):267–75.

20. Verdú E, Ceballos D, Vilches JJ, Navarro X. Influence of aging on peripheral nerve function and regeneration. Journal of the Peripheral Nervous System. 2000;5(4):191–208.

21. Cecchini T, Cuppini R, Ciaroni S, Barili P, Matteis RD, Grande PD. Changes in the number of primary sensory neurons in normal and vitamin-E-deficient rats during aging. Somatosensory & Motor Research. 1995;12(3–4):317–27.

22. Devor M, Govrin-Lippmann R. Neurogenesis in adult rat dorsal root ganglia: on counting and the count. Somatosensory and Motor Research. 1991;8(1):9–12.

23. Cruce WL, Lovell JA, Crisp T, Stuesse SL. Effect of aging on the substance P receptor, NK–1, in the spinal cord of rats with peripheral nerve injury. Somatosensory & Motor Research. 2001;18(1):66–75.

24. Chung YH, Kim D, Lee KJ, Kim SS, Kim KY, Cho D-Y, et al. Immunohistochemical study on the distribution of neuronal nitric oxide synthase-immunoreactive neurons in the spinal cord of aged rat. Journal of Molecular Histology. 2005;36(5):325–9.

25. Gagliese L, Melzack R. Age differences in nociception and pain behaviours in the rat.

Neuroscience & Biobehavioral Reviews. 2000;24(8):843–54.

26. Amenta F, Zaccheo D, Collier WL. Neurotransmitters, neuroreceptors and aging. Mechanisms of Ageing and Development. 1991;61(3):249–73.

27. Missale C, Govoni S, Croce L, Bosio A, Spano PF, Trabucchi M. Changes of β-endorphin and met-enkephalin content in the hypothalamus-pituitary axis induced by aging. Journal of Neurochemistry. 1983;40(1):20–4.

28. Galbavy W, Kaczocha M, Puopolo M, Liu L, Rebecchi MJ. Neuroimmune and neuropathic responses of spinal cord and dorsal root ganglia in middle age. PLoS ONE. 2015;10(8):e0134394.

29. Gao C, Wolf ME. Dopamine receptors regulate NMDA receptor surface expression in prefrontal cortex neurons. Journal of Neurochemistry. 2008;106(6):2489–501.

30. Latremoliere A, Woolf CJ. Central sensitization: a generator of pain hypersensitivity by central neural plasticity. The Journal of Pain. 2009;10(9):895–926.

31. Hotta H, Uchida S. Aging of the autonomic nervous system and possible improvements in autonomic activity using somatic afferent stimulation. Geriatrics & Gerontology International. 2010;10:S127–S36.

32. Seals DR, Esler MD. Human ageing and the sympathoadrenal system. The Journal of Physiology. 2000;528(3):407–17.

33. Burton AR, Fazalbhoy A, Macefield VG. Sympathetic responses to noxious stimulation of muscle and skin. Frontiers in Neurology. 2016;7:109.

34. Vierck Jr CJ. Mechanisms underlying development of spatially distributed chronic pain (fibromyalgia). Pain. 2006;124(3):242–63.

35. Yap QJ, Teh I, Fusar-Poli P, Sum MY, Kuswanto C, Sim K. Tracking cerebral white matter changes across the lifespan: insights from diffusion tensor imaging studies. Journal of Neural Transmission. 2013;120(9):1369–95.

36. Salat DH, Lee SY, van der Kouwe AJ, Greve DN, Fischl B, Rosas HD. Age-associated alterations in cortical gray and white matter signal intensity and gray to white matter contrast. NeuroImage. 2009;48(1):21–8.

37. Molton IR, Terrill AL. Overview of persistent pain in older adults. The American Psychologist. 2014;69(2):197–207.

38. Quiton RL, Roys SR, Zhuo J, Keaser ML, Gullapalli RP, Greenspan JD. Age-related changes in nociceptive processing in the human brain. Annals of the New York Academy of Sciences. 2007;1097(1):175–8.

39. Kuchinad A, Schweinhardt P, Seminowicz DA, Wood PB, Chizh BA, Bushnell MC. Accelerated brain gray matter loss in fibromyalgia patients: premature aging of the brain? The Journal of Neuroscience. 2007;27(15):4004–7.

40. Burgmer M, Gaubitz M, Konrad C, Wrenger M, Hilgart S, Heuft G, et al. Decreased gray matter volumes in the cingulo-frontal cortex and the amygdala in patients with fibromyalgia. Psychosomatic Medicine. 2009;71(5):566–73.

41. Edwards RR, Fillingim RB, Ness TJ. Age-related differences in endogenous pain modulation: a comparison of diffuse noxious inhibitory controls in healthy older and younger adults. Pain. 2003;101(1–2):155–65.

42. Rodriguez-Raecke R, Niemeier A, Ihle K, Ruether W, May A. Brain gray matter decrease in chronic pain is the consequence and not the cause of pain. The Journal of Neuroscience. 2009;29(44):13746–50.

43. Nir RR, Yarnitsky D. Conditioned pain modulation. Current Opinions in Supportive and Palliative Care. 2015;9(2):131–7.

44. Le Bars D. The whole body receptive field of dorsal horn multireceptive neurones. Brain Research Reviews. 2002;40(1–3):29–44.

45. Grashorn W, Sprenger C, Forkmann K, Wrobel N, Bingel U. Age-dependent decline of endogenous pain control: exploring the effect of expectation and depression. PLoS ONE. 2013;8(9):e75629.

46. Naugle KM, Cruz-Almeida Y, Vierck CJ, Mauderli AP, Riley JL. Age-related differences in conditioned pain modulation of sensitizing and desensitizing trends during response dependent stimulation. Behavioural Brain Research. 2015;289:61–8.

47. Naugle KM, Cruz-Almeida Y, Fillingim RB, Riley Iii JL. Offset analgesia is reduced in older adults. PAIN*. 2013;154(11):2381–7.

48. Grill JD, Coghill RC. Transient analgesia evoked by noxious stimulus offset. Journal of Neurophysiology. 2002;87(4):2205–8.

49. Keefe FJ, Porter L, Somers T, Shelby R, Wren AV. Psychosocial interventions for managing pain in older adults: outcomes and clinical implications†. BJA: British Journal of Anaesthesia. 2013;111(1):89–94.

50. Keefe FJ, Williams DA. A comparison of coping strategies in chronic pain patients in different age groups. Journal of Gerontology. 1990;45(4):P161–5.

51. Turk DC, Fillingim RB, Ohrbach R, Patel KV. Assessment of psychosocial and functional impact of chronic pain. The Journal of Pain. 2016;17(9, Supplement):T21–T49.

52. Larsson C, Ekvall Hansson E, Sundquist K, Jakobsson U. Kinesiophobia and its relation to pain characteristics and cognitive affective variables in older adults with chronic pain. BMC Geriatrics. 2016;16:128.

53. Aldwin CM. Does age affect the stress and coping process? Implications of age differences in perceived control. Journal of Gerontology. 1991;46(4):P174–80.

54. Gagliese L, Melzack R. Chronic pain in elderly people. Pain. 1997;70(1):3–14.

55. Casten RJ, Parmelee PA, Kleban MH, Powell Lawton M, Katz IR. The relationships among anxiety, depression, and pain in a geriatric institutionalized sample. Pain. 1995;61(2):271–6.

56. Meyer T, Cooper J, Raspe H. Disabling low back pain and depressive symptoms in the community-dwelling elderly: a prospective study. Spine (Phila Pa 1976). 2007;32(21):2380–6.

57. Hartvigsen J, Frederiksen H, Christensen K. Physical and mental function and incident low back pain in seniors: a population-based two-year prospective study of 1387 Danish Twins aged 70 to 100 years. Spine (Phila Pa 1976). 2006;31(14):1628–32.

58. Cedraschi C, Luthy C, Allaz AF, Herrmann FR, Ludwig C. Low back pain and health-related quality of life in community-dwelling older adults. European Spine Journal. 2016;25(9):2822–32.

59. Lukas A, Schuler M, Fischer TW, Gibson SJ, Savvas SM, Nikolaus T, et al. Pain and dementia. Zeitschrift für Gerontologie und Geriatrie. 2012;45(1):45–9.

60. Morrison RS, Siu AL. A comparison of pain and its treatment in advanced dementia and cognitively intact patients with hip fracture. Journal of Pain and Symptom Management. 19(4):240–8.

61. Pickering G, Jourdan D, Dubray C. Acute versus chronic pain treatment in Alzheimer's disease. European Journal of Pain. 2006;10(4):379.

62. Scherder E, Oosterman J, Swaab D, Herr K, Ooms M, Ribbe M, et al. Recent developments in pain in dementia. BMJ. 2005;330(7489):461–4.

63. Achterberg WP, Pieper MJC, van Dalen-Kok AH, de Waal MWM, Husebo BS, Lautenbacher S, et al. Pain management in patients with dementia. Clinical Interventions in Aging. 2013;8:1471–82.

64. Scherder E, Herr K, Pickering G, Gibson S, Benedetti F, Lautenbacher S. Pain in dementia. Pain. 2009;145(3):276–8.

65. Cole LJ, Gavrilescu M, Johnston LA, Gibson SJ, Farrell MJ, Egan GF. The impact of Alzheimer's disease on the functional connectivity between brain regions underlying pain perception. European Journal of Pain (London, England). 2011;15(6):568.e1–11.

66. Hofland SL. Elder beliefs: blocks to pain management. Journal of Gerontological Nursing. 1992;18(6):19–23.

67. Herr KA, Garand L. Assessment and measurement of pain in older adults. Clinics in Geriatric Medicine. 2001;17(3):457–vi.

68. Reid MC, Eccleston C, Pillemer K. Management of chronic pain in older adults. BMJ. 2015;350.

69. Kaye AD, Baluch A, Scott JT. Pain management in the elderly population: a review. The Ochsner Journal. 2010;10(3):179–87.

70. Abdulla A, Adams N, Bone M, Elliott AM, Gaffin J, Jones D, et al. Guidance on the management of pain in older people. Age and ageing. 2013;42 Suppl 1:i1–57.

71. Podichetty V, Mazanec D, Biscup R. Chronic non-malignant musculoskeletal pain in older adults: clinical issues and opioid intervention. Postgraduate Medical Journal. 2003;79(937):627–33.

72. Guidance on the management of pain in older people. Age and ageing. 2013;42(suppl_1):i1–i57.

73. Cook AJ. Cognitive-behavioral pain management for elderly nursing home residents. The Journals of Gerontology Series B, Psychological Sciences and Social Sciences. 1998;53(1):P51–9.

74. Cipher DJ, Clifford PA, Roper KD. The effectiveness of geropsychological treatment in improving pain, depression, behavioral disturbances, functional disability, and health care utilization in long-term care. Clinical Gerontologist. 2007;30(3):23–40.

75. Riddle DL, Keefe FJ, Nay WT, McKee D, Attarian DE, Jensen MP. Pain coping skills training for patients with elevated pain catastrophizing who are scheduled for knee arthroplasty: a quasi-experimental study. Archives of Physical Medicine and Rehabilitation. 2011;92(6):859–65.

76. Parker S, Vasquez R, Kahoe E, Henderson CR, Pillemer K, Robbins L, et al. A comparison of the arthritis foundation self-help program across three race/ethnicity groups. Ethnicity & Disease. 2011;21(4):444–50.

77. Middaugh SJ, Pawlick K. Biofeedback and behavioral treatment of persistent pain in the older adult: a review and a study. Applied Psychophysiology and Biofeedback. 2002;27(3):185–202.

78. Middaugh SJ, Woods SE, Kee WG, Harden RN, Peters JR. Biofeedback-assisted relaxation training for the aging chronic pain patient. Biofeedback and Self-regulation. 1991;16(4):361–77.

79. Latham NK, Bennett DA, Stretton CM, Anderson CS. Systematic review of progressive resistance strength training in older adults. The Journals of Gerontology Series A, Biological Sciences and Medical Sciences. 2004;59(1):48–61.

80. Ettinger WH, Jr., Burns R, Messier SP, Applegate W, Rejeski WJ, Morgan T, et al. A randomized trial comparing aerobic exercise and resistance exercise with a health education program in older adults with knee osteoarthritis. The Fitness Arthritis and Seniors Trial (FAST). JAMA. 1997;277(1):25–31.

81. Kendrick D, Kumar A, Carpenter H, Zijlstra GA, Skelton DA, Cook JR, et al. Exercise for reducing fear of falling in older people living in the community. The Cochrane Database of Systematic Reviews. 2014;(11):Cd009848.

82. Nelson ME, Rejeski WJ, Blair SN, Duncan PW, Judge JO, King AC, et al. Physical activity and public health in older adults: recommendation from the American College of Sports Medicine and the American Heart Association. Medicine and Science in Sports and Exercise. 2007;39(8):1435–45.

83. Hoffman MD, Shepanski MA, Ruble SB, Valic Z, Buckwalter JB, Clifford PS. Intensity and duration threshold for aerobic exercise-induced analgesia to pressure pain. Archives of Physical Medicine and Rehabilitation. 2004;85(7):1183–7.

84. Ishak NA, Zahari Z, Justine M. Muscle functions and functional performance among older persons with and without low back pain. Current Gerontology and Geriatrics Research. 2016;2016:10.

85. Liu C-j, Latham NK. Progressive resistance strength training for improving physical function in older adults. The Cochrane Database of Systematic Reviews. 2009;(3):CD002759.

86. Exercise prescription for older adults with osteoarthritis pain: consensus practice recommendations. A supplement to the AGS Clinical Practice Guidelines on the management of chronic pain in older adults. Journal of the American Geriatrics Society. 2001;49(6):808–23.

87. Wang C. Tai chi and rheumatic diseases. Rheumatic diseases clinics of North America. 2011;37(1):19–32.

88. Wolfe F, Ross K, Anderson J, Russell IJ, Hebert L. The prevalence and characteristics of fibromyalgia in the general population. Arthritis and Rheumatism. 1995;38(1):19–28.

89. Song R, Lee EO, Lam P, Bae SC. Effects of tai chi exercise on pain, balance, muscle strength, and perceived difficulties in physical functioning in older women

with osteoarthritis: a randomized clinical trial. The Journal of Rheumatology. 2003;30(9):2039–44.

90. Chen C-H, Yen M, Fetzer S, Lo L-H, Lam P. The effects of tai chi exercise on elders with osteoarthritis: a longitudinal study. Asian Nursing Research. 2008;2(4):235–41.

91. Backstrom KM, Whitman JM, Flynn TW. Lumbar spinal stenosis-diagnosis and management of the aging spine. Manual Therapy. 2011;16(4):308–17.

92. Katzman WB, Wanek L, Shepherd JA, Sellmeyer DE. Age-related hyperkyphosis: its causes, consequences, and management. The Journal of Orthopaedic and Sports Physical Therapy. 2010;40(6):352–60.

93. Moss P, Sluka K, Wright A. The initial effects of knee joint mobilization on osteoarthritic hyperalgesia. Manual Therapy. 2007;12(2):109–18.

94. French HP, Brennan A, White B, Cusack T. Manual therapy for osteoarthritis of the hip or knee – a systematic review. Manual Therapy. 2011;16(2):109–17.

95. Wang Q, Wang TT, Qi XF, Yao M, Cui XJ, Wang YJ, et al. Manual therapy for hip osteoarthritis: a systematic review

and meta-analysis. Pain Physician. 2015;18(6):E1005–20.

96. Cino K. Aromatherapy hand massage for older adults with chronic pain living in long-term care. Journal of Holistic Nursing. 2014;32(4):304–13; quiz 14–5.

97. Mok E, Woo CP. The effects of slow-stroke back massage on anxiety and shoulder pain in elderly stroke patients. Complementary Therapies in Nursing & Midwifery. 2004;10(4):209–16.

98. McFeeters S, Pront L, Cuthbertson L, King L. Massage, a complementary therapy effectively promoting the health and well-being of older people in residential care settings: a review of the literature. International Journal of Older People Nursing. 2016;11(4):266–83.

99. Meng CF, Wang D, Ngeow J, Lao L, Peterson M, Paget S. Acupuncture for chronic low back pain in older patients: a randomized, controlled trial. Rheumatology (Oxford, England). 2003;42(12):1508–17.

100. Grant DJ, Bishop-Miller J, Winchester DM, Anderson M, Faulkner S. A randomized comparative trial of acupuncture versus transcutaneous electrical nerve stimulation for chronic back pain in the elderly. Pain. 1999;82(1):9–13.

INDEX

Note: *Page number followed by f and t indicates figure and table respectively.*